AF327341

RETINOPATHY OF PREMATURITY: PROBLEM AND CHALLENGE

March of Dimes Birth Defects Foundation
Birth Defects: Original Article Series, Volume 24, Number 1, 1988

RETINOPATHY OF PREMATURITY: PROBLEM AND CHALLENGE

**Proceedings of a Symposium
Held at the National Institutes
Of Health, Bethesda, Maryland,
November 21–23, 1985**

Editors
John T. Flynn, MD
Bascom Palmer Eye Institute
University of Miami
Medical School
Miami, Florida

Dale L. Phelps, MD
Department of Pediatrics
University of Rochester
School of Medicine
Rochester, New York

ALAN R. LISS, INC., NEW YORK

To enhance medical communication in the birth defects field, the March of Dimes Birth Defects Foundation publishes the *Birth Defects Compendium (2nd Edition),* an *Original Article Series,* a *Reprint Series, Nursing Staff Development Modules, Genetics in Practice* (a quarterly newsletter), and provides a series of films and related brochures.

Further information can be obtained from:

Professional Education Department
March of Dimes Birth Defects Foundation
1275 Mamaroneck Avenue
White Plains, New York 10605

Published by:
Alan R. Liss, Inc.
41 East 11th Street
New York, New York 10003

Library of Congress Cataloging-in-Publication Data
Retinopathy of prematurity.
   (Birth defects, original article series ;
v. 24, no. 1)
   At head of title: March of Dimes Birth Defects
Foundation.
   Symposium jointly sponsored by the National
Children's Eye Care Foundation and the National
Eye Institute.
   Includes bibliographies and index.
   1. Retrolental fibroplasia—Congresses.
I. Flynn, John T., 1931–   . II. Phelps,
Dale L.   III. March of Dimes Birth Defects
Foundation.   IV. National Children's Eye Care
Foundation.   V. National Eye Institute.
VI. Series: Birth Defects: Original Article Series ;
v. 24, no. 1.   [DNLM: 1. Retinopathy of Prematurity—
Congresses. W1 BI966 v.24 no.1 / WW 270 R4398 1985]
RG626.B63 vol. 24, no. 1   616.04'3 s   88-6782
[RJ313]   [618.92'09773]
ISBN 0-8451-1068-3

Contents

Contributors

Soraya Abbasi, MD, Departments of Pediatrics and Obstetrics, University of Pennsylvania School of Medicine, Philadelphia, Pennsylvania 19104 **[219]**

Eduardo Bancalari, MD, Department of Pediatrics, Division of Neonatology, University of Miami Medical School, Miami, Florida 33101 **[41]**

Frank W. Bowen, MD, Departments of Pediatrics and Obstetrics, University of Pennsylvania School of Medicine, Philadelphia, Pennsylvania 19104 **[219]**

Peter A. Campochiaro, MD, Department of Ophthalmology, University of Virginia Medical School, Charlottesville, Virginia 22904 **[121]**

George Cassady, MD, Department of Pediatrics, University of Alabama at Birmingham, Birmingham, Alabama 35294 **[53]**

Steve Charles, MD, Vitreoretinal Research Foundation, Memphis, Tennessee 38119 **[287]**

John L. Davis, Jr., MD, Department of Ophthalmology, Johns Hopkins University, Baltimore, Maryland 21205 **[121]**

Eugene de Juan, Jr., MD, Department of Ophthalmology, Duke University Medical Center, Durham, North Carolina 27710 **[281]**

Robert W. Flower, Applied Physics Laboratory and Wilmer Ophthalmological Institute, Johns Hopkins University, Baltimore, Maryland 21205 **[129]**

John T. Flynn, MD, Bascom Palmer Eye Institute, University of Miami Medical School, Miami, Florida 33101 **[xiii,xvii,41,175,281]**

Robert Y. Foos, MD, Jules Stein Eye Institute, University of California at Los Angeles, Los Angeles, California 90024 **[73]**

Bert M. Glaser, MD, Department of Ophthalmology, Johns Hopkins University, Baltimore, Maryland 21205 **[121]**

Penny Glass, PhD, Division of Neonatology, Children's Hospital, National Medical Center, Washington, DC 20010 **[103]**

W. Richard Green, MD, Department of Ophthalmology, Duke University Medical Center, Durham, North Carolina 27710 **[281]**

Anita K. Harvey, PhD, Eli Lilly Co., Indianapolis, Indiana 46285 **[87]**

Helen M. Hittner, MD, Cullen Eye Institute, and Department of Pediatrics, Baylor College of Medicine, Houston, Texas 77030 **[147]**

Leonard M. Hjelmeland, PhD, Department of Ophthalmology and Biochemistry, University of California at Davis, Sacramento, California 95817 **[87]**

Lois Johnson, MD, Department of Pediatrics, University of Pennsylvania School of Medicine, Philadelphia, Pennsylvania 19104 **[219]**

The numbers in brackets are the opening page numbers of the contributors' articles.

Robert E. Kalina, MD, Department of Ophthalmology, University of Washington, Seattle, Washington 98105 **[185]**

Martin L. Katz, PhD, Department of Ophthalmology, University of Missouri School of Medicine, Columbia, Missouri 65212 **[237]**

Frank L. Kretzer, PhD, Cullen Eye Institute; and Department of Cell Biology, Baylor College of Medicine, Houston, Texas 77030 **[147]**

Burton J. Kushner, MD, Department of Ophthalmology, University of Wisconsin School of Medicine, Madison, Wisconsin 53706 **[193]**

Jerold F. Lucey, MD, Department of Pediatrics, University of Vermont, Burlington, Vermont 05404 **[37]**

Robert Machemer, MD, Department of Ophthalmology, Duke University Medical Center, Durham, North Carolina 27710 **[275, 281]**

Marie C. McCormick, MD, Joint Program in Neonatalogy, Brigham and Women's Hospital, Boston, Massachusetts 02115 **[3]**

Chari Otis, MS, Department of Biostatistics, University of Pennsylvania School of Medicine, Philadelphia, Pennsylvania 19104 **[219]**

Earl A. Palmer, MD, Department of Ophthalmology, Oregon Health Sciences University, Portland, Oregon 97201 **[255]**

Dale L. Phelps, MD, Department of Pediatrics, University of Rochester School of Medicine, Rochester, New York 14642 **[xiii, xvii, 209]**

Graham E. Quinn, MD, Department of Ophthalmology, University of Pennsylvania School of Medicine, Philadelphia, Pennsylvania 19104 **[219]**

W. Gerald Robison, Jr., PhD, Section of Ocular Pathology, National Eye Institute, National Institutes of Health, Bethesda, Maryland 21224 **[237]**

David Rutstein*, MD, Ridley Watts Professor of Preventative Medicine, Harvard Medical School, Boston, Massachusetts 02115 **[325]**

Misao Sato, MD, Department of Ophthalmology, Nippon University, Tokyo, Japan **[121]**

David B. Schaffer, MD, Department of Ophthalmology, University of Pennsylvania School of Medicine, Philadelphia, Pennsylvania 19104 **[219]**

William A. Silverman, MD, Columbia University College of Physicians and Surgeons, New York, New York 10032; present address: 90 La Cuesta Drive, Greenbrae, CA 94904 **[203, 297]**

Marshall Simonds, PC, c/o Goodwin, Procter, and Hoar, Exchange Place, Boston, Massachusetts 02109 **[325]**

John C. Sinclair, MD, Department of Pediatrics, McMaster University, Hamilton, Ontario, Canada L8N 3Z5 **[11]**

William Tasman, MD, Wills Eye Hospital, Jefferson Medical School, Philadelphia, Pennsylvania 19118 **[265]**

Stuart W. Teplin, MD, Clinical Center for the Study of Development and Learning, Child Development Institute, University of North Carolina at Chapel Hill, Chapel Hill, North Carolina 27514 **[301]**

Sally Zierler, DrPH, Department of Community Health, Division of Biology and Medicine, Brown University, Providence, Rhode Island 02912 **[23]**

*deceased.

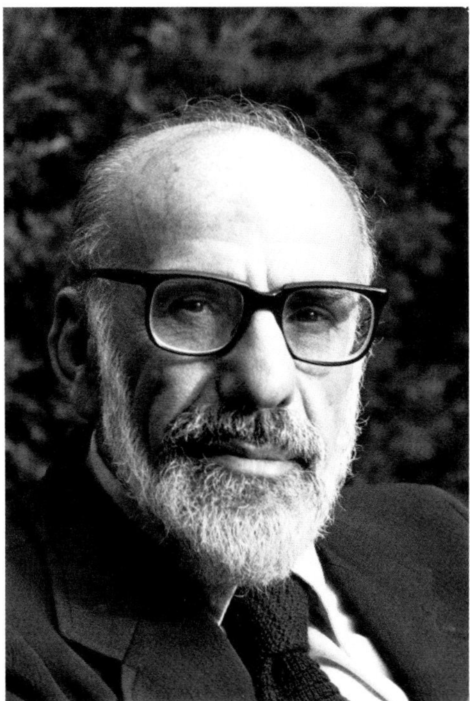

William A. Silverman

Dedication

One of our more pleasant tasks as editors has been the choice of whom to dedicate this book. William A. Silverman, M.D., needs no introduction to the vast majority of our readers. We honor him because of his contributions to our understanding of Retinopathy of Prematurity, a disease that has haunted his entire career, and because of his contributions in bringing the scientific method to perinatal research. To those for whom his name is not a household byword, we might best summarize his contributions to both neonatology and ophthalmology as well. Let us share some of his magic with you by telling how we first met him.

Our first contact arrived via U.S. mail. We received neat handwritten notes about a presentation or a manuscript he may have missed. Would we be willing to share it with him? Naturally, each of us was thrilled to find someone interested. The rest is history. Much to our utter astonishment, a reply came back, seemingly by return mail. It was a full review of our work. There was warm praise, sincere encouragement in a series of penetrating and perceptive questions about the study design and results, some of which we still ponder more than a decade later!

We didn't know it at the time, but we had become "adopted fellows" of Bill's, that is, he became an additional and very important mentor in our lives. We began to correspond, and received little notes appended to copies of interesting work. They asked, "Have you seen this?", or "Any thoughts?" Always, the article or thought was provocative, probing, or on occasion, just outrageously funny!

Bill is an insatiable reader and loves to quote our wise men through the ages. He made us aware of what Sir Peter Medawar taught, that "Science is the art of asking soluble questions." Bill has helped us both to do this, and to see problems in ways that allow the formation of answerable questions, testable hypotheses.

As the reader might imagine, we were early bitten by the bug that some have called "Silveromania," and began to ask ourselves, "Who is this guy?" As soon as we started to ask, of course, we learned from the many other students who have known him through the years that he was THE Dr. Silverman who had written one of the very special classics in perinatal medicine, the third edition of "Dunham's Premature Infants." This year 1979 brought a special time for those of us who admired and were insatiably curious about the man. He received the Virginia Apgar award at the American Academy of Pediatrics meeting in San Francisco, and we were treated to a full program all about Dr. Silverman, his life and his ideas.

He graduated from the University of California (San Francisco) School of Medicine in 1942 and moved to New York in 1944 where he completed his pediatric training. At the Babies Hospital, Columbia University, he was a student of Dr. Richard Day, the first Virginia Apgar awardee, who introduced him to the Premature Nursery, which he would later direct, and to statistical methods and the power of randomization, initially described by Sir Austin Bradford Hill.

First as a resident, and then as a private practitioner and part-time faculty member, and finally as a full-time faculty member and professor of Pediatrics, he exerted his considerable influence upon generations of young physicians, helping them to develop into physician/scientists.

His passion for using and teaching the randomized control trial grew, and he began to teach, increasingly, the need to question what we thought we knew, to examine the strength and the quality of the data that support our conclusions, and that we would be remiss to accept pronouncements merely because the speaker was an "authority."

His personal encouragement and support of those around him may seem surprising to the uninitiated, in light of his personal dedication to provoking dissent. Certainly he is always goading us to question each other, to doubt others and to demand the highest standards of evidence of data, to test our hypotheses. One of our favorites, of the many quotes he has sent us, is the one by the Reverend Robert Hall (1764–1831):

"The evils of controversy are transitory, while its benefits are permanent."

His students form a large informal "society" of current and former "Bill Silverman fellows." He also continued to write and has published several inspiring and encouraging articles and books on the Scientific Method and Human Experimentation.

It is with profound affection and respect for all his many contributions to our specialties, their subject matter, and most importantly, to ourselves as physicians and human beings that we dedicate this book.

John T. Flynn, M.D.
Dale L. Phelps, M.D.

Preface

The contents of this volume are based on the proceedings of a symposium on Retinopathy of Prematurity (ROP), held at the National Institutes of Health, November 21–23, 1985, jointly sponsored by the National Children's Eye Care Foundation, a private philanthropic foundation dedicated to supporting education and research in children's eye diseases, and the National Eye Institute. Surely no disease has caused such tragic acquired damage to vision early in life as ROP, striking as it does the youngest and smallest neonates. No disease has perplexed and baffled the physicians, both pediatricians and ophthalmologists, concerned with the care of these premature infants, as has ROP. It is paradoxical that today, in the midst of a true technical revolution in neonatal care, this blinding disease, long thought banished from the premature intensive care center, has reappeared in numbers not seen since the epidemic days of the 1940s and 1950s.

This volume covers a number of aspects of the ROP problem, ranging from the epidemiologic setting in which it occurs—the overall morbidity and mortality in the very low birthweight premature infants to the basic sciences concerned with the development of retinal blood vessels and cell membrane peroxidases to the psychologic problems of the family coping with a blind infant, and finally, to questions of malpractice, negligence, and expert witness testimony—all of which have become issues that this tragic condition has thrust to the forefront of the courtrooms of this country.

The audience we hope to reach is the interested professional—physician, nurse, social worker and family counselor. Within the covers of this volume we have tried to arrange our topics and presentations so that the reader may choose any one of a number of paths through the book. For some, perhaps only one or two issues hold interest. For others, with a deeper interest in the disease and its milieu, the whole book would be a suitable approach.

That such a spectrum of experience on a single entity could be encompassed in a book would seem a vain hope on anyone's part; yet we, as editors, believe it has been done successfully. That it has, is a tribute to the command of subject and range of interest of our contributors and the energy and enthusiasm they brought to the task. It is evident as one reads the individual chapters.

As we said at the outset, this book is an outgrowth of a symposium. But rather than treat it in the way these work products often get treated in print, we have interpolated a short précis of the discussion and the question and answer session that took place at each of the natural divisions of our subject. We take full editorial responsibility for this, for we felt it would indeed give the reader a flavor of the discussion the presentations aroused in the audience. It was a truly meaningful and memorable conference in that regard.

Finally, we wish to thank our staff editors, Natalie Paul and Tony Battle, from The March of Dimes and Alan R. Liss, Inc., respectively, and our manuscript typist, Mr. Frank Wilson, without whose tireless efforts on our behalf this book would not have seen the light of day.

John T. Flynn, M.D.
Dale L. Phelps, M.D.

I. THE LOW BIRTHWEIGHT INFANT

Significance of Low Birthweight for Infant Mortality and Morbidity

Marie C. McCormick, MD, SCD

Joint Program in Neonatology, Brigham and Women's Hospital, Boston, Massachusetts 02115

BIRTHWEIGHT: A MEASURE OF FETAL GROWTH

"Low birthweight" (LBW) has become a convenient, short-hand expression for a complex set of factors affecting the outcome of pregnancy, and, as is often the case with such conventions, a review of its genesis is worthwhile before discussing its implications. References to weighing babies and the special vulnerability of tiny babies can be found dating back to Biblical times. The idea that there was such a thing as a normal or expected birthweight did not emerge, however, until the end of the 17th century, with its great passion for measuring and quantifying the physical world, including man. Unfortunately, the first published norms were wrong. In his famous textbook, the eminent French obstetrician, Mauriceau, cited a normal birthweight of 15 pounds. At least in the English obstetric literature, these figures remained the standards until late in the 18th century, when the more accurate figures of 6–7 pounds were published. Not until the 1930s, however, did Yllpö, the Finnish pediatrician, suggest the use of the 2,500 gm cutoff to designate fetal growth so inadequate as to increase the risk of neonatal death. This cutoff point has been accepted and promulgated by a variety of sources, including World Health Organization statements [1,2].

Despite its widespread use, "low birthweight" has its limitations. Birthweight is but one measure of the adequacy of fetal development. Although highly correlated with birthweight, the duration of gestation is another. As the sophistication of diagnostic and therapeutic maneuvers in the perinatal period has increased, the combinations of these two measures have also increased in importance, giving rise to such distinctions as small- and

Based on an article in the *New England Journal of Medicine:* "The Contribution of Low Birthweight to Infant Mortality and Childhood Morbidity." N Engl J Med 312:82–90, 1985.

Birth Defects: Original Article Series, Volume 24, Number 1, pages 3–10
© 1988 March of Dimes Birth Defects Foundation

large-for-gestational age. In addition, 2,500 gm is but one point on a continuous distribution of birthweights, not a biologic marker. Indeed, birthweight distributions differ across different groups, raising questions about the applicability of a single cut-off weight for all births.

Nonetheless, LBW (and the more recent very low birthweight, VLBW; or 1,500 gm or less) has retained its usefulness as a measure of neonatal risk. In part, this utility stems from statistical issues; the continued use of a single standard facilitates comparisons between groups and over time. In addition, however, LBW does serve to distinguish a group of infants at increased risk for mortality and other health problems.

CONTRIBUTION TO MORTALITY

What, then, is the contribution of LBW to infant mortality? One answer to this question is an estimate of the extent to which being LBW increases the likelihood of infant death in comparison to normal birthweight infants; in other words, the relative risk of mortality associated with LBW. The answer to this question is that LBW confers a substantial increase in the risk of infant death in both the neonatal and the postneonatal periods. Compared to an infant born weighing more than 2,500 gm, an LBW infant is 40 times more likely to die in the neonatal period or the first month of life, a VLBW infant 200 times. The increased risk of death extends to the postneonatal period or remaining 11 months of the first year, albeit at lower levels, 5 and 20, respectively [3].

However, relative risk may be very high but only make a small contribution to mortality if it is a relatively rare event. We could then ask what proportion of all deaths occurs among LBW infants, or the attributable risk. The results are as follows: LBW infants account for 6–7% of all live births but over two-thirds of neonatal deaths and 20–30% of postneonatal deaths. Clearly, much of this is accounted for by VLBW infants, who make up 1% of all live births but 50% of all neonatal deaths and up to 25% of postneonatal deaths [3]. Moreover, these estimates are probably low. In areas where the neonatal death rate among normal birthweight infants is low, the proportion of deaths due to LBW infants is likely to be higher. By any standards, LBW confers a substantial risk for infant death.

CONTRIBUTION TO MORBIDITY

What are the implications of LBW for morbidity? The issues here are much less straightforward. For one thing, unlike the mortality data derived from vital statistics, no appropriate source of uniform data on infant and childhood morbidity is available. The discussions of the health problems of surviving infants must rely on a variety of clinical reports, often with varying definitions, ages at assessment, and types of observations. Second, since the first generation of children who have experienced modern intensive care are just entering middle childhood or school age, many of the long-term sequelae of perinatal events have not yet been described. Third, the full range of morbidity attributable to perinatal events is still being determined, and this would include complications of intensive care interventions. Also, the child is part of a social network, the most important unit of which is the family, and the effect of the birth and perinatal management of high-risk infants on young families is also being delineated. Finally, perinatal events represent only one determinant of child health, and disentangling the effects of birthweight alone or in conjunction with other determinants has proved difficult.

Within the bounds of these uncertainties, the risk for morbidity can be illustrated using two types of morbidity known to be associated strongly with birthweight. The first is neurodevelopmental handicap. The prevalence of cerebral palsy, hydrocephalus, mental retardation, sensorineural deficits, and seizures has been a primary focus in the follow-up studies of LBW infants since the first documentation of an increased risk among LBW infants for these problems in the 1950s. Of major concern has been the proportion of infants severely affected by such conditions, particularly among VLBW survivors, who appeared at greatest risk. Although studies from different sites may vary, about 2% of all LBW infants and 5–10% of VLBW infants can be characterized as severely affected, usually with some combination of cerebral palsy and/or mental retardation (or developmental delay).

Although less intensively studied, the increased risk for congenital malformations is also well documented. The rate of severe malformations is generally about 2%, and LBW infants appear to be about two times more likely to have such a malformation as normal birthweight infants.

Congenital malformations and neurodevelopmental handicap are not mutually exclusive occurrences. In our studies, 20–25% of VLBW infants had both. Because of this overlap and because of the association of both with perinatal events including LBW, we have combined them to provide an estimate of the relative and attributable risk of LBW for morbidity. The proportion of infants with one or both types of morbidity of all grades of severity ranges from 19% of normal birthweight infants to 42% of VLBW infants. At the more severe end, the percentages range from 2% to 14%. If we apply these figures to a population of surviving infants, the risks can be estimated as follows: LBW infants are 1.5 times more likely to experience a congenital malformation/developmental delay, VLBW infants 2.2 times. Moreover, the attributable risk is comparable to the distribution among all live births. Even for the severe forms of morbidity, the increase in risk is modest [3]. Thus we can conclude that LBW confers a much smaller risk for morbidity than for mortality.

RISK FACTORS FOR LBW MORBIDITY AND MORTALITY

As we well know, morbidity and mortality are not evenly distributed within populations. Factors known to increase the risk of LBW also are related to mortality, but in different ways. To illustrate some of the relationships, a subset of risk factors has been selected, and their relationship to neonatal and postneonatal mortality is discussed.

The first set of factors is labeled ''sociodemographic.'' More specifically, these factors are characteristics of many low-income or disadvantaged groups. These are well known risk factors for LBW. Adolescent mothers, black mothers, and mothers with less than high school education are about twice as likely to have an LBW infant as other mothers. As a result, they are also twice as likely to experience a neonatal death. What is of importance is that the risk of neonatal mortality is almost totally due to the risk of an LBW birth. In other words, controlling for birthweight virtually eliminates the differentials in neonatal mortality associated with these factors. However, controlling for birthweight does *not* eliminate differentials in postneonatal mortality [3].

Another set of factors may be considered ''reproductive'' risk factors. What these factors reflect is the mother's reproductive history independent of socioeconomic status. These factors act to increase the risk of neonatal mortality in two ways: first, by increasing the risk of LBW and, second, by increasing mortality independent of birthweight. The latter effect can be illustrated by the well established increased risk of older mothers having infants with malformations. As indicated, however, the risk is confined to the neonatal period [3].

What is being illustrated (and what is borne out by other studies) is that an infant may be doubly at risk, particularly coming from a low-income group. Not only is the risk of LBW increased but also this vulnerable infant returns to a milieu that places him/her at higher risk of other problems, eg, infectious illnesses, which are still the more frequent causes of postneonatal death, and, as suggested by other studies, environmental deprivation, resulting in failure to thrive and developmental delay.

CHANGES IN INFANT MORTALITY AND MORBIDITY IN RELATION TO LBW

In view of the importance of LBW in terms of infant mortality and morbidity, what do we know about the relationship between changes in infant mortality and changes in birthweight in the United States? To answer that question directly would require birth certificate data linked to infant death records for the country as a whole over time. The reason is that birthweight and maternal data, such as age and education, are on the birth certificate, whereas data on the infant's death are on the death certificate. Such information is not available. However, several types of studies permit some inferences.

At the turn of the century, the infant mortality rate was about 100 per 1,000 live births; that is, 10% of all infants died before their first birthday. By 1950, the rate was half that, or about 50 in 1,000. It is unlikely that changes in the proportion of LBW infants contributed much to this decline. Most of the decrease occurred in the postneonatal mortality rate and is attributed to improvements in sanitation and nutrition and to the control of infectious diseases [4].

By 1950, the infant mortality rate had arrived at its current configuration. Most infant deaths occurred in the neonatal period. As we have seen, most were related to LBW. And it stayed that way, at that level, for about 15 years [4]. This stagnation of the infant mortality rate generated a number of concerns.

–The limit in the reduction of infant loss had been reached, and no further reductions were possible for the most advantaged groups.
–Further reductions might be possible in disadvantaged (or low-income groups), but this would require massive social change.
–Attempts to improve the survivability of LBW infants were useless and costly.
–The technology was expensive; but, more importantly, the residual morbidity in survivors was extensive. Large studies documented the high rates of cerebral palsy and mental retardation. Of importance to this conference, this was also the period during which the risk of retrolental fibroplasia (or retinopathy of prematurity) was described [5].

Toward the end of the 1960s, the infant mortality rate began to decline, and it has continued to do so to the present. The decline has been substantial, to a level of about 12 per 1,000. The source of this change was not immediately evident, however, and much of the research over the past decade has been aimed at identifying the cause of this change and its implications. Briefly, changes in infant mortality could have occurred through three basic mechanisms.

1. The first is a reduction in the proportion of infants being born in high-risk groups, such as to teenage mothers and mothers with poor prior obstetric outcomes. The potential for this mechanism derived from the

availability of effective contraceptives (the pill and the IUD) and the subsequent decline in birth rate. The number of studies of the relationship of any shift in births among subgroups to changes in infant mortality are few, with the potential exception of adolescent mothers. These studies, however, do suggest some effect, but not a major effect. In all fairness, however, it is difficult to project "what might have been" statistically, since events that did not occur or were prevented cannot be measured. Nonetheless, most studies find a significant relationship between family planning services and infant mortality, but the relationship accounts for only a small part of the decline in infant mortality [6].

2. The second basic mechanism is to improve the outcome of pregnancy in high-risk groups through interventions in the antenatal period. Again, there was evidence for this mechanism. The Great Society programs had increased accessibility of medical care to the poor, and much research was going into making obstetric practice in the antenatal period more effective. In addition, perinatal services were being reorganized to bring this new technology to bear on high-risk women. However, the decreases in the proportion of infants born at LBW were small in comparison to the decreases in mortality. Moreover, the percentage of VLBW infants has remained constant at about 1%. The changes in LBW that did occur appeared to have occurred among those who started their prenatal care early. Also, the data available are not sufficient to determine whether those LBW babies being born were born in "better shape" because of prenatal interventions. However, changes in birthweight were not the major source in the decline in neonatal mortality [7].

3. This leaves the third mechanism: increased survivability of LBW infants because of hospital-based interventions in the perinatal period. This mechanism could be supported by process of elimination of other possibilities, but it is now also supported by a variety of studies. These include:

–clinical series from specific units over time, with increasing rates of survival of high-risk infants to attest to the increasing efficacy of perinatal care;
–studies that document differences in survival among high-risk infants born in centers with intensive care units and those without such units;
–studies documenting declines in neonatal mortality with the introduction of intensive care units into areas that previously had not had them;
–our own work, which shows that changes in delivery patterns to increase the referral of high-risk infants for delivery in specialized centers are associated with declines in mortality.

While this evidence is exciting in terms of the capacity of modern intensive care to save tiny babies, some disquiet arises when some of the adverse consequences are considered, namely, changes in postneonatal mortality and infant morbidity. Fewer studies address these issues. However, these studies appear to be converging on the following:

–Postneonatal mortality rates are higher among LBW infants, but this is not sufficient to offset the gains from the neonatal period. Moreover, the declines in neonatal mortality have not been accompanied by increases in postneonatal mortality rates.

–Morbidity related to antenatal and perinatal events occurs at higher frequency among LBW infants. As with postneonatal mortality, however, this is not sufficient to offset gains in survival. Moreover, morbidity may be decreasing as well [8].

WHAT OF THE FUTURE?

The enormous success of current perinatal care should not be minimized. However, it does raise several questions.

–Not the least of these is the cost. There is a general cost in terms of health care in the perinatal period, as well as additional costs for the minority of survivors with continued problems. There are also monetary and nonmonetary costs to young families just starting out that may affect their entire lives.

–It is not clear that technology can continue to reduce mortality at the same rate. Without invoking the ''biological limit'' argument of the 1950s, the most immature and tiniest infants present a management challenge to current intensivists.

–Most observers feel that continued declines in neonatal mortality will be achieved by decreasing the proportion of LBW infants, but, as was reviewed in a recent report from the Institute of Medicine [9], such reductions would require multiple different interventions tailored to the risk presented by the individual woman and substantial new resources put into prenatal care. Of particular concern are the real limits in the knowledge about managing preterm labor and in preventing the delivery of tiny infants. Although the report argues that such new investment would generate disproportionately larger savings from decreased need for intensive care, it is not clear in the current period where such resources would come from.

–Besides reducing funds available for new types of care, cost-containment strategies, both public and private, may threaten the arrangements that have contributed to decreases in mortality. Moreover, constraints on the availability of private and public funds may hamper research into the basic mechanisms of labor and fetal maturation and into improved techniques to manage high-risk newborns.

Such concerns are only reinforced by the fact that the rate of decline of infant mortality has begun to slow. From an annual rate of decline of about

4% per year, the rate has slowed to less than half that. Thus, although still declining, the infant mortality rate is declining more slowly, raising the fear of another period of stagnation. In reference to this conference, these considerations suggest the following:

–It is unlikely that the needs of the LBW infant with his or her problems will change rapidly. Although prenatal interventions hold great promise, much still has to be learned to prevent the delivery of tiny, immature infants. In any event, the 2–3% LBW rates experienced by our most advantaged mothers indicate that some infants will require intensive management for the foreseeable future.

–Efforts to support such infants require continuing investigation and innovation. Not only do appropriate management techniques appear to reduce mortality, they also appear to reduce subsequent morbidity as well. These efforts will increasingly focus on the tiniest babies, those most vulnerable to retinopathy of prematurity.

REFERENCES

1. Cone TE, Jr: De pondere infantum recens natorum: The history of weighing the newborn infant. Pediatrics 28:490–498, 1961.
2. Cone TE, Jr: "History of the Care and Feeding of the Premature Infant." Boston: Little, Brown and Company, 1985.
3. Shapiro S, McCormick MC, Starfield BH, Krischer JP, Bross D: Relevance of correlates of infant deaths for significant morbidity at 1 year of age. Am J Obstet Gynecol 136:363–373, 1980.
4. Shapiro S, Schlesinger ER, Nesbitt REL: "Infant, Perinatal, Maternal and Childhood Mortality in the United States." Cambridge, MA: Harvard University Press, 1968.
5. Silverman WA: "Retrolental Fibroplasia: A Modern Parable." New York: Grune & Stratton, 1980.
6. Hadley J: "More Medical Care, Better Health?" Washington, DC: The Urban Institute, 1982.
7. McCormick MC: The contribution of low birthweight to infant mortality and childhood morbidity. N Engl J Med 312:82–90, 1985.
8. McCormick MC, Shapiro S, Starfield BH: The regionalization of perinatal services: Summary of the evaluation of a national demonstration program. JAMA 253:799–804, 1985.
9. "Preventing Low Birthweight." Washington, DC: National Academy Press, 1985.

The Neonatal Intensive Care Unit: Organization of Care of the Low-Birthweight Infant

John C. Sinclair, MD

Department of Pediatrics, McMaster University, Hamilton, Ontario, Canada L8N 3Z5

The application of intensive care to the fetus and newborn infant is a relatively recent innovation [1]. Newer still is the regional organization of neonatal care. Regional programs for providing perinatal and neonatal intensive care have shown remarkable growth over the past 20 years [2]. It is the objective of this review to consider the operation of the neonatal intensive care unit (ICU) in the context of its place within a regional perinatal program.

REGIONAL ORGANIZATION OF PERINATAL/NEONATAL INTENSIVE CARE

I define a regional program in neonatal care as a cooperative, coordinated effort by health-care providers in a defined geographic region to intervene in the reproductive process so as to make available to every neonate a level of medical care that is commensurate with the risk of neonatal death or serious morbidity. Usually, and optimally, this program operates within the context of a regional perinatal program directed toward both mothers and newborns. Note that this definition is based on need and not on socioeconomic class or some other determinant of the utilization of health care.

Recommendations and guidelines for the organization and implementation of regional perinatal and neonatal programs have been published in the United States, Canada, and other countries. These recommendations recognize three levels of pregnancy risk requiring stepwise increments in the complexity and cost of health services: level I (about 85% of pregnancies), normal or low risk; level II (about 12% of pregnancies), moderate risk; and level III (about 3% of pregnancies), high risk. The proportion of live births requiring intensive care varies directly with the level of pregnancy risk; this proportion is about 3% in Ontario, Canada, and about 2% in Utah [3] (Table I). An additional 6% of births will require special care of moderate or

Birth Defects: Original Article Series, Volume 24, Number 1, pages 11–21
© **1988 March of Dimes Birth Defects Foundation**

TABLE I. Need for Neonatal Special Care (Utah, 1977)

	Babies		Days		Mean length of stay (days)
	No.	Percent	No.	Percent	
Special care					
Minimal	1,436	3.7	6,602	24	4.6
Intermediate	530	1.4	6,394	23	12.1
Intensive	715	1.8	14,443	53	20.3
Total special care	2,681	6.9	27,439	100	10.2
Total births	38,855	100			

Data from Jung and Streeter [3].

minimal intensity (about 5% in Utah). Given these estimates and current birth rates, one can estimate that, in the United States, about 100,000 babies per year will need intensive (level III) care and about 200,000 additional babies will need special care of level II intensity.

Typical indications [3,4] for the admission of newborns to ICUs include low birthweight (whether because of prematurity or intrauterine growth retardation), birth asphyxia, respiratory disease, infection, jaundice, malformations, and other conditions. The relative frequencies of the various reasons for admission are given for an English population in Table II along with the average length of stay [5]. The average length of stay in intensive care is determined by the degree of immaturity or illness and by the survival rate. As survival rate increases (especially among the most immature babies), the number of patient days for neonatal intensive care also increases.

EFFICACY OF NEONATAL INTENSIVE CARE

The efficacy of neonatal intensive care has been evaluated in controlled trials of a number of specific elements of neonatal care (Table III). Over 700 such trials had been performed by 1984 [6]. The application of the results of these studies has had an impact on the occurrence of retinopathy of prematurity (ROP) in two ways. First, studies have directly addressed the issue of causation of ROP (eg, the role of oxygen); the demonstration of a causal role for oxygen exposure led to a reduction in exposure and a reduction of incidence of ROP. Second, a much larger number of studies has addressed other aspects of neonatal care (eg, the thermal, respiratory, and nutritional aspects of management of premature infants). These studies have led to a substantially increased survival rate of premature infants, ie, of the population at risk of ROP. At first, this improvement in survival was seen mainly in infants of over 800 gm birthweight, but now the survival rate of

TABLE II. Admissions to Neonatal Intensive Care (Residents of Nottingham Health District, 1984)

Reason for admission	No.	Mean birth weight (gm)	Mean gestation (weeks)	Mean length of stay (days)	Deaths
Prematurity (without respiratory disease)	130	1940	33.7	15.0	0
Small for gestational age	37	1870	37.5	9.1	0
Asphyxia	25	2940	38.7	7.0	5
Respiratory disease	130	1700	31.9	31.3	24
Infection	8	3170	38.1	9.6	1
Jaundice	7	2730	38.3	6.3	0
Cerebral irritation	1	3760	40.0	1.0	0
Congenital anomaly	24	2660	37.4	9.8	11
Surgery not for congenital anomaly	4	2810	37.5	3.8	0
Observation	81	3290	39.4	3.5	0
Totals	447	2250	35.2	19.7	41

Data from Field et al [5].

even smaller liveborn infants is increasing substantially. As the limit of human viability is pushed downward to unprecedented levels, a new population at extreme risk of ROP (as concerns both incidence and severity) is being generated.

COMMUNITY EFFECTIVENESS OF NEONATAL INTENSIVE CARE

Community effectiveness is determined by five factors: efficacy of treatment, screening and diagnostic accuracy, physician compliance, patient compliance, and coverage [7]. An estimate of community effectiveness has been derived in the case of hypertension, based on independent estimates of each of these five factors (Table IV). The efficacy of antihypertensive drug treatment in reducing all morbid events (death, stroke, etc) has been determined in randomized trials under optimal conditions of diagnostic accuracy and patient and provider compliance and has been found to be very high. However, the impact at the community level is diluted because of problems of provider and patient compliance with therapeutic recommendations. In fact, only an estimated 37% of the efficacy is achieved in the community [7]. Can we make a comparable estimate in the case of neonatal intensive care of very-low-birthweight infants?

Neonatal intensive care consists of a number of specific elements, many

TABLE III. Randomized Controlled Trials of Efficacy of Neonatal Intensive Care: Major Subject Areas

Delivery room management
Screening and diagnosis
Thermal environment
Hydration
Feeding, content
Feeding, method
Vitamin supplementation
Mineral supplementation
Hyaline membrane disease, prevention and treatment
Intraventricular hemorrhage, prevention and treatment
Retinopathy of prematurity, prevention and treatment
Patent ductus arteriosus, prevention and treatment
Cardiorespiratory support, ventilation
Cardiorespiratory support, other aspects
Infection, prevention and treatment
Jaundice, prevention and treatment
Miscellaneous interventions

of which have been tested in randomized trials, as indicated previously. It is possible to estimate roughly the reduction in mortality risk when these elements are combined into a "package." In the early days of intensive care, Kitchen et al [8] carried out a controlled trial of intensive versus routine care in very-low-birthweight infants. The intensive care package consisted of arterial blood-gas monitoring, adjustment of oxygen concentration to maintain PaO_2 between 80 and 100 mm Hg, intravenous glucose and water, pH correction with bicarbonate, early enteral feeding, and daily monitoring of blood glucose, serum electrolytes, and bilirubin. Mechanical ventilation was not used. As is shown in Table V for the latter two years of this study, 35% of the control infants had died at 28 days compared to only 18% of the intensively treated infants, giving an efficacy in reducing neonatal mortality of 49% (difference in percentage incidence of neonatal mortality between control and intensively treated groups divided by the percent incidence in the control group).

Present-day neonatal ICUs, including our own, are experiencing mortality rates of only about 40% for infants weighing 500–1,000 gm at birth and only about 10% for those weighing 1,000–1,500 gm. Compared to birthweight-specific mortality rates of 90% and 50% for these two weight groups in the preintensive-care era, these figures translate into efficacies of 55% and 80% in the respective birthweight groups (Table VI). These latter calculated risk reductions for neonatal mortality may not be due entirely to the efficacy of neonatal intensive care (other changes have occurred that could affect the

TABLE IV. Calculation of Community Effectiveness: Hypertension

Efficacy	76%
Diagnostic accuracy	95%
Provider compliance	66%
Patient compliance	65%
Coverage	90%
Community effectiveness	28%
Percent of efficacy	37%
achieved in community	(28/76)

Data from Tugwell et al [7].

TABLE V. Efficacy of Neonatal Intensive Care in Reducing Neonatal Mortality (up to 28 days)[†]

	Died	Lived	Neonatal mortality (%)	Efficacy
Intensive care	11	49	18	$\dfrac{35 - 18}{35} = 49\%$
Routine care	21	39	35	

Data of Kitchen et al [8].
[†]Latter 2 years of clinical trial.

TABLE VI. Neonatal Mortality Before and After Neonatal Intensive Care

Birthweight class (gm)	Pre-intensive care (%)	Intensive care (%)	Efficacy in reducing neonatal mortality (%)
500–999	90	40	55
1,000–1,499	50	10	80

birthweight-specific mortality risk of newborns), but it is noteworthy that they appear to be in accord with (ie, credibly larger than) the risk reduction attributable to *limited* intensive care demonstrated by Kitchen et al [8] in the only experimental test of an intensive care package to date. The risk reductions of 55% (500–999 gm) and 80% (1,000–1,499 gm) will be taken as provisional estimates of the efficacy of present day neonatal intensive care in reducing mortality among very-low-birthweight infants.

The second determinant of community effectiveness is screening and diagnostic accuracy. After birth, the ascertainment of very-low-birthweight infants is virtually 100% accurate; all one has to do is weigh the baby. Before birth, the estimate is much less accurate, and errors in the prenatal estimation of gestational age or fetal weight occasionally lead to the unplanned delivery of very-low-birthweight babies outside of centers having neonatal intensive care facilities, and such babies could die in the first hours of life before admission to an ICU.

The third determinant of community effectiveness is provider compliance. This includes the decision to treat with intensive care as well as the treatment itself. Once the treatment decision is made, provider compliance in the highly regulated environment of the neonatal ICU is very high. However, not all very-low-birthweight infants can benefit from treatment, and a medical recommendation against instituting or continuing with intensive care may be made in the case of babies with extreme immaturity, lethal malformations, or profound brain damage. Moreover, an antepartum medical decision not to transfer a mother in preterm labor to a regional center may deprive the fetus of access to neonatal intensive care. A survey in Alabama [9] indicated that physicians who perform deliveries tend to underestimate the current potential for neonatal survival of premature infants. Moreover, when the physician considers a fetus to be nonviable, he is less likely to monitor the fetus, to perform a cesarean section for fetal distress, or to transfer the mother to be delivered in a perinatal center adjacent to a newborn ICU.

The fourth determinant of community effectiveness is patient compliance. Suppose that you are the parent of a newborn baby born very prematurely at 24 weeks and weighing 700 gm at birth. The neonatologist tells you that your baby, given intensive care, has a 50% chance of surviving and (if he survives) a 25% chance of having a significant handicap. Would you wish intensive care to be instituted? The structure of the decision to be taken is pictured in an idealized decision tree (Fig. 1), which shows two possible courses of action (ie, to initiate intensive care of this 700 gm infant or not) and three possible outcomes for each action (eg, survive intact, survive with handicap, or die in the early neonatal period). At each branchpoint where the outcome is determined not by choice but by chance (ie, at each "chance node"), one estimates numerically the probability of occurrence for each outcome. For each possible outcome, a utility value is determined. By multiplying the probability of occurrence of an outcome by its attendant utility, we obtain a score for that outcome. By adding the scores of the possible outcomes associated with an action, we obtain the expected utility of that action. The treatment plan that is preferred by the patient is the one whose prescription has the higher expected utility.

It will be apparent from this structure that differences between patients in the utilities they assign to the same health outcome might sometimes be pivotal in choosing the action that has the higher expected utility for that patient. At McMaster University, Torrance and coworkers [10] developed a four-attribute health state classification system that categorizes the health status of children according to physical function, role function, social-emotional function, and health problem. They asked a random sample of parents of Hamilton school children to value chronic handicapping states in childhood classified according to this system. They found considerable

Idealized Clinical Decision Tree

	Probability of occurrence		Utility of outcome (scale)	
Outcome 1	pA_1	x	(0-1)	Sum of scores
Action A Outcome 2	pA_2	x	(0-1)	=
Outcome 3	pA_3	x	(0-1)	Expected utility of Action A
Outcome 1	pB_1	x	(0-1)	Sum of scores
Action B Outcome 2	pB_2	x	(0-1)	=
Outcome 3	pB_3	x	(0-1)	Expected utility of Action B

Fig. 1. Decision tree illustrating a choice (choice node, open square) between two actions (eg, instituting intensive care or regular care) and indicating a chance (chance node, open circles) of three possible outcomes of each action (eg, survive intact, survive with handicap, die soon after birth). For each outcome, there is an estimated probability of occurrence and a health-state preference (conventionally measured on a utility scale extending from 1, normal health, to 0, dead; however, negative values are assigned for health states considered worse than death). This decision tree has been simplified for illustrative purposes; in most clinical situations, the possible actions and the possible consequences of each action are more numerous and the decision tree correspondingly more complex.

heterogeneity of values among the parents. This heterogeneity should warn us that the expected effect of an intervention, although valued as effective by most parents, may not be seen so by all. Indeed, 80% of parents in this survey identified one or more of the dysfunctional multiattribute health states as worse than death.

A description of the methods for the measurement of utility [11] is beyond the scope of this paper. The precision of utility measurement is such that it can be satisfactorily applied at the group level; unfortunately, the numerical quantification of preferences at the individual level is not particularly precise. The decision tree is shown more for conceptual reasons rather than as an applicable tool in the individual case. Nevertheless, it is sometimes clear that what the institution of neonatal intensive care *can* achieve is not preferred by some parents. These parental preferences may be pivotal in deciding to forego life-sustaining treatment.

Finally, community effectiveness is determined by coverage. Coverage refers to the extent to which an efficacious service is being utilized appropriately by all those who could benefit from it. In Canada, access to

TABLE VII. Admissions of Extremely-Low-Birthweight Infants to Intensive Care Units in Two Regions

	Ontario McMaster Health Region (1977–1980)[†]		Australia, State of Victoria (1978–1981)[‡]	
	No.	Percent	No.	Percent
Delivered at level III center	171	67	490	69
Delivered at community hospitals	84	33	221	31
Transfer neonate to level III center	42	16	105	15
No transfer	42	16	116	16
Total utilization of level III center	213	84	595	84
Total live births	255	100	711	100

[†]Ontario: Saigal et al [12].
[‡]Australia: Kitchen et al [13].

neonatal intensive care facilities is not restricted by socioeconomic class but may be restricted by geography.

Thus utilization of neonatal intensive care may be restricted by a number of factors as outlined above. We could measure the utilization of intensive care facilities by very-low-birthweight infants by calculating the proportion of live births of this weight and of a defined geographic area who are admitted to level III units. However, some relatively healthy babies under 1,500 gm may require only level II care. Therefore, we will estimate utilization by considering the proportion of babies of 500–1,000 gm birthweight who utilize level III care. This proportion has been estimated both in Ontario, Canada (McMaster Health Region), and in Australia (State of Victoria) [12,13]. In each region, the proportion is identical at 84% (Table VII). This is likely a slight underestimate of the extent of utilization, because appropriate utilization of level III care may not include a few infants included in the 500–1,000 gm weight group who are previable or who have lethal malformations such as anencephaly. Utilization is achieved in two ways, by delivery at the regional center or by transfer of the infant after delivery. Both in the McMaster Health Region and in Victoria, utilization occurs in remarkably similar ways: 67–69% of liveborn babies of extremely low birthweight are born in the level III centers, and 15–16% are born in level I or II units and transferred after birth.

What is the effectiveness of neonatal intensive care of these infants as measured at the community level? In the McMaster Health Region, we have already achieved a 46% survival rate among all 500–1,000 gm infants born to residents of the region [12] (Table VIII). Only 11% of such infants survived in this population in the preintensive-care era [14]. The reduction in

TABLE VIII. Survival Outcome of Neonatal Intensive Care for Extremely-Low-Birthweight Infants

Hospital of birth	Ontario, Canada (McMaster Health Region, 1977–1980)[†]		Victoria, Australia (1978–1981)[‡]	
	No.	Percent	No.	Percent
Delivered at level III center	92/171	54	167/490	34
Delivered at community hospitals	25/84	30	60/221	27
Transfer neonate to level III center	25/42	60	54/105	51
No transfer	0/42	0	0/116	0
Total survivors	117/255	46	227/711	32
Total livebirths	255		711	

[†]Ontario: Saigal et al [12].
[‡]Australia: Kitchen et al [13].

TABLE IX. Severe Functional Handicap Rate Among Extremely-Low-Birthweight Survivors at 2 Years (Victoria, Australia, 1979–1980 births)

	Handicapped/survivors	Percent handicapped
Delivered at level III center	16/71	23
Delivered at community hospitals	13/18	72
Transfer neonate to level III center	13/18	72
No transfer	no survivors	
Total	29/81	33

Data from Kitchen et al [15].

death rate from 89% to 54% comprises a risk reduction of 39% at the community level.

It is evident from population-based studies both in the McMaster Health region and in the State of Victoria in Australia that survival of extremely-low-birthweight infants is substantially higher among those delivered at the regional center than among those delivered at level I and II hospitals (Table VIII). This is not explained by differences in birthweight or gestational age [12,13] or maternal residence [12]. In the Australian survey [15], there was a three fold difference according to hospital of birth in the prevalence of handicap among survivors assessed at two years: 16 of 71 surviving extremely-low-birthweight infants born in 1980–1981 and delivered at level III units were handicapped vs 13 of 18 infants born in level I and II units and subsequently transferred to a level III unit for neonatal care (Table IX).

Table X shows the step-down from efficacy to community effectiveness for neonatal intensive care as compared with that for the treatment of hypertension. In the case of neonatal intensive care of extremely-low-

TABLE X. Efficacy and Community Effectiveness: Neonatal Intensive Care Versus Treatment of Hypertension

	Neonatal intensive care (500–999 gm) (%)	Hypertension (%)
Efficacy	55	76
Community effectiveness	39	28
Percent of efficacy achieved in community	70	37

birthweight babies, efficacy of neonatal intensive care in preventing death is estimated at 55% (Table VI). The observed community effectiveness (McMaster Health Region; Table VIII) is 39%. Thus, 70% of the efficacy is achieved in the community. In the case of the treatment of hypertension, there is a more marked step-down from efficacy to community effectiveness, largely because of suboptimal provider and patient compliance with diagnostic and therapeutic recommendations. Note that the efficacy of neonatal intensive care of babies of under 1,000 gm birthweight is less than the efficacy of the treatment of hypertension; however, at the community level, the effectiveness of neonatal intensive care is greater because of regional organization and, in a sense, a captive population of newborns who are readily ascertained as at risk. For babies of under 1,000 gm birthweight, further gains in efficacy of neonatal intensive care would appear to offer the greatest potential for gains in community effectiveness. Among babies born at 1,000–1,500 gm for whom efficacy of neonatal intensive care is already high (80%), future gains in community effectiveness will depend on maintaining high levels of compliance with program goals while striving for further improvement in efficacy of intensive care.

SUMMARY

A large and growing body of evidence based in large part on randomized clinical trials of therapy has established the efficacy of neonatal intensive care. The efficacy of neonatal intensive care is "leveraged" by highly efficient regional programs for ascertainment and referral of patients at risk. Thus the impact of neonatal ICUs is keenly felt in the community. The population incidence of ROP and its sequelae may be expected to rise as infants at highest risk—those at the border of viability—survive in increasing numbers.

REFERENCES

1. Hack M, Fanaroff AA, Merkatz IR: Current concepts: The low-birth-weight infant—Evolution of a changing outlook. N Engl J Med 301:1162–1165, 1979.

2. Butterfield LJ: Organization of regional perinatal programs. Semin Perinatol 1:217–233, 1977.

3. Jung AL, Streeter NS: Total population estimate of newborn special-care bed needs. Pediatrics 75:993–996, 1985.

4. British Paediatric Association and British Association for Perinatal Pediatrics: Categories of babies requiring neonatal care. Arch Dis Child 60:599–600, 1985.

5. Field DJ, Milner AD, Hopkin IE, Madeley RJ: Changing overall workload in neonatal units. Br Med J 290:1539–1542, 1985.

6. National Perinatal Epidemiology Unit, University of Oxford: "A Classified Bibliography of Controlled Trials in Perinatal Medicine 1940–84." Oxford: Oxford University Press, 1985.

7. Tugwell P, Bennett KJ, Sackett DL, Haynes RB: The measurement iterative loop: A framework for the critical appraisal of need, benefits and costs of health interventions. J Chronic Dis 38:339–351, 1985.

8. Kitchen WH, Ryan MM, Rickards A, et al: A longitudinal study of very low-birthweight infants: I: Study design and mortality rates. Dev Med Child Neurol 20:605–618, 1978.

9. Goldenberg RL, Nelson KG, Dyer RL, Wayne J: The variability of viability: The effect of physicians' perceptions of viability on the survival of very low birthweight infants. Am J Obstet Gynecol 143:678–684, 1982.

10. Torrance GW, Boyle MH, Horwood SP: Application of multiattribute utility theory to measure social preferences for health states. Operations Res 30:1043–1069, 1982.

11. Torrance GW: Preferences for health states. A review of measurement methods. In: "Clinical and Economic Evaluation of Perinatal Programs." Mead Johnson Symposium on Perinatal and Developmental Medicine, No. 20, 1982.

12. Saigal S, Rosenbaum P, Stoskopf B, Sinclair JC: Outcome in infants 501 to 1000 gram birth weight delivered to residents of the McMaster health region. J Pediatr 105:969–976, 1984.

13. Kitchen WH, Campbell N, Drew JH, Murton LJ, Roy RN, Yu VY: Provision of perinatal services and survival of extremely low birthweight infants in Victoria. Med J Aust 2:314–318, 1983.

14. Horwood SP, Boyle MH, Torrance GW, Sinclair JC: Mortality and morbidity of 500–1499 gram birth weight infants live-born to residents of a defined geographic region before and after neonatal intensive care. Pediatrics 69:613–620, 1982.

15. Kitchen W, Ford G, Orgill A, et al: Outcome of extremely low birth-weight infants in relation to the hospital of birth. Aust NZ J Obstet Gynaecol 24:1–5, 1984.

Causes of Retinopathy of Prematurity: An Epidemiologic Perspective

Sally Zierler, DrPH

Department of Community Health, Division of Biology and Medicine, Brown University, Providence, Rhode Island 02912

The purpose of this chapter is to provide a conceptual framework for the causes of retinopathy of prematurity (ROP) based on epidemiologic principles of causation [1] and related methodologic issues. Using these principles, a causal model is presented and applied to a database comprising information on over 3,000 premature infants who were originally assembled for a clinical trial on the management of patent ductus arteriosus.

PREMATURITY VERSUS OXYGEN

ROP is a disease of multifactorial origin, but two risk factors, usually referred to as prematurity and hyperoxia, are commonly thought to be the causes of most instances of this disease. There is considerable discussion in the literature regarding the relative contribution of these two factors, implying that these are two distinct hypotheses. However, this duality may reflect a confusion in concepts rather than ideas about nature. The following quotes from the literature are illustrative of the duality of hypotheses.

Statement I: "Oxygen has a long tradition of being implicated as a necessary and, when taken together with low birth weight, sufficient cause of acute RLF in the premature infant" [2].
Statement II: "It appears that prematurity per se may be responsible for many of the current causes of retrolental fibroplasia, in contrast to the overuse of oxygen which was the major cause during the epidemic of the early 1950s" [3].

The first statement asserts that, historically and currently, oxygen exposure is a necessary condition for ROP; furthermore, among low-birthweight infants, this exposure will inevitably lead to disease (if death or a preventive factor does not intervene). The second statement proposes that excessive

Birth Defects: Original Article Series, Volume 24, Number 1, pages 23–33
© **1988 March of Dimes Birth Defects Foundation**

exposure to oxygen used to be the major cause but, today, prematurity has acquired this status.

Both of these propositions recognize that prematurity has an important role. However, statement I claims that this role is effective only by circumstance, ie, in the presence of "oxygen," whereas statement II claims that prematurity has an independent and appreciable effect on disease occurrence. Both of these assertions, as stated, cannot be true, since the requirement for oxygen exposure described in I is implicitly refuted in II. I suspect, however, that these statements were not intended to be mutually exclusive. A review of the meaning of the terms "necessary and sufficient cause" and the distinction between operational and conceptual definitions of a causal factor may provide a basis for clarifying the interpretation of these statements and, more generally, for thinking about causes of ROP.

CAUSATION

The following discussion on concepts of causation is based on a model proposed by Rothman [1]. A more detailed discussion can be found in the original article. A cause is defined as that which brings about an effect. In an epidemiologic context, a cause is a characteristic of an environment, an individual, or an individual's behavior that acts either alone or, more commonly, in conjunction with other characteristics to bring about disease. Thus, what is commonly referred to as a cause, is more often a component cause, one of several (or many) components that act together to form a sufficient cause. A sufficient cause, then, by definition, is a set of component causes that brings about an effect (disease). A specific disease may result from any number of sufficient causes, and these sufficient causes may share some component causes, or they may be independent. Figure 1 is a simplified schema of three sufficient causes, each contributing to one-third of the disease occurrence. Also note that each of these causal pies has a different constellation, but all contain the component A. Factor A, then, must be the necessary cause, since without its contribution, every potential sufficient cause would be incomplete. Factor B is a component of two sufficient causes, and thus accounts for two-thirds of the disease (if we assume that each sufficient cause contributes equally to disease occurrence). Similarly, factor C accounts for two-thirds of the disease. The remaining component causes, D and E, together account for one-third of disease; since neither of these components appear in other sufficient causes, then we consider them to be completely synergistic. A synergistic effect is due to two or more factors acting together to bring about an effect that neither could result in alone.

A disease may have more than one necessary cause; for example, both the measles virus and a susceptible host are necessary causes of measles.

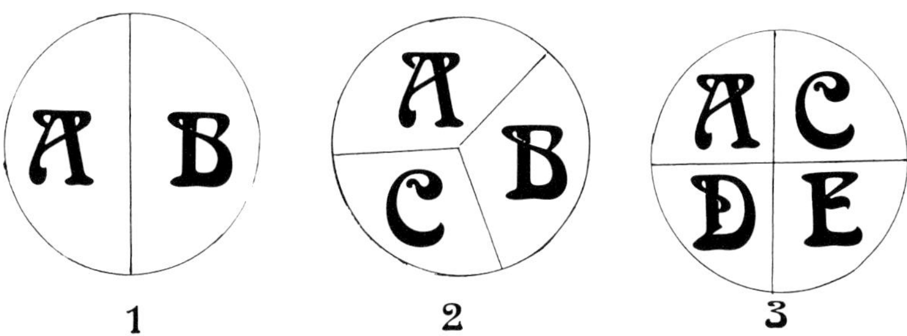

Fig. 1. Schema of three causes.

Eradication of the virus or of susceptibility would reduce the occurrence of measles by 100%. With respect to ROP, there is evidence to support the presence of immature retinal vasculature as a necessary cause. Animal experiments have demonstrated that vascular proliferative changes are not observed when fully developed retinal blood vessels are exposed to high levels of oxygen [4]. If this evidence is generalizable to humans, then immature retinal vasculature may be a necessary condition for the development of ROP. Operationally, this necessary component cause is often defined as prematurity, or low birthweight, because these easily recognizable characteristics are good indices of the theoretical causal factor, immature retinal vessels. It is important to remember, however, that gestational age and birthweight are only empirical measures of the presence or absence of a causal factor that in concept is immature vasculature. Appreciation of this distinction may explain, for example, observations of retinopathy in full-term infants, insofar as 9 months of gestation does not imply that retinal vasculature is necessarily mature. Were there evidence of retinopathy developing in infants observed at birth to have retinal vasculature developmentally normal for a full-term infant, then immature retinal vasculature could not be a necessary cause of this disease.

The hypothesis that oxygen is a cause of ROP developed during a time when hyperoxygenation of the sick premature infant was usual medical management. In that setting, oxygen management was a reasonable operational definition for exposure to excessive levels of oxygen. However, observations of retinopathy among infants managed at lower concentrations and infants who did not require any ventilatory support have raised questions about the credibility of the oxygen hypothesis [5]. Alternatively, these observations could raise questions about the validity of excessive oxygen management as the operational definition for hyperoxia, because this definition, today, fails to recognize the concurrent changes in oxygen management and the prevalence and degree of susceptibility to any extra-uterine oxygen exposure.

Today, we do not know what excessive oxygen means, but relative to 40 years ago, when concentrations of over 50% were routine, room air may deliver excessive oxygen to the very premature neonate [6]. Given the inevitability of postnatal exposure to oxygen levels that cannot be reduced without increasing risk of neurologic damage or death, there is limited usefulness in considering oxygen as a cause of ROP, except in instances when oxygen management clearly exceeds oxygen requirement. The oxygen hypothesis had an important contribution to identification of a *mechanism* for retinopathy. The hypothesis also led to empirical evidence that excessive oxygen administration initiated or potentiated the sequence of pathogenesis leading to acute proliferation of retinal vessels. To an epidemiologist, identification of a mechanism for the development of disease has a meaning very different from identification of a cause of disease. The former addresses the operative physiologic events underlying pathogenesis, whereas the latter relates to exogenous factors that initiate or promote this pathophysiologic sequence. Understanding disease mechanism on the biochemical level serves as a stimulus for identification of potential preventive factors (vitamin E is an example) that are capable of blocking an already sufficient cause. A cause, in the epidemiologic sense, is not a part of disease mechanism; rather, it is part of a sufficient cause that initiates or promotes this mechanism. Pragmatically, a cause should be susceptible to favorable manipulation so that the sufficient cause in which it is a member remains incomplete.

The two statements cited above can be applied to the causal model depicted in Figure 1. Statement I addresses an entire causal pie, and identifies factor A, the necessary cause, as ''oxygen.'' I can only speculate what this term is intended to represent, but if it means overuse of oxygen, then oxygen cannot be a necessary cause; in today's neonatal intensive care unit, relative to 40 years ago, overuse of oxygen is the exception rather than the rule. More importantly, in terms of the meaning of a necessary cause, retinopathy has been observed in infants who are not exposed to high concentrations of oxygen. On the other hand, if ''oxygen'' in this statement is interpreted as oxygen levels that are excessive relative to the developmental status of the infant (more precisely, of the retinal vasculature), but in absolute terms these levels are required for sustaining and nurturing life, then the oxygen hypothesis becomes void of any scientific meaning because it is untestable. Oxygen is a necessary and ubiquitous exposure. In concept and in fact, there is no living population that is not exposed to oxygen. Thus an epidemiologic design that might address this hypothesis would have to compare groups of infants exposed to different concentrations (the lowest being the oxygen level in room air) and durations of oxygen. However, these comparisons would be hopelessly confounded by the indication for oxygen supplementation, since the decision to administer oxygen, and the prescribed regimen, typically would be a function of lung maturation, and lung maturation is highly correlated with maturation of retinal vasculature. In other words, although the occurrence of retinopathy might be observed to increase with increasing duration of oxygen, one could not separate the effects of the underlying reason prompting higher or longer exposure from the exposure itself.

If, for the sake of argument, we assume that "oxygen" should be interpreted as overuse of oxygen, then factor B could be this component cause. With this conceptualization, Figure 1 explains how premature infants could be exposed to high oxygen concentrations and not develop retinopathy, because either these infants are lacking component C, which acts synergistically with A and B (in sufficient cause 2) or because of an unidentified preventive factor that blocks sufficient cause 1. Statement II is directly interpretable. "Prematurity" is represented by factor A, the necessary cause, and "overuse of oxygen" could be any of the other component causes, depending on how much disease would be attributed to this cause.

RELATIVE CONTRIBUTION OF A CAUSAL FACTOR

Statement II addresses the relative importance of prematurity and overuse of oxygen over two time periods. Figure 1 illustrates two reasons for a change in contribution of a causal factor to the occurrence of disease. First, if the prevalence of a component cause remains constant over time, then the strength of this factor will vary according to changes in the prevalence of the complementary components of the sufficient cause of which the factor is a member. With this reasoning, overuse of oxygen would account for less ROP if there were less exposure to any of the cofactors acting with oxygen to complete a sufficient cause. Similarly, the amount of disease attributed to prematurity would increase if its cofactors increased in prevalence. Second, the prevalence of the complements of a component cause could remain constant but the prevalence of the identified factor could change. Although an accurate description of the incidence of ROP over the last 40 years is not available, qualitative descriptions of disease occurrence suggest a U-shaped curve, with high incidence in the 1940s, a decreasing incidence over the next 20 years, and then an increasing incidence that today approaches a rate comparable to that of 40 years ago [7]. Applying the causal model, excessive oxygen exposure, once highly prevalent, caused a lot of disease. Reduction of this cause without an accompanying increase in other component causes or in other sufficient causes that were independent of oxygen exposure resulted

TABLE I. Hypothesized Determinants of ROP

Maternal factors	Neonatal factors
Alcohol	Acidosis
Anemia	Alkalosis
Diabetes	Anemia
Drugs	Apgar score
Duration of ruptured membranes	Apnea
Glucocorticoids	Birthweight
Multiple birth	Bradycardia
Threatened abortion	Bronchopulmonary dysplasia
Tobacco	Endotracheal intubation
Toxemia	Exchange transfusion
	Gestational age
	Hypotension
	Hyperoxia
	Hypoxia
	Intracranial hemorrhage
	Intrauterine growth retardation
	Indomethacin
	Light
	Patent ductus arteriosus
	Respiratory distress syndrome
	Sepsis
	Ventilatory support
	Vitamin E deficiency

in less disease. However, with increasing survival of the very low-birthweight infant, the prevalence of immature retinal vasculature increased, and the disease reappeared.

This resurgence could also suggest that the prevalence of other component causes has increased. In fact, in addition to prematurity and overuse of oxygen, a number of potential component causes have been suggested (Table I). Most of these agents are operational definitions for conceptual causes that could theoretically disrupt normal circulation and delivery of oxygen or affect (positively or negatively) maturation of retinal vasculature. In fact, many of these potential determinants may actually be confounded by the degree of prematurity and oxygen supplementation.

RETINOPATHY IN THE PATENT DUCTUS ARTERIOSUS (PDA)

A recent study by Purohit and colleagues [8] provides evidence that many variables considered as risk factors for ROP have no association with the disease after controlling for the effects of prematurity and hyperoxia. The infants enrolled in this study were originally monitored for entry into a

TABLE II. Selection Criteria for Three Studies of Acute Proliferative Retinopathy of Prematurity

	Flynn [9]	Kalina and Karr [10]	Purohit et al [8] (PDA cohort)
Birthweight (gm)	600–1,500	≤ 2,000	500–1,750
Vital status	Survived 28 + days	Survived hospitalization	Survived hospitalization (avg. dur. 44 days)
Study period	1/1/75–12/31/81	1968–1980	4/79–4/81
Location	Jackson Memorial Hospital, Florida	University Hospital, Seattle	12 Participating, U.S. hospitals
No. eligible	1,115	1,849	3,099
No. examined for ROP	639	1,849	3,025

TABLE III. Estimates of Cumulative Incidence (%) of Acute Proliferative Retinopathy of Prematurity

Birthweight (gm)	Flynn [9] Examined (n = 639)	All (n = 1,115)	Purohit et al [8] (n = 3,025)	Birthweight (gm)	Kalina and Karr [10] (n = 1,849)	Purohit et al [8] (n = 3,025)
600–999	66	33	28	750	54	43
1,000–1,299	34	19	15	750–999	38	26
1,300–1,500	11	7	5	1,000–1,249	16	15
				1,250–1,449	6	7
				1,500–1,750	3	3
Total	29	16	11		10	11

clinical trial on the management of PDA. The selection criteria for the retinopathy study are listed in Table II and are compared with the eligibility criteria in two other recent and independent studies [9,10] of other infant populations who were monitored expressly for acute proliferative vascular changes. The birthweight-specific incidence of acute proliferative retinopathy among the 3,025 survivors of the PDA cohort is shown in Table III. These rates are compared with rates estimated from the other two studies. The Florida series probably overestimates the incidence, since these infants were examined only if they had survived at least 28 days in the neonatal intensive care unit. The investigator recognized that these infants were younger and sicker than the general population of premature infants and cautioned that these rates may be inflated. The second column in Table III shows the rates when all infants ever admitted to the nursery were included, with the assumption that, had they been examined, they would have been free of disease. [This assumption is essentially correct. Discharge from the nursery occurred before they could be examined—Ed.] These adjusted rates, and those estimated from the Seattle series and from the PDA cohort, are remarkably comparable. The Seattle series may be the most accurate measure, since these rates were derived from a population routinely screened for acute proliferative changes in retinal vasculature among infants born weighing 2,000 gm or less.

APPLICATION OF THE CAUSAL MODEL

With some basis for supporting the validity of the retinopathy experience among infants in the PDA cohort, some examples of identified risk factors for ROP, based on this cohort, will be presented. The proportion of disease attributed to these factors was estimated in two ways: 1) the amount of disease attributed to a given factor among infants exposed to that factor [technically known as the attributable risk percent among the exposed $(AR_e\%)$] and 2) the amount of disease that this factor caused in the total population [known as the population attributable risk (PAR) or etiologic fraction].

The role of prematurity and duration of oxygen use was evaluated in this cohort to estimate the amount of disease associated with these determinants. Note that duration of oxygen use could be the operational definition for two causes, excessive exposure to oxygen and immature retinal vasculature, since the need for long-term ventilatory support is highly correlated with the degree of prematurity of the infant. In concept, it is not clear what duration of oxygen supplementation actually represents. It should be perfectly clear that duration of oxygen supplementation and hyperoxia are not the same, although they could be. Premature infants on oxygen for the longest duration may have the lowest oxygen levels measured in their arterial blood.

Based on the data from the Purohit et al study used in Table III, ROP would be reduced by 54% if infants weighing between 500 and 1,500 gm at birth were 250 gm heavier. Furthermore, among infants weighing less than 1,500 gm at birth, ROP would be reduced by 80% if these infants weighed 1,500–1,750 gm. Finally, in the total population of infants weighing 1,750 gm or less, the rate of retinopathy would be expected to be 3%, a reduction of 73% in total incidence if the weights were shifted by aliquot amounts.

The frequency of ROP in terms of duration of ventilatory support (intermittent mandatory ventilation or continuous positive airway pressure) is shown in Table IV. If the distribution of days on the ventilator was shifted, so that infants on support for 2 weeks or more actually were ventilated for 5–13.9 days, and those in the latter category were ventilated for less than 5 days, and so on, then ROP would be reduced by 65%. Had no ventilatory

TABLE IV. Rate of ROP According to Duration of Ventilatory Support (CPAP or IMV)

Duration of O_2	No. of infants	Percent ROP
14+ days	390	41
5–13.9 days	459	15
1 hr–4.9 days	834	7
No CPAP/IMV	1,335	3

TABLE V. Oxygen Management, Birthweight, and Retinopathy of Prematurity

< 750 gm	Duration of ventilatory support unrelated to risk of ROP
750–999 gm	Duration of ventilatory support unrelated to risk until at least two weeks on oxygen, then risk increases fourfold
1,000–1,249 gm	Risk triples as duration of support increases from 0 duration to next category (1 hr–4.9 days), then doubles with each successive category
1,250–1,750 gm	Risk low and relatively constant until at least 5 days support, then risk increases two- to threefold

support been required, ROP would be reduced by 82% among infants who were ventilated; among all infants, the rate would fall by 73%.

The amount of disease attributed to each of these causes implies that at least 73% of the sufficient causes include one or both of these factors. In fact, if these factors truly reflect different causes, and together account for 100% of disease occurrence, then at least 46% of the sufficient causes must include both of these factors, since the total contribution of all sufficient causes cannot exceed 100%.

Table V summarizes the additional contribution of oxygen management to risk, beyond the contribution of prematurity. The data on which these estimates are based are described elsewhere [8]. In general, these results suggest that the effect of ventilatory support decreases as birthweight decreases. For infants born weighing under 750 gm, the occurrence of retinopathy is unrelated to duration of oxygen supplementation, whereas, among infants born weighing 1,000 gm or more, risk increases with any ventilatory support, particularly after 5 days. The question remains, however, whether this overall pattern suggests an added, independent effect of oxygen, or does it suggest that duration of support is a sensitive index of degree of immaturity. As birthweight increases, does it become a less accurate index of immaturity? Again, we are confronted with the possibility of confounding by indication for oxygen management. Infants born weighing over 1,000 gm requiring oxygen support may be developmentally less mature than infants in the same weight category who do not require ventilation.

TABLE VI. Maternal Diabetes and ROP

	Diabetes	Diabetes, Insulin	Diabetes, No Insulin	No Diabetes
No. of infants	55	23	32	2,870
Rate of ROP (%)	16	13	19	11
AR[†](%)	35	18	42	
PAR[‡] (%)	1			

[†]AR, attributable risk among infants exposed to maternal diabetes.
[‡]PAR, population attributable risk.

TABLE VII. Maternal Antihistamine Use Within 2 Weeks of Delivery

	Antihistamine use	No antihistamine use
No. of infants	86	2,940
Rate of ROP (%)	22	11
AR[†] (%)	50	
PAR[‡] (%)	2	

[†]AR, attributable risk among infants exposed to antihistamine.
[‡]PAR, population attributable risk.

Two risk factors, among others, that were found to be associated with retinopathy after controlling for the effects of other suspected factors were maternal diabetes and maternal antihistamine use within 2 weeks of delivery [8]. The data summarizing their individual contributions to disease occurrence are given in Tables VI and VII. Because both these component factors are rare, they account for only a small proportion of disease in the total population of premature infants. However, among infants exposed to either of these factors, the attributable risk is considerably greater. For example, less than 2% of the population comprised infants of diabetic mothers. Although 1% of the observed retinopathy in the total population could be attributed to maternal diabetes (were this factor truly causal), over one-third of the exposed infants developed retinopathy because of maternal diabetes. Note, incidentally, that this contribution increases if management of diabetes during pregnancy did not include insulin treatment.

About 3% of mothers used antihistamines within 2 weeks of delivery. Twenty-two percent of the exposed infants developed retinopathy, and half of these infants developed the disease because of antihistamine exposure. However, in the total population, only 2% of the disease would be attributed to antihistamine use (again, assuming that this factor was truly causal).

SUMMARY

This chapter presents a strategy for integration of the current thinking about the causes of ROP. Application of these concepts assumes that results of any etiologic study are derived from valid methods. Discussion of principles of validity in epidemiologic studies is beyond the scope of this paper. However, reference was made to two sources of invalidity in studies of the causes of ROP: 1) the empirical or operational definition and measurement of the conceptual cause, and 2) confounding by degree of immaturity of retinal vasculatures, particularly with regard to interpretation of duration of ventilatory support as a cause of ROP.

The distinction was made between an agent that initiates or promotes disease mechanism and a cause. Failure to appreciate this distinction has contributed to the confusion about the role of oxygen in the pathogenesis of retinopathy. Apart from settings of oxygen mismanagement, oxygen per se is part of the mechanism for development of disease. Certainly there are other biochemical requirements in addition to oxygen that set the stage for full-blown disease. Factors that are associated with the disruption of normal development of retinal vasculature and are susceptible to manipulation (either by reduction or elimination) during the prenatal and postnatal period may be more useful component causes to investigate.

REFERENCES

1. Rothman KJ: Causes. Am J Epidemiol 104:587–592, 1976.
2. Flynn JT: Retrolental fibroplasia: Old problems, new challenges. Adv Perinatal Med 4:189–228, 1985.
3. Patz A: Retrolental fibroplasia (retinopathy of prematurity). (Editorial). Am J Ophthalmol 94:552–554, 1982.
4. Patz A: Current concepts of the effect of oxygen on the developing retina. Curr Eye Res 3:159–163, 1984.
5. Lucey JF, Dangman B: A reexamination of the role of oxygen in retrolental fibroplasia. Pediatrics 73:82–96, 1984.
6. Johnson L: Retrolental fibroplasia: A new look at an unsolved problem. Hosp Pract 16:109–121, 1981.
7. Phelps DL: Retinopathy of prematurity: An estimate of vision loss in the United States— 1979. Pediatrics 67:924–926, 1981.
8. Purohit DM, Ellison RC, Zierler S, Miettinen OS, Nadas AS: Risk factors for retrolental fibroplasia: Experience with 3,025 premature infants. National Collaborative Study on Patent Ductus Arteriosus in Premature Infants. Pediatrics 76:339–344, 1985.
9. Flynn JT: Acute proliferative retrolental fibroplasia: Multivariate risk analysis. Trans Am Ophthalmol Soc 81:549–591, 1983.
10. Kalina RE, Karr DJ: Retrolental fibroplasia: Experience over two decades in one institution. Ophthalmology 89:91–95, 103, 1982.

II. THE LOW BIRTHWEIGHT INFANT: SPECIFIC PROBLEMS IN MANAGEMENT

Perinatal Intracranial Hemorrhage and Retinopathy of Prematurity: Currently Nonpreventable Complications of Premature Birth?

Jerold F. Lucey, MD, FAAP

Department of Pediatrics, University of Vermont, Burlington, Vermont 05404

Periventricular-intraventricular hemorrhage (IVH) is the most important of the several types of perinatal intracranial hemorrhage that can occur in the premature infant. It is the most common and the most serious.

DIAGNOSIS

Prior to 1978, this diagnosis was made only on clinical grounds in the severest cases and confirmed postmortem. It is important to realize this, as any study done prior to 1978 will have grossly underestimated the true incidence of intracranial bleeding. When the computerized tomography (CT) and real-time ultrasound scans were introduced into neonatal care, the whole picture changed. It became possible to see small hemorrhages and to follow their course with these noninvasive techniques. Papille et al [1] proposed a simple classification system in which the smallest superficial subependymal hemorrhages were classified as grade 1 and the severest, which involved brain parenchyma, as grade 4.

It was quickly established that approximately 30–40% of infants of less than 32 weeks gestational age or under 1,500 gm of birthweight had intracranial hemorrhages. The incidence did seem to vary between research centers and debates have occurred over the explanations for these differences.

Ultrasound technology is changing very rapidly. It is now apparent that the size of the hemorrhage is not of major prognostic significance. Research techniques such as positron emission tomography (PET) and magnetic resonance imagery (MRI) have established that around each area of hemorrhage there is a hypoxic lesion of quite variable size. The blood, which is seen on ultrasound, is not a reliable sign of the size of the more serious

Birth Defects: Original Article Series, Volume 24, Number 1, pages 37–40
© **1988 March of Dimes Birth Defects Foundation**

hypoxic lesion; however, PET and MRI are not available in most nurseries. The leaders in the field point out that the hemorrhages seen on ultrasound are merely markers of more serious damage caused by the hypoxic lesions [2].

NATURAL HISTORY

In general, it can be said that if you have about 100 infants with hemorrhages one-fifth of the patients will die. These are the ones we used to diagnose clinically prior to 1978. The other infants follow a variable course, 50% resolving spontaneously and 20% having some change in ventricular size—half of these, 10%, arrest spontaneously, and the other 10% progress and require neurosurgical decompression. It is not necessary to remind the reader of the ''problems'' that a condition with a highly variable natural course can cause.

The first thing that became apparent is that the incidence not only *varied* but, since it has been studied, *it is going down*. The reasons for this decline are hotly debated, but in some units today only 20–30% of infants have hemorrhages. The reasons for this decrease in incidence and severity remain obscure.

One thing that has become obvious is that the incidence of hemorrhages is highly affected by gestational age; 60–80% of all infants of less than 28 weeks or 1,000 gm will have such hemorrhages, but only 20% of larger premature infants have a hemorrhage.

RELATIONSHIP TO RETINOPATHY OF PREMATURITY (ROP)

We have recently learned several things about the etiology of hemorrhages. Lou et al [3] have pointed out that asphyxiated newborn infants have lost their ability to regulate cerebral blood flow. With a small group of asphyxiated newborns, they demonstrated that cerebral blood flow was pressure-passive, which means that as you decrease or increase blood pressure, cerebral blood flow also varies. Neonatal brain capillaries are therefore exposed to surges of blood pressure that can cause them to rupture. This lack of cerebral blood flow control probably results in marked changes in retinal and choroidal blood flow. The brain and retina of sick infants are therefore exposed to erratic blood flow patterns resulting in either under- or overperfusion of the retina. A better term for ROP might be ''shock eye.''

Perlman et al [4] have recently given us an important new insight into the pathogenesis of this deranged cerebral and retinal circulation. They demonstrated a striking association between a fluctuating pattern of cerebral blood flow velocity on the first day of life and the occurrence of IVH in a series of infants requiring assisted ventilation for respiratory distress syndrome. This

TABLE I. Important Risk Factors for IVH-ROP

Extreme prematurity
Duration of oxygen administration
Duration of assisted ventilation
Apneic spells
Blood transfusions
Seizures

fluctuating pattern was related to the infant breathing out of synchrony with the ventilator.

Continuous monitoring of blood oxygen has taught us a great deal. We now realize the absolute futility of trying to describe ''an arterial O_2.'' The sick infant exists with a constantly changing arterial oxygen tension. Along with these fluctuations, which we cannot control or avoid, occur changes in arterial blood pressure, cerebral blood flow, and probably retinal blood flow and intracranial pressure.

Many of the ordinary care events in the life of an infant result in hypoxemia [5]. This in turn may result in or contribute to the lack of cerebral blood and retinal blood flow regulation, resulting in hypoperfusion or hyperperfusion injury to the eye and brain.

It is this deranged system of oxygen delivery to the brain and eye that makes it impossible to judge whether an elevated or a depressed oxygen concentration in a *peripheral* artery is the ''cause of retinopathy.'' It should be obvious that our continued fixation of measuring a single substance (O_2) at one point in time in a peripheral artery and trying to claim that this is the only cause of brain or retinal damage is not going to be productive.

Recent articles demonstrating an association between a risk factor and retinopathy all really demonstrate one thing, and that is that it is the sickest, smallest infants, who require the most care and are at the highest risk for every adverse outcome [6]. This is particularly obvious when one compares the risk factors for IVH and for ROP (Table I). Several studies have pointed out that this association is highly significant [7–9]. It is highly likely that ROP is of multifactoral etiology. The risk factors are all capable of causing a deranged retinal blood flow, with the eye responding to ''hypoxia'' by developing retinopathy.

SUMMARY

There is now considerable evidence that the control of cerebral circulation in sick small infants is sometimes seriously deranged and subject to wide fluctuations during neonatal care. Our current preoccupation with looking at oxygen administration and peripheral arterial oxygen tensions as the *only* cause of ROP is not likely to be productive. Until we know more about the causes of cerebral blood flow fluctuation, IVH, asphyxia, and their effects on the retinal circulation, we are not apt to make much progress.

There is a strong association between retinopathy and IVH in premature infants. With our current knowledge, we are unable to prevent or to treat either IVH or ROP. The public should be better informed that both of these conditions are usually unavoidable complications of premature birth.

REFERENCES

1. Papile LA, Burstein J, Burstein R, Koffler H: Incidence and evolution of subependymal and intraventricular hemorrhage: A study of infants with birthweights less than 1500 gm. J Pediatr 92:529–534, 1978.
2. Volpe JJ, Herscovitch P, Perlman JM, Raichle ME: Positron emission tomography in the newborn: Extensive impairment of regional cerebral blood flow with intraventricular hemorrhage and hemorrhagic intracerebral involvement. Pediatrics 72:589–601, 1983.
3. Lou HC, Lassen NA, Friis-Hansen B: Impaired autoregulation of cerebral blood flow in the distressed newborn infant. J Pediatr 94:118–121, 1979.
4. Perlman JM, Goodman S, Kreusser KL, Volpe JJ: Reduction in intraventricular hemorrhage by elimination of fluctuating cerebral blood flow velocity in preterm infants with respiratory distress syndrome. N Engl J Med 312:1353–1357, 1985.
5. Long JG, Philip AG, Lucey JF: Excessive handling as a cause of hypoxemia. Pediatrics 65:203–207, 1980.
6. Lucey JF, Dangman B: A reexamination of the role of oxygen in retrolental fibroplasia. Pediatrics 73:82–96, 1984.
7. Hungerford J, Stewart A, Hope P: Ocular sequelae of preterm birth and their relation to ultrasound evidence of cerebral damage. Br J Ophthalmol 70:463–468, 1986.
8. Brown DR, Milley JR, Ripepi UJ, Biglan AW: Retinopathy of prematurity—Risk factors in a five-year cohort of critically ill premature neonates. Am J Dis Child 141:154–160, 1987.
9. Bancalari E, Flynn J, Goldberg RN, Bawol R, Cassady J, Schiffman J, Feuer W, Roberts J, Gillings D, Sim E: Influence of transcutaneous oxygen monitoring on the incidence of retinopathy of prematurity. Pediatrics 79:663–669, 1987.

Respiratory Physiology, Oxygen Therapy, and Monitoring: Report of a Clinical Trial of Constant Monitoring

Eduardo Bancalari, MD, and John T. Flynn, MD

Department of Pediatrics, Division of Neonatology (E.B.), and Bascom Palmer Eye Institute, (J.T.F.), University of Miami Medical School, Miami, Florida 33101

The purpose of this chapter is twofold. The first section deals with the ventilatory problems of the premature infant and their therapy. The second section deals with preliminary results of a clinical trial of constant transcutaneous oxygen monitoring in the prevention of retinopathy of prematurity (ROP).

NURSERY PRACTICES
Respiratory Physiology

The respiratory function of the newborn undergoes a series of adaptive changes after birth that are required for normal transition from fetal respiration to air breathing. Within a few seconds of birth, the respiratory system of the infant must replace the placenta as the gas exchange organ in order to preserve normal tissue respiration. A number of problems can occur during this period of adaptation, which explains the high incidence of respiratory failure during the first few hours of life. This is even more striking in the preterm infant, in whom the development of the respiratory system is not complete at birth. The following are some of the most important characteristics of the respiratory system in preterm infants that make them more susceptible to respiratory failure.

Preterm infants have a high incidence of periodic breathing and apneic episodes that are due to incomplete development and maturation of the respiratory control mechanisms. The incidence of apnea increases at lower gestational age and it occurs in approximately 50% of infants delivered at under 32 weeks of gestation [1]. These episodes produce hypoxemia and hypercapnia and are usually associated with bradycardia and decreased arterial blood pressure. When apneic episodes are severe, the infant may not

Birth Defects: Original Article Series, Volume 24, Number 1, pages 41–52
© 1988 March of Dimes Birth Defects Foundation

resume respiration spontaneously and requires physical stimulation or artificial ventilation. The lack of resumption of spontaneous ventilation is in part due to the paradoxical response to hypoxemia that is observed during the first 2 weeks of life in the preterm infant [2]. Whereas the adult responds with hyperventilation when exposed to a low arterial oxygen tension, the premature infant responds with a depression of ventilation and apnea when his arterial oxygen tension falls below a critical level for more than a few minutes.

Another characteristic of the preterm infant that makes him or her susceptible to respiratory failure is a highly compliant chest wall [3], which produces respiratory instability whenever there is an increase in respiratory load. In addition, the preterm infant has an increased tendency to develop respiratory muscle fatigue, leading to hypoventilation or apnea when the work of breathing is increased secondary to lung disease or airway obstruction. Finally, the lung of the preterm infant is not fully developed, and the alveolar surface may be insufficient to sustain normal gas exchange. Moreover, the thickness of the alveolar wall is increased, thereby limiting the diffusion of oxygen from the alveolar space to the capillary blood [4]. The preterm infant may also have functional immaturity of the lungs, characterized by a decreased synthesis of surfactant, increased alveolar surface tension, and progressive alveolar collapse. This produces the respiratory distress syndrome, one of the most common causes of respiratory failure in the preterm infant. The incidence of this problem also increases with lower gestational age, and it occurs in more than 20% of infants born before 28–30 weeks of gestation [5].

Infection of the amniotic fluid may be associated with premature delivery; therefore, many premature infants are exposed to prenatal colonization with bacteria, placing them at high risk of developing pneumonia [6,7] and contributing to the high incidence of respiratory failure during the first few days of life.

Oxygen Therapy

Indications. Because of the frequency of respiratory failure in the preterm infant, a very high proportion of these patients require supplemental oxygen in the first weeks of life. The most frequent indications for oxygen therapy are hypoxemia secondary to respiratory distress syndrome or neonatal pneumonia. In addition, a large number of infants weighing under 1,300 gm at birth develop chronic lung disease secondary to damage produced by the mechanical ventilation and high inspired oxygen concentrations used during the acute respiratory failure. In these infants, the hypoxemia lasts many weeks, and thus they require oxygen therapy for long periods of time. Very small preterm infants, because of the morphologic immaturity of their lungs, also require long periods of oxygen therapy to keep their arterial oxygen tension within acceptable limits.

Methods. Oxygen therapy consists of increasing the inspired and the alveolar oxygen concentration to produce a larger gradient between the alveolar gas and the pulmonary capillaries. This increased gradient allows more oxygen to diffuse across the alveolar capillary membrane and improves oxygenation of the arterial blood. The inspired oxygen concentration must be adjusted according to the needs of each infant at a given time to maintain normal arterial oxygenation. This is accomplished by using mixers that blend air and oxygen to obtain the necessary inspired O_2 concentration. The inspired gas must be humidified, especially when the oxygen-enriched mixture is given through an endotracheal tube that bypasses the upper airway. Proper humidification reduces insensible water loss and prevents airway damage and drying of secretions in the airway. Because of the tendency of the preterm infant to lose heat and develop hypothermia, it is also essential that the inspired gas be heated to a temperature close to that of the infant.

There are different methods to provide an increased oxygen concentration in the inspired gas. This can be accomplished by increasing the O_2 concentration in the incubator; however, it is difficult to maintain a stable concentration, especially when the incubator is opened to care for the infant. It is also difficult to obtain concentrations above 60–70% inside the incubators. In infants who are breathing spontaneously, oxygen can be administered through a plastic hood that covers the entire head, allowing the infant to move the head within the hood while the inspired oxygen concentration remains stable. During transport, oxygen can be administered by face mask. In infants who require oxygen for long periods of time, this can be administered through nasal canulae, but, with this method, it is difficult to control and to measure the inspired oxygen concentration. Finally, in those neonates who require mechanical ventilation, the inspired oxygen concentration is provided through the endotracheal tube by the ventilator.

Complications. There are several complications of O_2 therapy that can result from the administration of high inspired oxygen concentrations. Because the oxygen has to be given through a humidification system and at increased temperatures, there is a risk of bacterial contamination and respiratory infection.

Improper humidification of the inspired gas produces an increase in water loss and may also result in drying of the respiratory secretions and airway damage. When the gas is not heated, thermal losses increase, and the infant may develop hypothermia. This is especially important when oxygen is being given through a hood that covers the head because of the rich perfusion and the large surface area of the head in proportion to the rest of the body in small infants.

Finally, a high inspired oxygen concentration given for several days produces acute oxygen toxicity in the lung. This is characterized by damage of the bronchial and alveolar epithelium and alterations of the capillary endothelium that may lead to pulmonary edema and fibrosis. It is possible that some of the antioxydant enzyme systems are not fully developed in the preterm infant, making them more susceptible to oxygen toxicity [8–10]. In premature infants, prolonged oxygen administration has also been associated with an increased incidence of ROP. This will be discussed below.

Oxygen Monitoring

Inspired oxygen concentration (FIO$_2$). The FIO$_2$ is usually measured using oxygen analyzers, with the sensor placed in the inspiratory line of a ventilator, inside the incubator or the oxygen hood. Most oxygen analyzers can be used continuously, and they have alarms that indicate when the oxygen concentration is outside a preset range.

Arterial oxygen. Arterial oxygenation can be monitored by measuring the partial pressure of oxygen in the arterial blood (PaO$_2$), the saturation of oxygen in the hemoglobin, and the total oxygen content per volume of blood. The most common method of evaluating oxygenation in the newborn is to measure arterial oxygen tension. The oxygen saturation of the blood is determined by the oxygen tension in a relationship that is defined by the oxygen affinity of the hemoglobin. Although the oxygen content determines the amount of oxygen that is available for diffusion into the cells, this measurement is not used in clinical practice.

Whereas, in the adult or older pediatric patient, it is possible to use the presence or absence of cyanosis to determine the adequacy of oxygenation, this is not a useful sign in the newborn. Because of the poor peripheral circulation in sick infants, it is common to have cyanosis even with normal PaO$_2$. On the other hand, because of the higher oxygen affinity of the fetal hemoglobin, cyanosis in the neonate appears at lower PaO$_2$, closer to the level at which oxygen delivery to the tissues may be insufficient.

Arterial oxygen tension. This is the most common method to evaluate arterial oxygenation. Partial pressure of oxygen can be measured directly in a small sample of blood using a Clark electrode. The advantages of this method are its accuracy and the fact that the analysis can be done in a few seconds. Its limitations are that it provides only intermittent measurements and requires a blood sample obtained through an arterial line or by an arterial puncture. Umbilical or radial lines are used in the neonate to obtain these samples. These methods are invasive and carry a significant risk of infection, thrombosis, and hemorrhage. Arterial punctures are difficult to perform in small infants, and they usually induce crying or apnea that results in an acute change in the arterial oxygen tension. Blood samples can also be obtained through a peripheral puncture in a heel or finger tip that has been prewarmed to produce arterialization of the capillary blood. This is also a traumatic procedure that produces a reaction in the infant. Although capillary samples allow an accurate measurement of pH and $PaCO_2$, they are less reliable when the peripheral perfusion is impaired, such as in shock or in cold stress. In these cases, the PaO_2 in the capillary samples can be significantly lower than in the arterial blood. Moreover, because there is always some degree of venous admixture into the sample, the capillary PO_2 is lower than arterial PO_2. This is more striking at higher arterial PO_2 values because of the larger difference between venous and arterial PO_2 [11–14].

Transcutaneous PO_2 electrode. This system was introduced a few years ago and was developed in Germany by Lübbers [15] and by Huch et al [16]. It has become one of the most valuable tools in the clinical management of neonatal respiratory failure. It is based on a small PO_2 electrode that is applied to the skin and has a heating element that produces vasodilatation and increases perfusion to the area where the electrode is placed. The oxygen diffuses from the skin capillaries through a membrane into the electrode and gives a signal that is proportional to the arterial oxygen tension. The advantages of this system are that it is noninvasive, allows continuous measurements of transcutaneous oxygen tension ($TcPO_2$), and does not require blood samples to measure oxygenation. Most systems are also equipped with recording devices that allow the evaluation of oxygenation over a long period of time. These monitors are equipped with alarms that indicate when transcutaneous oxygen tension is outside of a preset range. The major limitation of this device is that the $TcPO_2$ depends very much on skin blood flow. Conditions characterized by poor peripheral perfusion and decreased skin blood flow such as shock or administration of drugs such as tolazoline produce a significant deterioration in the correlation between the transcutaneous oxygen measurement and the arterial PO_2 [17–20]. The heating element normally produces hyperemia and sometimes a first-degree skin burn. To prevent this, it is necessary to reposition and recalibrate the electrode every 2–4 hours. In some cases, the electrode produces mild skin burns and a small scar that may persist for years [21].

Oxygen saturation. Oxygen saturation can be measured directly in blood samples obtained through arterial lines or by arterial punctures. This method requires a relatively large amount of blood, and, although it is used in cardiac catheterization laboratories, it is not a common method for evaluation of oxygenation in neonatal intensive care units.

Transcutaneous oxygen saturation monitor. Recently, a new system for monitoring transcutaneous oxygen saturation in the newborn has become available. This system is based on the differences in light transmission across the tissue of a small finger or toe that are produced by different hemoglobin O_2 saturations. It has advantages similar to the transcutaneous oxygen tension monitors but is less sensitive to skin perfusion and therefore can be used in infants with poor cardiovascular function [22,23]. It is extremely simple to operate; does not need reposition of the sensors, which are disposable; and does not need calibration; the values are very similar to those obtained in arterial blood. The only drawback of this system is that the clinicians have to adapt their thinking to oxygen saturation rather than arterial oxygen tension. Because of the shape of the hemoglobin O_2 dissociation curve, at higher PaO_2, relatively large changes in PaO_2 result in only small changes in saturation. As the PaO_2 approaches values of 40–50 mm Hg, the changes in saturation per mm Hg PaO_2 become much larger. Also, with PaO_2 above 80–90 mm Hg, O_2 saturation is close to 100%; therefore, higher PaO_2 values will not be accompanied by changes in saturation.

In very active infants, it may be difficult to keep the sensor in place to obtain an accurate reading. This is a minor limitation, since most infants who require continuous oxygen measurements are severely ill and are not very active. This instrument also provides a reading of heart rate that allows the monitoring of cardiovascular function simultaneously with oxygenation. The system is equipped with alarms that can be set at any oxygen saturation and can be connected to a recorder to register oxygen saturation continuously.

TRANSCUTANEOUS OXYGEN MONITORING AND ROP: REPORT OF A CLINICAL TRIAL

For a number of years, there has been evidence relating oxygen therapy to ROP [24–27]. Although it is likely that this is a multifactorial disease [28], several studies have suggested a correlation between the duration of oxygen exposure and the development of ROP [24,29]. Attempts to relate different inspired oxygen concentrations with the disease so far have been inconclusive [24,29,28]. Although it has been mentioned for many years that ROP is probably related to the levels of arterial oxygen tension, several attempts to define the relationship between specific levels of arterial oxygen tension and ROP have been unsuccessful [29,30]. It has been postulated that the reason why this relationship has not been established is because of the intermittent nature of the arterial oxygen measurements. It is possible that between arterial samples the infants were exposed to abnormal arterial oxygen tensions that could not be detected by intermittent blood sampling.

The introduction of continuous oxygen monitoring devices opened the door for testing again the hypothesis that ROP is related to abnormal arterial oxygen tensions. Although it has been suggested that continuous oxygen monitoring may reduce the incidence of ROP [31], this has not been demonstrated in a prospective, controlled study. To answer these questions and to define the role of continuous oxygen monitoring in the incidence of ROP, a prospective, controlled study was done at the University of Miami/Jackson Memorial Hospital between the years 1982 and 1984. The principal aim of the study was to investigate whether, by continuous transcutaneous oxygen monitoring during oxygen therapy, it is possible to reduce the incidence of ROP. The second aim was to evaluate whether continuous monitoring could shorten the exposure to oxygen and mechanical ventilation in infants with respiratory failure. The third aim of this study was to define the relationship between the exposure to different TcPO$_2$ levels and the development of ROP. This paper describes the results related to the first two aims.

Materials and Methods

All infants born at Jackson Memorial Hospital during the study period with birth weights between 550 and 1,300 gm and who required oxygen therapy at some time during the first 7 days of life were eligible for the study. A total of 438 infants under 1,300 gm were born during the study period. Out of these, 296 infants were enrolled in the study. Of the 142 not enrolled, 74 were in critical condition at birth and expired before parental consent could be obtained, 42 did not require oxygen therapy, and in 11 cases parents did not consent to the study. Five infants had severe congenital anomalies, two had hydrops fetalis, one was born to a mother with suspected AIDS, and in one there was an error in admission criteria. The other six cases were not randomized because monitors were not available at the time they became eligible for the study. Infants enrolled in the study were assigned, during the first 12 hours of oxygen therapy, to a continuous monitoring (CM) or a standard care (SC) group, using a random list of numbers.

To ensure even distribution of weights in the two groups, infants were randomized to the CM or SC groups according to their birthweight using two strata, one from 500 to 899 gm and the other from 900 to 1,300 gm. Before randomization, all infants receiving oxygen were monitored continuously. After randomization, infants in the CM group were kept on a transcutaneous oxygen monitor as long as they required any additional oxygen in the inspired gas to maintain their PaO$_2$ above 50 mm Hg. Infants assigned to the SC group were monitored only during the more acute stage of their disease subject to availability of monitors in the unit.

In both groups, arterial oxygen tension was measured intermittently in blood samples obtained through umbilical arterial lines or peripheral arteries according to the unit protocol, usually every 4 hours while the infant was on

TABLE I. Physical Characteristics of All Infants Enrolled

	500–899 gm		900–1,300 gm	
	CM (n = 43)	SC (n = 45)	CM (n = 105)	SC (n = 103)
Birthweight (gm)	746 ± 95	741 ± 88	1093 ± 114	1106 ± 123
Gestational age (weeks)	27.6 ± 2.0	27.4 ± 2.0	29.9 ± 2.0	30.2 ± 1.2
SGA	13	9	6	3
Male/female	21/22	24/21	53/52	57/46
Black/white	35/8	33/12	70/35	64/39

mechanical ventilation and less frequently after the infants were weaned from the ventilator. In all infants, an attempt was made to keep arterial oxygen tension between 50 and 70 mm Hg by adjusting the inspired oxygen concentration or the settings on the ventilator. The transcutaneous monitors on the CM infants had visual and audible alarms that were set at 50 mm Hg for the low and 70 mm Hg for the high limit.

Management was otherwise identical in both groups. Eye examinations were done in all infants by a pediatric ophthalmologist using indirect ophthalmoscope. The examinations were begun when the infant reached 32 weeks of conceptual age and was in stable clinical condition, and they were repeated every 2–4 weeks until the baby was discharged from the hospital. ROP was diagnosed when one eye examination or more was positive prior to discharge [32].

Results

Of the 296 infants enrolled in the study, 214 were discharged alive from the hospital. Of these, 202 had a conclusive eye examination and could be classified as either ROP or non-ROP. In 12 infants, four in the CM and eight in the SC group, ROP could not be definitely diagnosed or ruled out. These infants were excluded from the analysis of ROP incidence. The physical and clinical characteristics of the infants enrolled in both groups are shown in Tables I and II. There were no differences in birthweight, gestational age, sex distribution, or race between CM and SC infants in any of the birthweight strata. A larger proportion of infants weighing over 900 gm in the CM group had 5-minute Apgar scores of 4 or less than infants in the SC group. Although more infants developed sepsis and expired in the CM group than in the SC group, the differences did not reach statistical significance. The duration of hospitalization was also similar in the two groups. Table 3 shows the number of hours of oxygen therapy and mechanical ventilation in the survivors in the two groups and the median hours that the two groups spent on continuous oxygen monitor during the first 28 days of life. The median

TABLE II. Clinical Data on All Infants Enrolled

	500–899 gm		900–1,300 gm	
	CM (n = 43)	SC (n = 45)	CM (n = 105)	SC (n = 103)
5 Min Apgar ≤ 4	8	10	16*	4
RDS	36	39	73	62
PDA	21	27	34	33
Apnea	37	38	81	88
CNS hemorrhage	20	22	43	36
Sepsis	18	14	23	14
NEC	2	2	15	13
CLD	19	17	15	16
Exchange transfused	11	9	10	9
PRBC transfused (ml)	134 ± 92	145 ± 136	99 ± 101	98 ± 100
Survived	22	24	79	89

*P < 0.01 CM vs SC.

TABLE III. Respiratory Therapy and O$_2$ Monitoring Over First 28 Days [median (ranges)]

	500–899 gm		900–1,300 mg	
	CM (n = 22)	SC (n = 24)	CM (n = 79)	SC (n = 89)
Hours of O$_2$ therapy	466 (85–659)	410 (2.8–672)	89 (0.8–672)	109 (0.2–672)
Hours of IPPV	236 (59–672)	161 (11–672)	49 (0–672)	33 (0–473)
Hours of TcPO$_2$ monitoring (during O$_2$ therapy)	456* (82–644)	56 (1–287)	84* (0.7–672)	35 (0.2–343)
No. of arterial blood gas measurements	69 (38–206)	67 (13–136)	33 (0–123)	31 (1–200)

*P < 0.005, CM vs SC.

number of hours of oxygen therapy was similar in both groups. The duration of mechanical ventilation was longer in the CM group infants, but the difference is not significant because of the large individual variation. As expected, the time on transcutaneous monitoring was significantly greater in infants in the CM group than in the SC group. The number of arterial blood gas determinations was similar in both groups. The incidence of ROP in the two study groups is shown in Table IV. Four infants in the CM group developed cicatricial ROP; five in the SC group had cicatricial ROP. The overall incidence of ROP was similar in the two groups, 54% in CM and 64% in SC infants.

TABLE IV. ROP Incidence (Survivors)[†]

	500–899 gm		900–1,300 gm	
	CM (n = 22)	SC (n = 24)	CM (n = 79)	SC (n = 89)
ROP total (%)	19 (86)	22 (92)	33 (44)	45 (56)
ROP cicatricial (%)	4 (18)	3 (12.5)	0 (0)	2 (2.5)
Indefinite	0	0	4	8

[†]%ROP excluding indefinites.

Discussion

The overall incidence of ROP in this study was higher than that reported for similar gestational-age infants in previous publications [33,34]. This is most likely related to the fact that infants were examined repeatedly during their hospital stay, allowing the detection of mild forms of the disease that may be missed when infants are examined only once at the time of discharge from the hospital. As in previous reports, there was a clear relationship between ROP and birthweight, with over 80% of infants weighing under 1,000 gm developing some form of the disease. The incidence of cicatricial ROP was similar to that reported previously, and all cases except one occurred in infants under 1,000 gm. The results did not confirm the hypothesis that continuous monitoring could reduce the incidence of ROP in preterm infants who require oxygen therapy. Although there were more infants with ROP among patients with birthweights above 1,100 gm in the SC group, this can be explained by the fact that these infants had a more protracted respiratory course and received oxygen for longer periods of time. Although this longer exposure to additional oxygen may have been influenced by the lack of monitoring, this seems unlikely because transcutaneous monitoring did not influence the duration of oxygen exposure in the smaller infants. There are several possible explanations for the lack of effect of transcutaneous monitoring on the incidence of ROP. It is possible that in the more immature infants factors other than arterial oxygen tension are more important in the development of ROP. Another possibility is that the selected PaO_2 range of 50–70 mm Hg is too high for these very immature infants. Finally, in many infants, especially in those with periodic breathing and frequent apneic episodes, there are fluctuations in arterial oxygen tension that take the PaO_2 below 50 mm Hg and over 70 mm Hg, and these fluctuations cannot be avoided in spite of using continuous oxygen monitoring.

It is difficult to interpret the effect of continuous monitoring on the evolution of the respiratory disease because of the very large individual variation in oxygen requirements and mechanical ventilation among patients.

Although infants in the continuous monitoring group spent more time on mechanical ventilation, this difference was not statistically significant.

These results show no evidence that continuous monitoring has an impact on the incidence of ROP in infants weighing under 1,300 gm, except in infants with birthweights greater than 1,100 gm. Certainly it does not reduce the incidence in small infants, in whom this complication occurs more frequently and is more severe [32]. The lack of effect of continuous monitoring suggests that factors other than arterial oxygen tension may be more important in the development of ROP. It is also possible that, in spite of the continuous monitoring, arterial oxygen tension may still reach levels that are damaging to the immature retina.

REFERENCES

1. Henderson-Smart DJ: The effect of gestational age on the incidence and duration of recurrent apnea in newborn babies. Aust Paediatr J 17:273–276, 1981.
2. Rigatto H, Brady JP, de la Torre Verduzco R: Chemoreceptor reflexes in preterm infants: I. The effect of gestational and postnatal age on the ventilatory response to inhalation of 100% and 15% oxygen. Pediatrics 55:604–613, 1975.
3. Gerhardt T, Bancalari E: Chestwall compliance in full-term and premature infants. Acta Paediatr Scand 69:359–364, 1980.
4. Burri PH, Weibel ER: Ultrastructure and morphometry of the developing lung. In Hodson WA (ed): "Development of the Lung." New York: Marcel Dekker, Inc., 1977, pp 215–268.
5. Hjalmarson O: Epidemiology and classification of acute, neonatal respiratory disorders. A prospective study. Acta Paediatr Scand 70:773–783, 1981.
6. Garite TJ, Freeman RK: Chorioamnionitis in the preterm gestation. Obstet Gynecol 59:539–545, 1982.
7. Naeye RL: Factors that predispose to premature rupture of fetal membranes. Obstet Gynecol 60:93–98, 1982.
8. Frank L, Groseclose EE: Preparation for birth into an O$_2$-rich environment: The antioxidant enzymes in the developing rabbit lung. Pediatr Res 18:240–244, 1984.
9. Frank L: Effects of oxygen on the newborn. Fed Proc 44:2328–2334, 1985.
10. Gerdin E, Týden O, Eriksson UJ: The development of antioxidant enzymatic defense in the perinatal rat lung: Activities of superoxide dismutase, glutathione peroxidase, and catalase. Pediatr Res 19:687–691, 1985.
11. Gandy G, Grann L, Cunningham N, Adamsons K Jr, James LS: The validity of pH and PcO$_2$ measurements in capillary samples in sick and healthy newborn infants. Pediatrics 34:192–197, 1964.
12. Banister A: Comparison of arterial and arterialized capillary blood in infants with respiratory distress. Arch Dis Child 44:726–728, 1969.
13. Glasgow JFT, Flynn DM, Swyer PR: A comparison of descending aortic and "arterialized" capillary blood in the sick newborn. Can Med Assoc J 106:660–662, 1972.
14. Karna P, Poland RL: Monitoring critically ill newborn infants with digital capillary blood samples: An alternative. J Pediatr 92:270–273, 1978.
15. Lübbers DW: Theoretical basis of the transcutaneous blood gas measurements. Crit Care Med 9:721–733, 1981.

16. Huch R, Huch A, Albani M, Gabriel M, Schulte FJ, Wolf H, Rupprath G, Emmrich P, Stechele U, Duc G, Bucher H: Transcutaneous PO_2 monitoring in routine management of infants and children with cardiorespiratory problems. Pediatrics 57:681–690, 1976.
17. Versmold HT, Linderkamp O, Holzmann M, Strohhacker I, Riegel KP: Limits of $tcPO_2$ monitoring in sick neonates: Relation to blood pressure, blood volume, peripheral blood flow and acid base status. Acta Anaesthesiol Scand 68 [Suppl]:88–90, 1978.
18. Swanström S, Elisaga IV, Cárdona L, Cardenes A, Mendez-Bauer C, Rooth G: Transcutaneous PO_2 measurements in seriously ill newborn infants. Arch Dis Child 50:913–919, 1975.
19. Peabody JL, Gregory GA, Willis MM, Tooley WH: Transcutaneous oxygen tension in sick infants. Am Rev Respir Dis 118:83–87, 1978.
20. Rome ES, Stork EK, Carlo WA, Martin RJ: Limitations of transcutaneous PO_2 and PCO_2 monitoring in infants with bronchopulmonary dysplasia. Pediatrics 74:217–220, 1984.
21. Golden SM: Skin craters—A complication of transcutaneous oxygen monitoring. Pediatrics 67:514–516, 1981.
22. Deckardt R, Steward DJ: Noninvasive arterial hemoglobin oxygen saturation versus transcutaneous oxygen tension monitoring in the preterm infant. Crit Care Med 12:935–939, 1984.
23. Fanconi S, Doherty P, Edmonds JF, Barker GA, Bohn DJ: Pulse oximetry in pediatric intensive care: Comparison with measured saturations and transcutaneous oxygen tension. J Pediatr 107:362–366, 1985.
24. Kinsey VE: Retrolental fibroplasia: Cooperative study of retrolental fibroplasia and the use of oxygen. Arch Ophthalmol 56:481–543, 1956.
25. Gordon HH, Lubchenco L, Hix I: Observations on the etiology of retrolental fibroplasia. Bull Johns Hopkins Hosp 94:34–44, 1954.
26. Lanman JT, Guy LP, Dancis J: Retrolental fibroplasia and oxygen therapy. J Am Med Assoc 155:223–226, 1954.
27. Patz A, Hoeck LE, DeLaCruz E: Studies on the effect of high oxygen administration in retrolental fibroplasia: I. Nursing observations. Am J Ophthalmol 35:1248–1253, 1952.
28. Lucey JF, Dangman B: A reexamination of the role of oxygen in retrolental fibroplasia. Pediatrics 73:82–96, 1984.
29. Kinsey VE, Arnold HJ, Kalina RE, Stern L, Stahlman M, Odell G, Driscoll JM Jr, Elliott JH, Payne J, Patz A: PaO_2 levels and retrolental fibroplasia: A report of the cooperative study. Pediatrics 60:655–668, 1977.
30. Yu VY, Hookham DM, Nave JR: Retrolental fibroplasia—controlled study of 4 years' experience in a neonatal intensive care unit. Arch Dis Child 57:247–252, 1982.
31. Yamanouchi I, Igarashi I, Ouchi E: Successful prevention of retinopathy of prematurity via transcutaneous oxygen partial pressure monitoring: In Huch ER, Huch A (eds): "Continuous Transcutaneous Blood Gas Monitoring." New York: Marcel Dekker, Inc., 1983, pp 333–340.
32. Bancalari E, Flynn JT, Goldberg R et al: Influence of transcutaneous oxygen monitoring on the incidence of retinopathy of prematurity. Pediatrics 79:663–669, 1987.
33. Kalina RE, Karr DJ: Retrolental fibroplasia: Experience over two decades in one institution. Ophthalmology 89:91–95, 1982.
34. Campbell PB, Bull MJ, Ellis FD, Bryson CQ, Lemons JA, Schreiner RL: Incidence of retinopathy of prematurity in a tertiary newborn intensive care unit. Arch Ophthalmol 101:1686–1688, 1983.

Relation Between Persistent Patency of the Ductus Arteriosus and Retinopathy of Prematurity

George Cassady, MD

Department of Pediatrics, University of Alabama at Birmingham, Birmingham, Alabama 35294

Galen was aware of the presence of an anatomic channel between aorta and pulmonary artery in the fetus as early as 200 AD [1]. More than 1,400 years later, Harvey described unidirectional flow of blood from venous to arterial systems through this structure in the fetus and suggested a purpose for it before birth [2]. Two more centuries passed before clinicians became commonly aware that failed closure of the structure after birth often accompanied other structural defects of the heart. It was in 1907 when Monroe first suggested surgical closure in selected instances [1,2]. The first successful surgical closure was recorded by Gross and Hubbard 32 years later [3]. Details of the events surrounding normal postnatal closure of the duct were reported from studies of more than 100 babies during the 20 years that followed [4–9]. Thus, by 1960, students of perinatal physiology understood the vital role of this structure during fetal life as well as many of the consequences of its persistence after birth. Recent technologic advances have provided increasingly complex and precise descriptions of postnatal closure, and an accurate timetable for ductal closure in both normal term and ill preterm infants is now available [10,11].

There were clues as early as the mid-1800s that delayed ductal closure often accompanied premature birth. Direct evidence that this was so and that persistent ductal patency might be of clinical harm was only recently obtained, however. Clinical observations were made in Australia by Burnard of a persistent murmur in some preterm babies with breathing problems [12,13]. Cardiac catheterization data from Rudolph and coworkers in Boston, which showed sizable left-to-right shunts through a persistently patent ductus arteriosus (PDA) in preterm babies with respiratory distress, were published about the same time [14]. These findings led Clement Smith to observe in 1960 that ''there is considerable evidence to indicate that

Birth Defects: Original Article Series, Volume 24, Number 1, pages 53–65
© **1988 March of Dimes Birth Defects Foundation**

respiratory distress is accompanied by left-to-right shunt through the ductus arteriosus'' [15]. Unfortunately, ductal ligation failed to reverse a worsening clinical course in a single baby on whom this procedure was later performed at Harvard [1], and Smith's concept of a role for the ductus in neonatal respiratory problems was doubted. For several years, the role of cardiac failure in the respiratory distress syndrome (RDS) was debated, and not all management schemes included measures to correct congestive failure. It was nearly a decade later that a flood of reports appeared claiming better outcomes for babies with RDS who had PDA ligation. Subsequent development of prostaglandin blockers and their clinical availability prompted a second wave of descriptive reports claiming benefit for babies with RDS who had ''medical closure'' of their PDAs with indomethacin. Before we examine these reports in more detail, it is important to note that authors from this era first suggested PDA treatment only for babies with a clinically diagnosed, ''symptomatic'' PDA who also had respiratory distress. It is only recently that early treatment has been proposed for ''asymptomatic'' PDAs in babies with RDS or that the consequence of ''prophylactic treatment'' for particularly vulnerable babies, regardless of whether cardiac or pulmonary symptoms are detected, has been examined. Most literature data therefore pertain to ''clinically diagnosed'' PDAs in babies with prior, usually severe, pulmonary problems. Since treatment based on clinical diagnosis begs the question of the accuracy, reproducibility, sensitivity, specificity, and predictive power of the diagnostic tests available at that time, it is appropriate to begin with a discussion of these factors.

DIAGNOSTIC METHODS

Several clinical signs may provide good evidence for persistent ductal patency. Such signs fail, however, to provide an accurate estimate of shunt size. Furthermore, absence of these clinical signs does not preclude presence of a large shunt; two-thirds or more of the large shunts may be clinically ''silent'' [10,11,16,17]. Since a baby with a loud murmur, bounding pulses, widened pulse pressure, and a precordial/suprasternal thrill may well have a small, clinically inconsequential shunt, whereas another baby without any of these signs may have a huge shunt, prevalence estimates in groups of low-birthweight babies as well as definitive diagnosis in individual babies are likely to be inaccurate when based solely on such clinical criteria.

Both aortographic and sonographic estimates of left atrial (LA) size have failed to help much. The functional meaning of retrograde flow after high-pressure aortic radiocontrast injections is unclear [18,19]. The LA/aortic root ratio, despite early enthusiasm about its clinical usefulness [20], has been shown more recently to be a poor predictor of shunt size, especially for tiny babies on ventilators [10,21–23]. Two-dimensional echocardiography is noninvasive and currently provides quick, accurate information about ductal patency and direction of ductal flow [24]. Clinical management of the PDA is currently based on this technique in most centers in this country. Since the technique fails to provide consistently accurate estimates of shunt size, however, its current popularity as a diagnostic tool in individual patients may be misplaced.

Two recent diagnostic methods show real promise. One of these combines Doppler flow methods with the commonly used 2-D echocardiographic technique [25–27]. The other tracks and quantitates pulmonary and systemic flows using computer-analyzed radionuclide techniques [28–30]. Because both are time consuming, require expensive capital equipment investments, and demand considerable personnel expertise in interpretation, widespread clinical application of these techniques has been slow in coming. Limited data suggest that they both provide results that compare favorably with the ''gold standard'' of cardiac catheterization, and both have been shown to be clinically feasible to use in busy neonatal intensive care settings.

The bottom line is that there are serious limitations in the accuracy of most diagnostic methods commonly used to determine the direction and amount of shunt through the PDA. Decisions correctly based on estimates of shunt size have been uncertain because of these limitations in available diagnostic techniques. These same factors also have limited the certainty of our knowledge about the pathophysiology of ductal patency.

We have discovered with reasonable certainty, however, that ductal closure is delayed in prematurely born babies, that shunts through this structure may have great clinical significance, and that these problems are magnified in direct proportion to the smallness, immaturity, and severity of illness of our tiny patients. We have found also that those babies with PDA shunts have worse outcomes—specifically more death, chronic lung disease, intracranial hemorrhage, necrotizing enterocolitis (NEC), and retinopathy— than do their weight and maturity peers without evidence of PDA. It is therefore appropriate to discuss at this point certain of these observations in more detail.

CLINICAL RELATIONSHIPS

Why is all this important? What relevance is there between a ''developmental malformation'' in the cardiovascular system and retinopathy of prematurity (ROP)? The baby whose lung is flooded with blood, shunted from aorta to pulmonary artery through a PDA, suffers many problems. The lungs, turgid with double, triple, or more their usual volume of blood, become less compliant (or stiffer) and harder to inflate [31,32]. As the work of breathing increases and pulmonary elasticity diminishes, the baby's breathing falters, intermittent apneic episodes appear and become progressively more common, CO_2 retention progresses, and hypoxemia ultimately occurs as hypoventilation progresses [33]. Wide fluctuations in blood gases may occur as the baby struggles to breathe with increasingly stiff lungs. These same problems occur in the baby on the ventilator as the PDA opens and left-to-right shunting progresses. For the ventilated baby, the consequences are even more ominous, however, since the stiffening lungs prevent getting the baby off the ventilator, and the harmful effects of prolonged positive-pressure ventilation become inevitable as time passes [34,35].

There are problems upstream and downstream as well. Pulse pressure widens and pulsatility increases in cerebral as well as systemic arterial vessels. Distal aortic blood flow, and perhaps cerebral flow as well, is dramatically reduced as a consequence of the ductal "steal" of blood through the ductus [36]. The widely fluctuating vascular pressures in the brain may increase the risk of intraventricular bleeding [37–41]. Mesenteric blood flow may be reduced to the point where ischemic mucosal necrosis occurs in the intestines [42]. It is not difficult to imagine why the literature consistently links such conditions as bronchopulmonary dysplasia (BPD), intraventricular hemorrhage (IVH) and NEC, and ROP with PDA in these fragile, labile, ultraimmature premies.

Especially pertinent here are observations of the Vanderbilt group [43]. They examined the role of the PDA in babies with birthweights of 1,500 gm or less who lived 3 or more days after birth and who were admitted to their unit in 1975. Outcome was ultimately much worse in those babies with PDAs. Survival was reduced from 85% (48/56) to 61% (27/44). Even more striking were the differences in morbidity. Literally *all* the babies with BPD, NEC, IVH, and scarring retinopathy were in the PDA group. Conversely, *none* of these complications were detected in the babies without PDAs. These observations have subsequently been confirmed and amplified by a multitude of observational studies from other U.S. centers. In response to these findings, a variety of management schemes have been proposed and implemented and their results examined. A closer examination of these attempts to counter or prevent the harmful consequences of ductal patency and shunting is therefore appropriate at this point.

TREATMENTS
Surgery

Anecdotal reports of ductal ligation in single babies, small groups of infants, or large groups of preterm babies had flooded the literature by the 1970s. These reports shared several common features: All were enthusiastic about clinical benefits, all claimed low surgical risks, and all concerned primarily premature babies with respiratory distress. All used "clinical criteria" of "significant" PDA shunting, often "confirmed" by what now have been proved to be insensitive and nonspecific diagnostic tests. Unfortunately, these studies were generally flawed by so many other errors in experimental design that proper interpretation of their conclusions is not possible in most instances. Most were descriptive exercises, not hypothesis-testing, "risk-taking," clinical experiments. Criteria for selection of subjects were inconstant from report to report, making it impossible to compare results between studies. Other problems of subject selection were common in most. Diagnostic methods used differed, and a "gold standard" was seldom employed. Additionally, reproducibility and precision of the diagnostic techniques employed were seldom provided. Most of the diagnostic schemes employed were qualitative at best and provided no quantitative information about shunt size. Nearly all the studies were characterized by the total absence of appropriate comparison or control groups. Precise details of the intervention (surgery) were usually not provided, and methods employed to reduce surgical risks unique to these tiny babies were incompletely spelled out. Other supportive care management employed was uncertain, was rarely detailed, and, when provided, varied considerably in most of these reports. Clinical descriptions of concurrent conditions that might have affected outcome in these babies were scarce and incomplete in nearly all these reports. Finally, outcome criteria employed to judge what was "good" or "best" were inconstant and variable.

Despite these problems, some observations from this era—again, particularly those from the Vanderbilt group—are of special and continued value [44]. They studied 25 babies of 1,500 gm birthweight or less who were on mechanical ventilation for RDS and were diagnosed as having a symptomatic PDA refractory to at least 48 hours of "medical management" [43]. The babies were randomly assigned to two management schemes about 1 week after birth. Medical management was continued in one group of 15 babies; surgical ligation of the PDA was performed in another group of 10 babies. In addition to some of the design flaws noted above, the small number of babies in this study limited the "power" of its conclusions considerably. Nevertheless, some valuable differences between the groups were found, and the study provides perhaps the most persuasive clinical evidence available in the literature for the value of surgical intervention. Death was a bit less frequent in the surgery group (1/10 or 10% vs 3/12 or 25%). There were bigger differences in morbidity. Babies in the ligated group had *no* NEC, but 20% (3/15) of those in the control/medical management group developed the condition. All but one of the five babies with ROP and all but one of the four babies with BPD were in the control group. BPD was therefore half as common and ROP only one-third as common in the ligated babies as in the control group. The small sample size precluded a "statistical" significance for these sizable clinical differences; one can calculate that it would have required from 30 (for the differences in NEC) to 110 patients (for the differences in BPD) in each treatment group to "prove statistically" that these very sizable and important clinical differences were "real." A dramatic reduction in the duration of ventilator dependence in the surgical group was significant, however. Ten days after entry into the study, about three-fourths of the ligated babies were extubated and off the ventilator. In contrast, more than three-fourths of the control babies were still intubated and on the ventilator at the same time. As an associated finding, hospital costs were significantly less for the surgical group.

Less optimistic were results from Denver about that time [45] concerning smaller babies of less than 1,000 gm birthweight. During a 3-year period (1976–1978), 47 of 106 such babies lived. In 30 of the survivors, a PDA was diagnosed and "medical management" begun. About half (14) improved, and for these no information is given about outcome. Of the 16 who failed to improve and were surgically ligated about 1 week (mean) after birth, BPD occurred in 81% and ROP in 60%. Higher altitude, different methods of care, and lower birthweights may be among the factors that explain these grim figures. Nevertheless, these kinds of observations, as well as the lack of surgical expertise at many neonatal care centers and the many and often unique risks of PDA ligation in these "ultrasmall premies," set the stage for an enthusiastic reception of a new drug, indomethacin, for treatment of the condition.

Indomethacin

As the role of prostaglandins in ductal closure became known, use of indomethacin became popular [46,47]. A new flood of descriptive, uncontrolled, enthusiastic, inconclusive, and badly flawed studies inundated the literature. Reports concerning use of this drug in nearly 1,500 infants are now available [48]. Again, most studies included too few babies for any definitive conclusions. Information is now available, however, from a collaborative study sponsored by the National Institutes of Health that included about 400 babies from 13 institutions in the United States [49–54]. This study examined the results of different methods of treatment. Babies who weighed 1,750 gm or less at birth and were found to have a "hemodynamically significant" PDA were randomly assigned to one of two treatment schemes: "medical treatment" alone or "medical treatment" with indomethacin. Treatment failures were then again randomly assigned to one of two treatment groups: either indomethacin or surgical ligation was provided as "back-up treatment." Results from this study are noteworthy not only for the number of babies involved but also because random treatment allocation was employed. In addition, an intravenous preparation of the drug was used, and plasma concentrations of the drug were measured. These features of the study design ensured that more predictable and appropriate drug levels could be achieved consistently with enteral preparations, both important factors in assessment of response to treatment. Results confirmed the effectiveness of indomethacin when used under conditions of the study. Ductal closure was (ultimately) obtained with 79% success in the drug group and in but 35% of the placebo group. Results from those babies with lowest birthweight and at highest risk (<1,000 gm) were less impressive (54% vs 26%), but the differences were still remarkable. Unfortunately, there were but 41 babies in this critical low-birthweight group (28 placebo and 13 indomethacin), and several clinically startling advantages in the indomethacin group were not "statistically significant." It is nevertheless important to point out that there was *no* IVH, NEC, or scarring retinopathy in the indomethacin-treated babies, whereas there were six babies with IVH (21%) and three each with NEC and severe ROP (11%) in the placebo group. To prove these important clinical differences statistically would have required many more patients. The incidence of BPD was no different in the two groups (46% vs 43%). Since treatment/intervention was begun so late in this study—only 145 of the total of 405 babies (36%) in the group were treated within 4 days of birth— this lack of pulmonary advantage was predictable.

A puzzling feature was a higher frequency of scarring retinopathy (grades III and IV) in the babies who failed medical treatment and were then ligated (14/142, or 10%) than in those whose "back-up treatment" was indomethacin instead of surgery (6/139, or 4%). A similar high incidence was observed in those babies who failed initial indomethacin treatment and were then ligated (12/79, or 15%) when contrasted with those who received a second treatment with the drug (3/75, or 4%). These data are difficult to interpret in that the surgically ligated babies were clearly a highly selected group of treatment failures. The lack of detail provided concerning the surgical management(s) employed (and their possible variations), and the lessening of these differences (to a point of statistical insignificance) at later follow-up, also makes it difficult to understand the clinical importance of these variations in visual outcome in the different treatment groups. Looked at in yet another way, the (increased) rate of cicatricial ROP in the surgically treated babies "was similar to that reported recently as the usual rate in premature infants with the same clinical characteristics" [51], an observation that suggests that early indocin treatment may have reduced ROP in a vulnerable population. This is a particularly important point since theoretical [55] as well as animal data [56,57] suggest that tampering with the prostaglandin cascade may have harmful effects on the retina. Anecdotal observations of ROP in three babies who received indomethacin—and the implication of a cause and effect relationship between the drug and the outcome—are of limited value since the babies described were in a high-risk group by virtue of their birthweights and gestational ages (970–1,200 gm; 26–29 weeks), and no control or comparison groups were provided. Observations of a sixfold increase in ROP in babies who weighed less than 1,000 gm at birth and whose PDAs were treated with indomethacin (9/26 or 35% vs 3/49 or 6%) are also difficult to understand [58,59]. Final details of this (abstracted) study have yet to be made available, but preliminary data suggest that there were important differences in duration of oxygen therapy and of hyperoxia (PaO_2) between the two groups. It is also unclear what alternative treatment was used in the comparison group for their (presumably comparably severe) hemodynamically significant PDAs. Although it may be appropriate to maintain a high degree of continued suspicion about a relation between indomethacin treatment and ROP [60], the most complete and convincing data currently available indicate that the drug does not increase the risk of retinopathy in susceptible babies [53,61].

Indomethacin has clearly been proved an effective drug in many babies with PDAs. Unlike surgery, it is "79% rather than 100% effective" and may be even less so in the smallest babies who are at highest risk, if we are to believe the 54% success figure from the collaborative study [51]. Nevertheless, convincing if not conclusive evidence for reduced intensity of ventilator support [35], duration of ventilator dependence, and BPD [35,62,63] as well as direct pulmonary function studies appear to confirm that the same improvements in lung compliance observed after ductal ligation also follow indomethacin therapy [64,65]. Despite worrisome effects of the drug on platelet function [48,66], its use appears actually to reduce the risks of ventricular hemorrhage in susceptible infants [67–71]. In a similar fashion, the risk of NEC may also be lessened [51] despite drug-related effects on gastrointestinal perfusion and function [48].

CONCLUSIONS AND SUMMARY

Our current clinical concept of the very tiny premie, born 3 or more months early at a birthweight of 1 kg or less, is a picture painted in precise detail with sophisticated methods available only in the past few years. The hazards of developmental immaturity in these ultrapremies are now clearly understood not to be limited only to the pulmonary system. Vascular flow changes from fetal to adult channels more slowly and less certainly in these babies than in their term brothers and sisters. These developmental disturbances in the cardiovascular system are interdependent with and inseparable from concurrent pulmonary events. Thus, the lungs of the baby with RDS may stiffen first with the diffuse atelectasis of surfactant deficiency (RDS or hyaline membrane disease), and then, literally as quickly as they recover from the RDS, they again stiffen, this time with pulmonary engorgement of blood progressively shunted from aorta to pulmonary artery through the open PDA. These events are often overlooked or misinterpreted as a perverse ''failure to wean from ventilation'' and are commonly treated inappropriately with continued pulmonary/ventilatory interventions. The baby improves from RDS by day 2 or 3, worsens from the PDA shunt on days 4 and 5, ventilation is continued but the shunt is not corrected, and, in the worst possible (but all too common) case, lung damage has occurred by the end of the first week and the outcome is then determined by the course of a new, iatrogenic lung disease—bronchopulmonary dysplasia (BPD).

Other organ systems are also affected. Widened pulse pressures hammer preductal organs—the brain and eyes, for instance—with quantitatively and qualitatively altered blood flow. Diversion (''run-off'' or ''steal'' and actually reversed direction of flow) of forward-flowing aortic blood at the ductus causes ischemic compromise (at best) and varying degrees of temporary or permanent functional and structural damage (at worst) to such postductal organs as gut and kidneys. NEC is the likely result of such gut compromise. Some degree of renal failure is common, and the consequently impaired handling of salt and water further worsens compromised perfusion by the now faltering heart.

Add to all this the fluctuations and aberrations of oxygenation and gas exchange that even our most thoughtful, meticulous, careful, and skillful attempts at mechanical ventilation impose on these tiny patients, and it becomes clear why a cluster of morbidities—RDS, PDA, BPD, IVH, ROP, NEC—are so common and why they are so often associated the one with the other. It also becomes clear why successful attempts to counter a single one of these disorders so often result in a reduced prevalence or morbidity from the others.

Current efforts to prevent RDS in babies who will ''inevitably'' be born months too early clearly reduce the risks of a PDA. Stated another way, a PDA is found in virtually all these tiny patients who have RDS. Babies in this smallest weight/lowest developmental maturity group who do not have RDS or PDA have less intracranial hemorrhage. They also probably have less retinopathy and fewer gastrointestinal problems. Certainly, the overwhelming consensus in the literature is that treatment schemes that reduce the frequency or provide early, prompt correction for the pathophysiologic consequences of PDA in these patients are consistently accompanied by evidence of a reduced frequency and/or severity of ROP. Thinking this way makes it much easier to understand the bottom line of this discussion—that is, to understand why a PDA has unmistakable causal as well as incidental associations with ROP—and to understand why prevention or early correction of the PDA seems to reduce prevalence and severity of ROP in these developmentally vulnerable babies. Hopefully, this approach makes clear the reasons why details about the frequency, presence, and management of PDA are essential ingredients of any report about ROP, and why frequency of ROP may vary from place to place—or from one treatment to another—in relation to these associated factors. Finally, this chapter tries to explain why attempts to examine the advantages or disadvantages of new approaches to treatment or prevention must include complete and detailed analyses of these clinically and pathophysiologically associated disorders, most particularly of the PDA.

REFERENCES

1. Casteñada AR: Patent ductus arteriosus: A commentary. Ann Thorac Surg 31:92–96, 1981.
2. Cassels DE, Bharati S, Lev M: The natural history of the ductus arteriosus in association with other congenital heart defects. Perspect Biol Med 18:541–572, 1975.
3. Gross RE, Hubbard JP: Surgical ligation of a patent ductus arteriosus: Report of first successful case. J Am Med Assoc 112:729–731, 1939.
4. Prec KJ, Cassels DE: Dye dilution curves and cardiac output in newborn infants. Circulation 11:789–798, 1955.
5. Rowe RD, James LS: The normal pulmonary arterial pressure during the first year of life. J Pediatr 51:1–4, 1957.
6. James LS, Rowe RD: The pattern of response of pulmonary and systemic arterial pressures in newborn and older infants to short periods of hypoxia. J Pediatr 51:5–11, 1957.
7. Adams FH, Lind J: Physiologic studies on the cardiovascular status of normal newborn infants (with special reference to the ductus arteriosus). Pediatrics 19:431–437, 1957.
8. Moss AJ, Emmanouilides G, Duffie ER: Closure of the ductus arteriosus in the newborn infant. Pediatrics 32:25–30, 1963.
9. Cassels DE (ed): "The Heart and Circulation in the Newborn and Infant." New York: Grune & Stratton, 1966, p 526.
10. Daniels O, Hopman JC, Stoelinga GB, Busch HJ, Peer PG: Doppler flow characteristics in the main pulmonary artery and the LA/Ao ratio before and after ductal closure in healthy newborns. Pediatr Cardiol 3:99–104, 1982.
11. Dudell GG, Gersony WM: Patent ductus arteriosus in neonates with severe respiratory disease. J Pediatr 104:915–920, 1984.
12. Burnard ED: A murmur from the ductus arteriosus in the newborn baby. Br Med J 1:806–810, 1958.
13. Burnard ED: The cardiac murmur in relation to symptoms in the newborn. Br Med J 1:134–138, 1959.
14. Rudolph AM, Drorbaugh JE, Auld PAM, Rudolph AJ, Nadas AS, Smith CA, Hubbell JP: Studies on the circulation in the neonatal period. The circulation in the respiratory distress syndrome. Pediatrics 27:551–566, 1961.
15. Smith CA: Circulatory factors in relation to idiopathic respiratory distress (hyaline membrane disease) in the newborn. J Pediatr 56:605–611, 1960.
16. Thibeault DW, Emmanouilides GC, Nelson RJ, Lachman RS, Rosengart RM, Oh W: Patent ductus arteriosus complicating the respiratory distress syndrome in preterm infants. J Pediatr 86:120–126, 1975.

17. McGrath RL, McGuinness GA, Way GL, Wolfe RR, Nora JJ, Simmons MA: The silent ductus arteriosus. J Pediatr 93:110–113, 1978.

18. Thibeault DW, Emmanouilides GC, Dodge ME, Lachman RS: Early functional closure of the ductus arteriosus associated with decreased severity of respiratory distress syndrome in preterm infants. Am J Dis Child 131:741–745, 1977.

19. Higgins CB, DiSessa T, Kirkpatrick SE, Ti CC, Edwards DK, Kelley MJ, Friedman WF, Kurlinski J: Assessment of patent ductus arteriosus in preterm infants by single lateral film aortography. Radiology 135:641–647, 1980.

20. Silverman NH, Lewis AB, Heymann MA, et al: Echocardiographic assessment of ductus arteriosus shunt in premature infants. Circulation 50:821–825, 1974.

21. Purohit DM, Caldwell CC, Webb HN, et al: Effects of assisted ventilation on echocardiographic findings in two infants with patent ductus arteriosus. J Thorac Cardiovasc Surg 72:294–295, 1976.

22. Valdes-Cruz LM, Dudell GG: Specificity and accuracy of echocardiographic and clinical criteria for diagnosis of patent ductus arteriosus in fluid-restricted infants. J Pediatr 98:298–305, 1981.

23. Ellison RC, Peckham GJ, Lang P, Talner NS, Lerer TJ, Lin L, Dooley KJ, Nadas AS: Evaluation of the preterm infant for patent ductus arteriosus. Pediatrics 71:364–372, 1983.

24. Smallhorn JF, Huhta JC, Anderson RH, Macartney FJ: Suprasternal cross-sectional echocardiography in assessment of patent ductus arteriosus. Br Heart J 48:321–330, 1982.

25. Stevenson JG, Kawabori I, Guntheroth WG: Pulsed Doppler echocardiographic diagnosis of patent ductus arteriosus: Sensitivity, specificity, limitations, and technical features. Cathet Cardiovasc Diagn 6:255–263, 1980.

26. Huhta JC, Cohen M, Gutgesell HP: Patency of the ductus arteriosus in normal neonates: Two-dimensional echocardiography versus Doppler assessment. J Am Coll Cardiol 4:561–564, 1984.

27. Vick GW 3rd, Huhta JC, Gutgesell HP: Assessment of the ductus arteriosus in preterm infants utilizing suprasternal two-dimensional/Doppler echocardiography. J Am Coll Cardiol 5:973–977, 1985.

28. Vick GW 3rd, Satterwhite C, Cassady G, Philips J, Yester MV, Logic JR: Radionuclide angiography in the evaluation of ductal shunts in preterm infants. J Pediatr 101:264–268, 1982.

29. Parker JA, Treves S: Radionuclide detection, localization, and quantitation of intracardiac shunts and shunts between the great arteries. Prog Cardiovasc Dis 20:121–150, 1977.

30. Treves S, Fyler D, Fujii A, Kuruc A: Low radiation iridium 191m radionuclide angiography: Detection and quantitation of left-to-right shunts in infants. J Pediatr 101:210–213, 1982.

31. Lees MH, Way RC, Ross BB: Ventilation and respiratory gas transfer of infants with increased pulmonary blood flow. Pediatrics 40:259–271, 1967.

32. Griffin AJ, Ferrara JD, Lax JO, et al: Pulmonary compliance: An index of cardiovascular status in infancy. Am J Dis Child 123:89–95, 1972.

33. Kitterman JA, Edmunds LH Jr, Gregory GA, et al: Patent ductus arteriosus in premature infants. Incidence, relation to pulmonary disease and management. N Engl J Med 287:473–477, 1972.

34. Brown ER: Increased risk of bronchopulmonary dysplasia in infants with patent ductus arteriosus. J Pediatr 95:865–866, 1979.

35. Jacob J, Gluck L, DiSessa T, Edwards D, Kulovich M, Kurlinski J, Merritt TA, Friedman WF: The contribution of PDA in the neonate with severe RDS. J Pediatr 96:79–87, 1980.

36. Spach MS, Serwer GA, Anderson PA, Canent RV Jr, Levin AR: Pulsatile aortopulmonary

pressure-flow dynamics of patent ductus arteriosus in patients with various hemodynamic states. Circulation 61:110–122, 1980.

37. Ellison P, Eichorst D, Rouse M, Heimler R, Denny J: Changes in cerebral hemodynamics in preterm infants with and without patent ductus arteriosus. Acta Paediatr Scand 311 [Suppl]:23–27, 1983.

38. Perlman JM, Hill A, Volpe JJ: The effect of patent ductus arteriosus on flow velocity in the anterior cerebral arteries: Ductal steal in the premature newborn infant. J Pediatr 99:767–771, 1981.

39. Martin CG, Snider AR, Katz SM, Peabody JL, Brady JP: Abnormal cerebral blood flow patterns in preterm infants with a large patent ductus arteriosus. J Pediatr 101:587–593, 1982.

40. Lipman B, Serwer GA, Brazy JE: Abnormal cerebral hemodynamics in preterm infants with patent ductus arteriosus. Pediatrics 69:778–781, 1982.

41. Bejar R, Merritt TA, Coen RW, Mannino F, Gluck L: Pulsatility index, patent ductus arteriosus, and brain damage. Pediatrics 69:818–822, 1982.

42. Strange M, Crouse D, Godoy G, Pacifico A, Kirklin J, Kirklin J, Joiner C, Philips J, Cassady G: Early ductus arteriosus ligation reduces risk of necrotizing enterocolitis. Pediatr Res 20:362A, 1986.

43. Cotton RB, Stahlman MT, Kovar I, Catterton WZ: Medical management of small preterm infants with symptomatic ductus arteriosus. J Pediatr 92:467–473, 1978.

44. Cotton RB, Stahlman MT, Bender HW, Graham TP, Catterton WZ, Kovar I: Randomized trial of early closure of symptomatic patent ductus arteriosus in small preterm infants. J Pediatr 93:647–651, 1978.

45. Kilbride HW, Whitfeld JM, Vigneswaran R: Outcome following closure of PDA in preterm infants [letter]. J Pediatr 96:1121–1122, 1980.

46. Friedman WF, Hirschklau MJ, Printz MP, et al: Pharmacologic closure of patent ductus arteriosus in the premature infant. N Engl J Med 295:526–529, 1976.

47. Heymann MA, Rudolph AM, Silverman NH: Closure of the ductus arteriosus in premature infants by inhibition of prostaglandin synthesis. N Engl J Med 295:530–533, 1976.

48. Roberts RJ: Prostaglandins, prostaglandin inhibitors, and vitamin E. In "Drug Therapy in Infants: Pharmacologic Principles and Clinical Experience." Philadelphia: W.B. Saunders Co., 1984, pp 250–283.

49. Nadas AS: Indomethacin and the patent ductus arteriosus [editorial]. N Engl J Med 305:97–98, 1981.

50. Ellison RC, Peckham GJ, Lang P, Talner NS, Lerer TJ, Lin L, Dooley KJ, Nadas AS: Evaluation of the preterm infant for patent ductus arteriosus. Pediatrics 71:364–372, 1983.

51. Gersony WM, Peckham GJ, Ellison RC, Miettinen OS, Nadas AS: Effects of indomethacin in premature infants with patent ductus arteriosus: Results of a national collaborative study. J Pediatr 102:895–906, 1983.

52. Peckham GJ, Micttinen OS, Ellison RC, Kraybill EN, Gersony WM, Zierler S, Nadas AS: Clinical course to 1 year of age in premature infants with patent ductus arteriosus: Results of a multicenter randomized trial of indomethacin. J Pediatr 105:285–291, 1984.

53. Purohit DM, Ellison RC, Zierler S, Miettinen OS, Nadas AS: Risk factors for retrolental fibroplasia: Experience with 3,025 premature infants. National Collaborative Study on Patent Ductus Arteriosus in Premature Infants. Pediatrics 76:339–344, 1985.

54. Cunningham MD, Ellison RC, Zierler S, Kanto WP Jr, Miettinen OS, Nadas AS: Perinatal risk assessment for patent ductus arteriosus in premature infants. Obstet Gynecol 68:41–45, 1986.

55. Schrager GO: PDAs, prostaglandins, and RLF [letter]. Pediatrics 62:860–861, 1978.

56. Chemtob S, Beharry K, Rex J, Laudignon N, Aranda JV: Effect of PGE_1 on ocular blood flow in the newborn piglet. Pediatr Res 19:169A, 1985.
57. Flower RW, Blake DA, Wajer SD, Egner PG, McLeod DS, Pitts SM: Retrolental fibroplasia: Evidence for a role of the prostaglandin cascade in the pathogenesis of oxygen-induced retinopathy in the newborn beagle. Pediatr Res 15:1293–1302, 1981.
58. Lindemann R, Blystad W, Egge K: Retrolental fibroplasia in premature infants with patent ductus arteriosus treated with indomethacin. Eur J Pediatr 138:56–58, 1982.
59. Sun S, Baldomerio A, Caputo A, Aranda Z: Indomethacin, patent ductus arteriosus (PDA) and retinopathy of prematurity (ROP). Pediatr Res 17:124A, 1983.
60. Flower RW: Indomethacin and retrolental fibroplasia [letter]. J Pediatr 104:326, 1984.
61. Procianoy RS, Garcia-Prats JA, Hittner HM, Adams JM, Rudolph AJ: Use of indomethacin and its relationship to retinopathy of prematurity in very low birthweight infants. Arch Dis Child 55:362–364, 1980.
62. Cotton RB, Hickey DE, Graham TP, Stahlman MT: Effect of early indomethacin (I) on ventilatory status of preterm infants with symptomatic patent ductus arteriosus (sPDA). Pediatr Res 14:442A, 1980.
63. Merritt TA, Harris JP, Roghmann J, Wood B, Campanella V, Alexson C, Manning J, Shapiro DL: Early closure of the patent ductus arteriosus in very-low-birth-weight infants: A controlled trial. J Pediatr 99:281–286, 1981.
64. Yeh TF, Thalji A, Luken L, Lilien L, Carr I, Pildes RS: Improved lung compliance following indomethacin therapy in premature infants with persistent ductus arteriosus. Chest 80:698–700, 1981.
65. Naulty CM, Horn S, Conry J, Avery GB: Improved lung compliance after ligation of patent ductus arteriosus in hyaline membrane disease. J Pediatr 93:682–684, 1978.
66. Setzer ES, Smith M, Goulding PJ, Bandstra TE: Severity of platelet dysfunction induced by prophylactic indomethacin in the premature. Pediatr Res 18:346A, 1984.
67. Setzer ES, Morse BM, Goldberg RN, Smith M, Bancalari E: Prophylactic indomethacin and intraventricular hemorrhage (IVH) in the premature. Pediatr Res 18:345A, 1984.
68. Maher P, Lane B, Ballard R, Piecuch R, Clyman RI: Does indomethacin cause extension of intracranial hemorrhages: A preliminary study. Pediatrics 75:497–500, 1985.
69. Mahony L, Carnero V, Brett C, Heymann MA, Clyman RI: Prophylactic indomethacin therapy for patent ductus arteriosus in very low-birth-weight infants. N Engl J Med 306:506–510, 1982.
70. Mahony L, Caldwell RL, Girod DA, Hurwitz RA, Jansen RD, Lemons JA, Schreiner RL: Indomethacin therapy on the first day of life in infants with very low birthweight. J Pediatr 106:801–805, 1985.
71. Sola A, Lezama C, Urman J: Should prophylactic indomethacin (PROPH INDO) be used in VLBW infants with hyaline membrane disease (HMD)? Pediatr Res 18:348A, 1984.

Commentary and Questions: Session I

The aim of the first module was to put the low-birthweight infant, at risk for the development of ROP, in perspective. This was particularly so with regard to other morbidity in survivors. As was pointed out by Dr. McCormick, low birthweight itself in the absence of other complicating factors, confers a modest risk of morbidity. One wonders if this is also true for ROP, although there is no a priori reason to suspect that it is not.

The delivery of care to the neonate, particularly the high-risk neonate, was covered succintly by Dr. Sinclair. The inherent logic of the system has led to a partitioned level of care that is probably the envy of all medical delivery care systems on this continent, or should be if it isn't. Although not free of defects and glitches, it nevertheless has led to the rational distribution of care according to need rather than on any other basis.

Finally, Dr. Zierler explored the knotty problem of causality in ROP and how difficult it is to unravel the risks associated with a number of component causes, no one of which may represent either a necessary or sufficient cause of ROP. Even low birthweight, long linked to ROP in the putative chain of causality, is only the second-hand measure for immaturity of retinal blood vessels, the real but as yet unmeasurable variable of interest.

In the question session, the audience sought to explore further these concepts of causality with Dr. Zierler. For example, given the complicated nature of many interacting cofactors, is it in fact possible to approach ROP by means of a collaborative study? Could "robust statistics" untangle the enigma of the disease?

In answer to this query, Dr. Zierler seemed to indicate that, rather than consider statistical technique being capable of isolating "the" cause, the event (ROP) might be conceived of as having occurred as a result of a series of determinants, such as poor prenatal care, very low birthweight, very immature retinas, and the like, all of which gave rise to the phenomenon of ROP. On still another point, the notion of causality introduced by Dr. Zierler needed further explanation and clarification for the audience. With regard to this question, Dr. Zierler defined a sufficient cause as the set of component causes that work together either sequentially or concurrently to bring about an effect, in this case ROP. A necessary cause is the component cause common to all sufficient causes. Thus, without this necessary component

Birth Defects: Original Article Series, Volume 24, Number 1, pages 67–69
© **1988 March of Dimes Birth Defects Foundation**

cause, disease will not occur. In her way of thinking, this necessary cause is immaturity of the retinal vasculature. What we understand by this is something different than what we understand by low birthweight, although the two may be, and usually are, related. Component causes that work together may very well be independent of one another. A comment by Dr. Silverman is relevant here to the effect that physicians are prone to wield Occam's razor, the fewest possible cause(s) related to a given condition. This is best exemplified by the idea of infectious diseases. However, even with that model, we recognize that we do not cover, by any means, the component causes. Robust statistics and their use will not solve the problem for us either.

In the second panel of this first session, intraventricular hemorrhage (IVH), patent ductus arteriosus (PDA), and respiratory therapy and its monitoring were explored. The first two provide a milieu of serious disease in which ROP seems to thrive. Respiratory therapy and its monitoring, particularly with modern transcutaneous monitors, seem to provide a means, however crude, at this stage to begin quantitative measurements of the oxygen variable as it relates to ROP.

There are still many uncertainties surrounding not so much the diagnosis of IVH or PDA as the estimates of their severity. In both instances, the current diagnostic modalities, ultrasound and computed tomography, although orders of magnitude better than clinical signs or symptoms, nevertheless fail in many instances to estimate properly the severity of these diseases accurately. Although no special therapy exists for IVH today (nor for ROP), one cannot close that option. With PDA, estimates of severity are critical to decisions of when to intervene and with what modality, medication or surgery. The technical problems of accurate monitoring of oxygen levels in the blood have, in part, been solved in the premature infant. The technique is not without its unreliable aspects, as was pointed out by Dr. Bancalari. Nevertheless, monitoring served as the basis of a randomized study of its usefulness in the prevention of ROP. It did not prevent ROP.

From the audience came the question of whether IVH could be due to hypoxia or hyperoxia? According to Dr. Lucey, the answer is not clear. Following up on the previous question regarding hypoxia and hyperoxia, and their relation to IVH, Dr. Lucey elaborated on the possibility that multiple hyperoxic episodes result in the IVH getting larger. Two questions then arose. Does IVH occur in utero? and why is IVH decreasing? It seems that IVH does occur in utero, and nobody knows why IVH seems to be decreasing in its overall incidence.

Another questioner raised the possibility that Dr. Bancalari, in fact, demonstrated a real difference between the transcutaneous-monitored babies in the heavier birthweight strata. Dr. Bancalari responded that, although there was some preliminary evidence, one must carefully control all other variables in this weight group, such as the possibility that the infants monitored on the standard care regime were, in fact, a sicker group of infants.

Several questions arose from the study of Dr. Bancalari. In particular, guidelines for the use of the transcutaneous monitor. As Dr. Bancalari pointed out, at the start of this study, guidelines were set to maintain the infants' transcutaneous PO_2 between 50 and 70 mm Hg. This proved impossible in infants who were breathing on their own. In fact, the infants could be maintained between these levels only 60% of the time. The mechanism of transcutaneous monitoring control used in this study was a servocontrolled mechanism with a long time delay. This proves particularly unstable when one tries to manipulate it.

Finally, the ultimate topic of the possibility of prevention of prematurity came up for discussion. In France, a concerted effort has been made to limit the number of premature births. Commenting on these data, Dr. McCormick felt that the effort did not hold up under scrutiny, particularly among Algerian French, who have the highest incidence of premature labor and delivery. The program, which was designed to prevent premature labor and delivery, did not, in fact, prevent it in this population.

III. THE PREMATURE RETINA

Pathologic Features of Retinopathy of Prematurity

Robert Y. Foos, MD

Jules Stein Eye Institute, University of California at Los Angeles, Los Angeles, California 90024

This chapter summarizes over a decade of experience with the pathology of the vitreoretinopathy associated with premature birth in man, adapting the information where possible to fit the recently published clinical classification of the disease[1–4]. The term vitreoretinopathy is preferred since, as will be demonstrated, the alterations of the vitreous body in this condition are critically important in the retinal detachment that leads to blindness. Since an understanding of the process of normal retinal vasculogenesis is necessary to appreciate the earlier stages of the retinopathy, this will be discussed first. This chapter considers the interactions of the retinal lesions and those of the vitreous body in the more advanced stages and concludes with a description of the retinal detachment, which has many unique features in the disorder.

RETINAL VASCULOGENESIS

Retinal vascularization in man begins at approximately the fourth lunar month of gestation and with rare exceptions is complete before birth; ''mature'' is a better descriptive term than ''complete''; normally in the adult there is a 1–3 mm zone behind the ora serrata that is devoid of vessels. More importantly, only the immature vasculature is subject to injury, which is the basis for the proliferative retinopathy to be described. Beginning at the optic disc, a vasculogenic wave sweeps in the inner retina toward the periphery [5]. This wave, which is visible macroscopically in the laboratory, contains two active zones on microscopic examination (Fig, 1): The *vanguard*, which is most anterior, contains principally primitive spindle-shaped cells of mesenchymal origin, and the *rear guard*, in which the mesenchymal cells differentiate into endothelial cells (upon transforming, the vanguard cells become factor VIII-positive). These endothelial cells then aggregate into cords, which subsequently lumenize and become the primordial capillaries.

The superficial aspect of the avascular retina anterior to the vanguard

Birth Defects: Original Article Series, Volume 24, Number 1, pages 73–85
© **1988 March of Dimes Birth Defects Foundation**

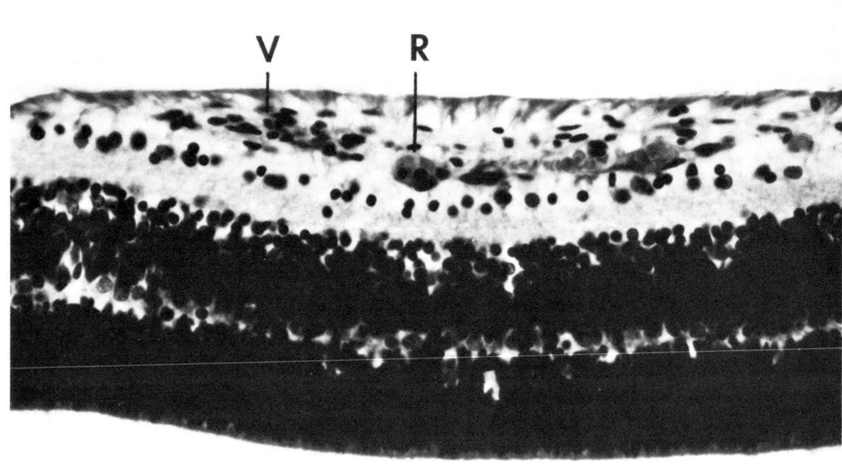

Fig. 1. Advancing vasculature in nerve fiber layer of retina in premature stillborn infant (birthweight 920 gm). Anteriorly, the vanguard (V) contains a thin layer of primitive spindle-shaped mesenchymal cells. In the rear guard (R), immediately posterior, the mesenchymal cells have differentiated into endothelial cells, lumenized, and formed the primordial capillaries. Photoreceptor cells are poorly developed. (H & E×540).

contains intercommunicating cystic spaces, which appear microscopically as superficial blebs bordered by Mueller cells [1]. While I have always wondered why these ''spaces'' were confined to the avascular retina, I have dismissed them as autolytic artefacts. Flower et al, on the other hand, have ascribed especial importance to these spaces and the adjacent Mueller cells, suggesting that they play a physical and perhaps a biochemical role in retinal vasculogenesis in lower animals [6].

Because of the nasally eccentric position of the optic nerve and the greater distance the vasogenic tissue must travel temporally, the primitive vasculature reaches the temporal periphery and matures later than in the nasal quadrants. Remodeling of the primitive ''chicken wire'' capillary meshwork into the adult form takes place over the ensuing months and is usually complete 2–3 months after birth [7].

The concept of vasogenic mesenchymal cells originating from the disc and proliferating peripherally as a vanguard for the primitive retinal vasculature has been questioned recently by Flower and coworkers [6]. They found in the dog that endothelial cells arose from primitive precursors (angioblasts),

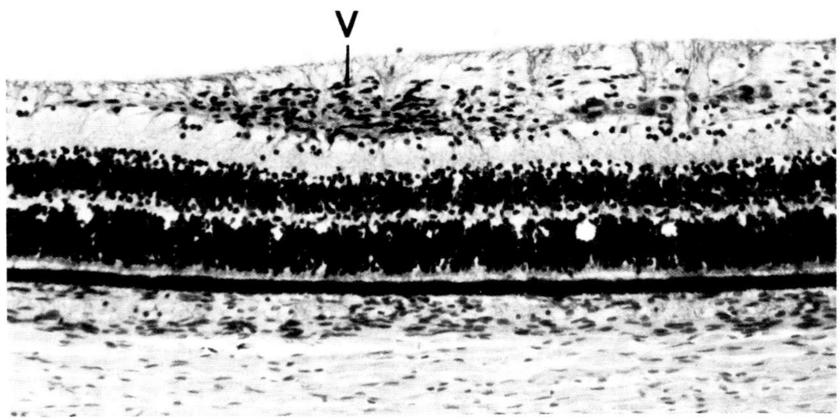

Fig. 2.   ROP stage 1. Retina is notably thickened (demarcation line) as a result of hyperplasia of vanguard mesenchymal cells (V). (H & E × 250).

which were resident in the superficial retina at the time of birth. If confirmed, this information will impact significantly on the use of lower animals as a model of the retinopathy in man and perhaps also on our understanding of the fundamental aspects of this disease.

STAGE 1 RETINOPATHY

Stage 1, the first of the acute phases of retinopathy, is a proliferative response of the vasogenic tissue following injury, at least one injurious factor being hyperoxia [8]. Macroscopically, this stage is characterized by a *demarcation line* within the retina, representing a thickened exaggeration of the line of the normal advancing vasculature [2]. Posterior to the demarcation line, retinal vasodilation is evident.

Microscopically, the demarcation line corresponds to hyperplasia of the primitive spindle-shaped mesenchymal cells of the vanguard (Fig. 2). This change is present in succeeding stages, and becomes progressively more severe in the advanced stages, sometimes extending anteriorly as a wide translucent apron as far as the ora serrata (see below). Since the nasal retinal vasculature is usually mature at the time of injury, most retinal lesions (of all stages) are found temporally where maturation is normally delayed.

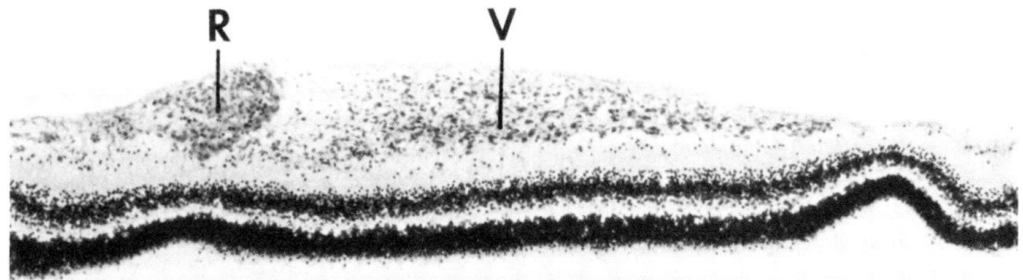

Fig. 3. ROP stage 2. Mesenchymal cells in vanguard (V) have proliferated to form a thick layer tapering anteriorly. Posteriorly, the endothelial cells of the rear guard (R) also have proliferated to form a globular aggregate in meridional profile. Together, the proliferating vanguard and rear guard layers progressively thicken the retina to form the ridge that clinically is recognized as stage 2. (H & E × 250).

STAGE 2 RETINOPATHY

Stage 2, the second of the acute phases, is a response to continuing injury and is characterized macroscopically by the development of a *ridge* within the retina [2]. The ridge represents a further thickening of the line in stage 1, but in addition a thin white line appears behind and separated from the vanguard by a lucent line of approximately equal width. Again, in this and subsequent stages, the vanguard may extensively involve the nonvascularized retina anterior to the ridge. Occasionally, circular discontinuities or "holes" occur in the sheet of vanguard cells, creating a cribriform pattern [3]. Since it corresponds topographically to the normal advancing vasculature, the ridge has a circumferential (or radial) orientation, although only rarely is it observed to involve 360° of the fundus in pathological specimens. Microscopically, the vanguard tissue is more hyperplastic than in stage 1, and a new feature is added, proliferation of the endothelial cells of the rear guard zone, which corresponds to the thin white line noted macroscopically (Fig. 3). The lucent line noted grossly behind the vanguard is a region of relative hypocellularity. Inflammation is conspicuously lacking in this and subsequent stages.

Within this stage, the ridge may show progressive thickening, although the retinal surface remains intact. The ridge also may become conspicuously hyperemic (Fig. 4), a complication that has been characterized clinically with fluorescein angiography as an arteriovenous shunt [9–11]. Retinal vasodilation posterior to the ridge is more exaggerated in this stage, and serous exudation into the vitreous body over the ridge may be found. It is important to understand that, in the vast majority of stage 1 and 2 cases, the retinal lesions arrest and regress, leaving behind no residual scars.

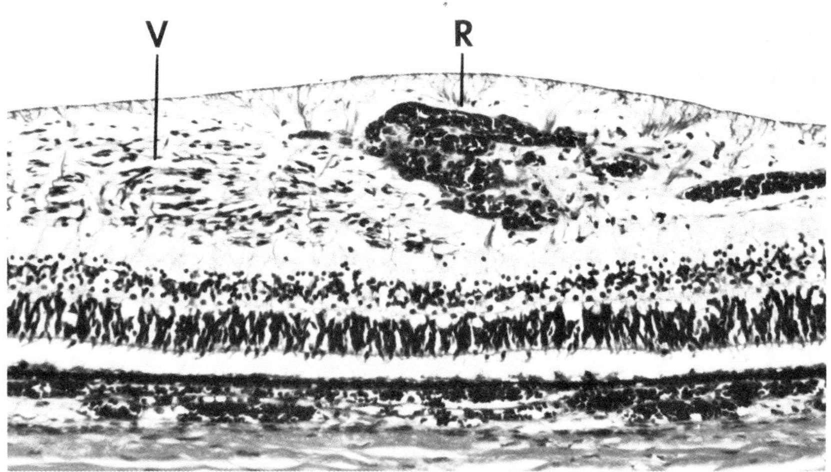

Fig. 4.   ROP stage 2. The rear guard region (R) shows conspicuous hyperemia, the intraretinal portion of the complication that has been characterized clinically as an arteriovenous shunt [9–11]. V, vanguard. (H & E × 300).

STAGE 3 RETINOPATHY

Stage 3 is characterized by extraretinal vascularization (ERV), which takes three distinct forms: placoid, polypoid, or pedunculated [3]. The placoid form, which occurs in the region of the ridge (and therefore has a circumferential orientation), is by far the most common and, by virtue of its relationship to the early stages of retinal detachment (see below), is the most important type of ERV. Polypoid ERV is uncommon and occurs as isolated hemispherical mounds on the retinal surface behind but in the same quadrant as the ridge. The pedunculated type of ERV is rare and arises on a delicate stalk from the retina behind the ridge; in form, it may resemble a frond, palm tree, or sea fan and may lie fairly close to the retinal surface or extend high into the vitreous body.

Microscopically, ERV occurs from the region of the rear guard or the more posterior aspect of the ridge, with proliferation of cords of endothelial cells without lumina or more commonly delicate, thin-walled vessels through the retinal surface into the vitreous cavity (Fig. 5). Thus, these vessels are derived from proliferating endothelial cells and not from vasoformative mesenchymal cells as in normal retinal angiogenesis. This has been confirmed in our laboratory with factor VIII preparations.

Some eyes with highly active and elevated ridges have extremely delicate

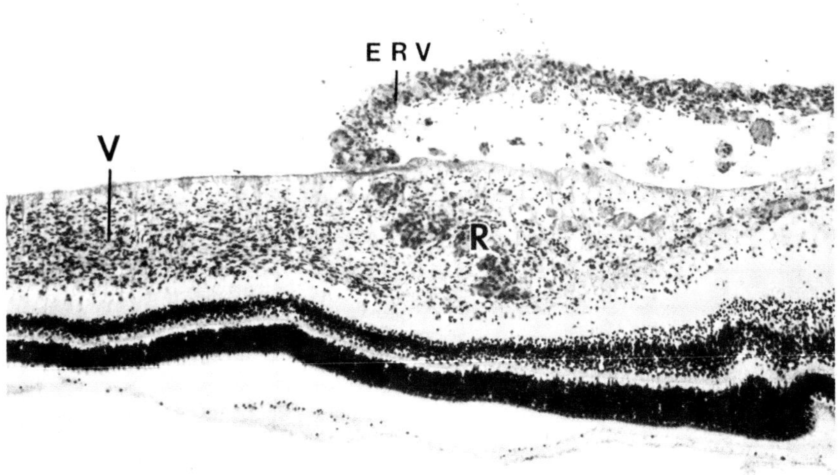

Fig. 5. ROP stage 3. All three pathological phases are shown, including proliferation of vanguard (V), rear guard (R), and extraretinal vascularization (ERV), the latter forming a plaque on the retinal surface. Buckling of retina is evident, which often heralds the onset of retinal detachment and stage 4. (H & E × 60).

vessels bridging from the more posterior retina to the summit of the ridge. The infrequent branches of these vessels are often obtuse and occasionally either angulate posteriorly or deviate downward to reinsert into the underlying retina. The basis for these extraretinal vessels is unclear. Most appear to have been dragged upward and out of the plane of the retina by the elevation of the ridge or by folding of the retina anteriorly (see below). Others arise far posterior to the ridge, and no evidence of retinopathy is present in the vicinity of their apparent origin. Most observers agree, however, that they have no prognostic significance and that, in the clinical setting, where the retina is transparent (and the media sometimes hazy), these vessels should not be misinterpreted as being within a detached retina [12].

Beginning with stage 3, the vitreous body undergoes significant and occasionally profound changes. These take two major forms, synchysis and condensation. Synchysis produces sometimes large pockets in the vitreous body over the ridge; this is found usually over arrested lesions (see below). It seems probable that synchytic destruction of the vitreous body is related to release of lytic substances by incompetent vessels, either in the retina or in the vitreous body. Condensation becomes manifest as sheets and strands extending high into the vitreous body, usually angulating anteriorly toward the equator of the lens. It seems likely that condensation of the vitreous body over the ridge is related to depolymerization of hyaluronic acid and collapse of the collagenous framework into optically visible structures [13]. Condensation of the vitreous body usually is associated with retinal buckling, which often heralds the onset of retinal detachment (stage 4). In the later stages, the vitreous body usually shows severe central synchysis, and condensed sheets are attached to the surface of the detached retina. It is not clear at present whether these changes in the vitreous body represent sequential changes or whether they reflect preexisting individual differences in the vitreous body. Nonvascular proliferative extraretinopathy, usually in the form of glial strands from the retinal surface, can sometimes be found at this stage [13–15].

STAGE 4 RETINOPATHY

Retinal detachment is the characteristic feature of stage 4. The detachment may have several features that are potentially of prognostic importance, and a committee with international representation has recently published a classification reflecting these features to refine further the clinical classification [14] of this stage. The detachment may be *exudative* or *tractional*. The exudative type has a serous (or less often hemorrhagic) retroretinal exudate, is dome-shaped, and has a relatively smooth retinal surface. The tractional type is caused by either horizontal or vertical tractional forces, is peaked, and has an irregular retinal surface [15–22]. It may be *subtotal* or *total*. Subtotal detachment (stage 4) involves only a portion or portions of the fundus; total detachment involves the entire retina, with residual attachments only at the disc and ora serrata (stage 4).

Detachment may be *segmental* or *circumferential*. Segmental detachment involves only a small segment of the fundus; circumferential detachment involves a larger region with a circumferential or radial orientation. It may be *macular* or *extramacular*. Macular detachment is found only when injury occurs very early and the developing vasculature is parapapillary and involves the macula (zone I); in extramacular detachments, the proliferative vasogenic tissue involves zones II and III (more peripheral fundus). Because of residual retinal attachments at the disc and ora serrata, when detachment is total, the retina resembles a funnel, the base or mouth of the funnel being anterior. The funnel may be *open* or *closed* (either anterior, posterior, or along its entire length). These features may be *visible* or *not visible* depending clinically on the amount and density of tissue in the retrolental space.

A group of clinical signs and symptoms apparently relating to the ''activity'' of the disease may also have prognostic importance. These include active vs atrophic (largely based on the diameter of vessels in retina

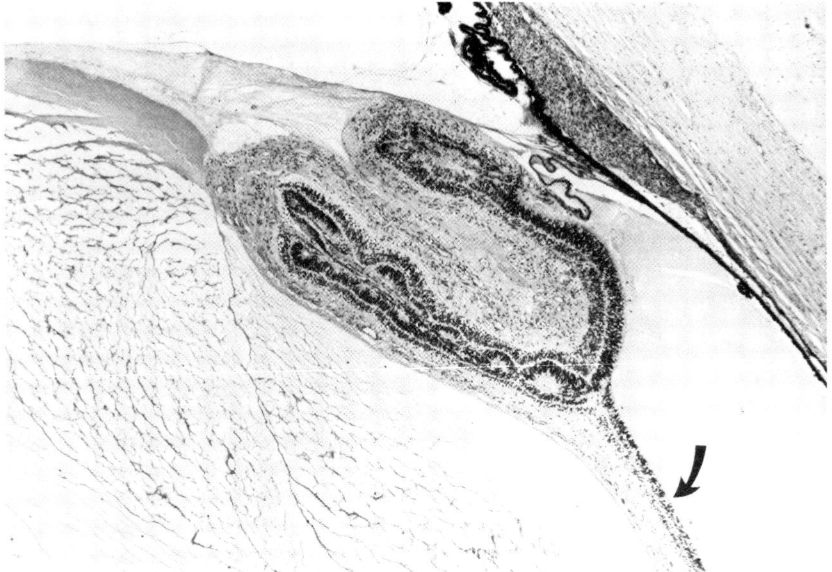

Fig. 6. ROP stage 4. Anterior retina is folded and rolled like a scroll, which has foreshortened and detached the retina posteriorly (arrow). Serous exudate is notable in vitreous and in retroretinal space. (H & E×60).

and iris), exudate (type, location, and amount), appearance of proliferative tissue (gelatinous vs white), and hemorrhage (retinal, vitreous, or retroretinal).

The pathologic features of the retinal detachment in this condition are unique. Detachment is initiated when repeated or continuing injury results in buckling of the retina in the region of the ridge (Fig. 5). Thereafter, the retina becomes folded and progressively "drawn" anteriorly. When viewed in meridional profile, the retina becomes pleated or rolled like a scroll, resulting in meridional foreshortening and progressive detachment from the underlying pigment epithelium throughout the fundus (Fig. 6). The retroretinal space at this stage contains a serous exudate of varying density, although serous retinal detachment also may occur earlier, without obvious traction, and may be self-limiting. Subsequently, the "V" or funnel shape of the detachment becomes altered in shape by closure anteriorly, posteriorly, or totally (Fig. 7) [16–23]. The vitreous body at this stage is present as condensed sheets (with conspicuous stranding) on the retinal surface and in the retrolental space. Posterior vitreous detachment is found only in those eyes that have had significant vitreous hemorrhage. Complications related to persistence of the

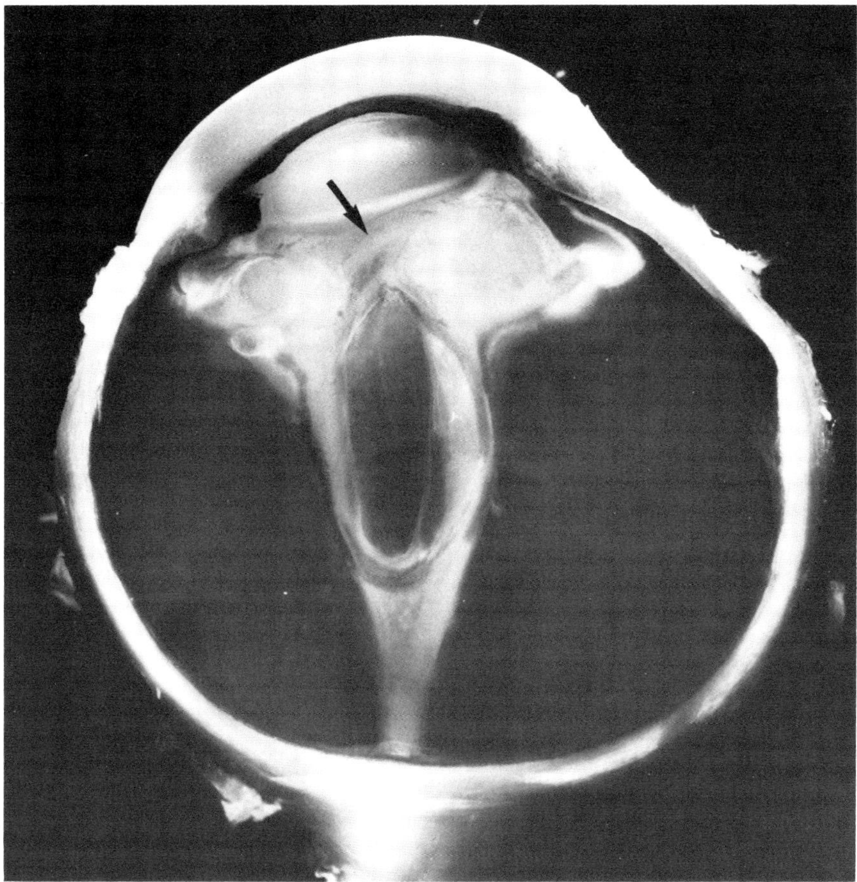

Fig. 7.   ROP stage 4. Peripheral retina is folded, and total retinal detachment is present. The funnel of detached retina is almost closed posteriorly and is filled anteriorly with retrolental fibrous tissue of moderate density (arrow). ($\times 5$.)

hyaloid system are extremely rare. Extrapapillary vascularization occurs occasionally but only very late in the course of the disease process.

Although sometimes subtle, extraretinal proliferation of *nonvascular* tissue is usually present at this stage [15]. Such tissue is manifest as delicate tufts or strands extending into the vitreous body from the retinal surface. Usually, these lesions occur in clusters from the nonvascularized retina, but they may be more widely scattered or occur posterior to the extraretinal vascularization.

Microscopically, the detached retina shows the customary degeneration of outer and inner segments of the photoreceptor cells and mild, largely superficial gliosis. The latter is more conspicuous anteriorly, where the retina has folded. Epiretinal membranes are uncommon until the very late stages [15]. Retroretinal membranes, however, are relatively common, and they are frequently pigmented, sometimes recapitulating the underlying pigment epithelium [4]. Pigmented retroretinal membranes result from colonization of undersurface of the retina by cells that have migrated via the retroretinal fluid from the underlying pigment epithelium. Other retroretinal membranes are nonpigmented and are clearly related to proliferation of retinal glia; these are occasionally found in the postequatorial fundus. Anteriorly, in the region of retinal folding and extraretinal vascularization, proliferating vascular tissue and stellate or spindle-shaped cells resembling fibroblasts may be found along condensed vitreous strands or sheets, sometimes high in the overlying vitreous body.

ARRESTED AND REACTIVATED RETINOPATHY

As was mentioned above, the vast majority of retinal lesions in ROP not only arrest but also regress without residua. However, inactive scars as well as reactivated retinal lesions have been found in our autopsy material, although at present they have not been fully characterized [3]. Some of the regressed lesions appear as white, linear scars of the retina, marking the topographical location of the intraretinal proliferative tissue when injury occurred. Others show more severe scarring, with white, irregularly thickened retinal folds, scattered retinal pigmentation, and marked changes of the overlying vitreous. The severe cases apparently represent those that had advanced to stage 3 or beyond at the time of arresting. Reactivation of retinopathy after arresting also has been shown. In such cases, the site of initial injury is marked by either intraretinal or both intraretinal and extraretinal scars. All such cases show evidence of renewed retinal vascularization following arrest, with subsequent reinjury and recurrence of retinopathy more anterior in the fundus.

DISCUSSION

Prognostically, the most important of the constellation of lesions associated with ROP is retinal detachment, especially when detachment is related to traction. The type of detachment seen in ROP is unique and results from progressive changes in the peripheral retina. After the appearance of the circumferential (stage 2) and extraretinal vascularization intervenes (stage 3), the retina buckles and progressively is "drawn" anteriorly toward the equator of the lens. Thereafter, the retina becomes folded, pleated, and rolled like a scroll, the retina throughout the fundus becoming detached as a result of foreshortening. It is important to recognize that there is no tissue behind the lens or bridging across the vitreous cavity (eg, along detached posterior hyaloid) during this process as in the cell-mediated proliferative vitreoretinopathy associated with rhegmatogenous retinal detachments in adults. The fundamental cause (or causes) of these progressive changes is presently poorly understood, but most likely the process is multifactorial.

Intraretinal factors must include the vanguard tissue, which in most advanced cases constitutes a considerable mass of mesenchyme in the superficial retina. Like most other cells, the vanguard cells probably contain contractile proteins, and this may be a factor in the initial meridional buckling and inward folding of the retina. Likewise, the progressive elevation of the ridge may result in part from contraction of the narrow band of rear guard endothelial cells, which would result in radial traction. Astrogliosis of the superficial retina is an additional intraretinal factor that must be considered, although this process becomes conspicuous only in the later phases, when folding is already developed [24].

Extraretinal factors responsible for the folding and rolling of the peripheral retina are more conspicuous. Contraction of the extraretinal vasoproliferative tissue is the most obvious theoretical factor, and it is important to note that buckling, folding, and rolling do not occur in the absence of extraretinal vascularization. Recognition of the synergistic interaction of the vitreous body and vessels is also important; the extraretinal vessels (or cords of endothelial cells) frequently extend along planes established by synchytic destruction or condensation of the vitreous body. Thus the vitreous body appears at the very least to provide a vehicle for the traction exerted by other extraretinal tissue. Synchysis itself is probably related to lytic substances released during the extraretinal vasoproliferative stages that cause destruction of the overlying vitreous body. It is uncertain whether this represents simply depolymerization of the hyaluronic acid substrate of the vitreous body and subsequent condensation of the collagenous framework as has been described by Balazs, [13] or perhaps actual destruction of both hyaluronate and collagen by catabolic enzymes. Since it has implications far beyond its application to the retinopathy associated with prematurity, the more important question is whether the collagenous framework of the vitreous body can foreshorten and thereby cause traction on the retina. Although there has been no laboratory confirmation of this, the weight of circumstantial evidence from the present study suggests that the tractional forces so generated are biophysically active and not passive.

Most investigators agree that the bulk of stage 1 and 2 lesions regress and leave little if any residua. However, the morphologic features of residual lesions following the arrest of more severe retinopathy have not been fully characterized, although they must be recognized clinically. It would be important to know if any of the lesions are progressive and threaten vision later in their course, since this not only would change the prognosis but also would suggest the need for prophylactic therapy. In addition, the characterization of residual lesions is potentially important in the differential diagnosis of the many developmental, degenerative, and postinflammatory conditions of the fundus. Perhaps even more important is the recognition that reinjury can reactivate retinopathy following arrest. This has been documented by the clinical team at our institution in several cases, one of which was published [3]. Again, there is a need for more information concerning this phenomenon, especially regarding the need and the frequency with which one must follow cases that arrest.

REFERENCES

1. Foos RY, Kopelow SM: Development of retinal vasculature in paranatal infants. Surv Ophthalmol 18:117–127, 1973.
2. Foos RY: Acute retrolental fibroplasia. Albrecht von Graefes Arch Klin Exp Ophthalmol 195:87–100, 1975.
3. Foos RY: Chronic retinopathy of prematurity. Ophthalmology 92:563–574, 1985.
4. Flynn JT: An international classification of retinopathy of prematurity: Clinical experience. Ophthalmology 92:987–994, 1985.
5. Ashton N: Oxygen and the growth and development of retinal vessels: In vivo and in vitro studies. Am J Ophthalmol 62:412–435, 1966.
6. Flower RW, McLeod DS, Lutty GA, Goldberg B, Wajer SD: Postnatal retinal vasculature development of the puppy. Invest Ophthalmol Vis Sci 26:957–968, 1985.
7. Cogan DG: Development and senescence of the human retinal vasculature. Trans Ophthalmol Soc UK 83:465–489, 1963.
8. Lucey JF, Dangman B: A reexamination of the role of oxygen in retrolental fibroplasia. Pediatrics 73:82–96, 1984.
9. Cantolino SJ, Curran JS, Van Caden TC, Edwards W: Acute retrolental fibroplasia: Classification and objective evaluation of incidence, natural history and resolution by fundus photography and intravenous fluorescein angiography. Perspect Ophthalmol 2:175–187, 1978.
10. Flynn JT, O'Grady GE, Herrera J et al: Retrolental fibroplasia: I. Clinical observations. Arch Ophthalmol 95:217–223, 1977.
11. Kushner BJ, Essner D, Cohen IJ, Flynn JT: Retrolental fibroplasia: II. Pathologic correlation. Arch Ophthalmol 95:29–38, 1977.
12. Kingham JD: Acute retrolental fibroplasia. Arch Ophthalmol 95:39–47, 1977.
13. Balazs EA: The molecular biology of the vitreous. In McPherson A (ed): "New and Controversial Aspects of Retinal Detachment." New York: Harper and Row, 1968, pp 3–15.
14. Committee for the Classification of Retinopathy of Prematurity: II. The classification of retinal detachment. Arch Ophthalmol 105:906–912, 1987.
15. Foos RY: The spectrum of nonvascular proliferative extraretinopathies. In Nicholson DH (ed): "Ocular Pathology Update." New York: Masson, 1980, pp 107–114.
16. Tasman W: Late complications of retrolental fibroplasia. Ophthalmology 86:1724–1740, 1979.

17. Charles S: Vitreous surgery for retinopathy of prematurity (ROP). In "Retinopathy of Prematurity Conference Syllabus." Washington, DC: 1981, pp 858–863.

18. Lightfoot D , Irvine AR: Vitrectomy in infants and children with retinal detachments caused by cicatricial retrolental fibroplasia. Am J Ophthalmol 94:305–312, 1982.

19. McPherson AR, Hittner HM, Lemos R: Retinal detachment in young premature infants with acute retrolental fibroplasia: Thirty-two new cases. Ophthalmology 89:1160–1169, 1982.

20. Machemer R: Closed vitrectomy for severe retrolental fibroplasia in the infant. Ophthalmology 90:436–441, 1983.

21. Schepens CL: "Retinal Detachment and Allied Diseases." Philadelphia: WB Saunders, 1983, p 703.

22. Patz A: Current therapy of retrolental fibroplasia: Retinopathy of prematurity. Ophthalmology 90:425–427, 1983.

23. Trese MT: Surgical results of stage V retrolental fibroplasia and timing of surgical repair. Ophthalmology 91:461–466, 1984.

24. Foos RY, Gloor BP: Vitreoretinal juncture; healing of experimental wounds. Albrecht von Graefes Arch Klin Exp Ophthalmol 196:213–230, 1975.

Growth Factors: Soluble Mediators of Wound Repair and Ocular Fibrosis

Leonard M. Hjelmeland, PhD, and **Anita K. Harvey**, PhD

Department of Ophthalmology and Biochemistry, University of California at Davis, Sacramento, California 95817 (L.M.H.); Eli Lilly, Co., Indianapolis, Indiana 46285 (A.K.H.)

Several authors discussing the pathophysiology of the proliferative retinopathies have commented on similarities with the physiology of mesenchymal wound repair [1,2]. The presence of myofibroblastic cells and the contraction of cellular membranes found either in the vitreous body or on the inner or outer surfaces of the retina directly parallel cellular events found in the granulation tissue of maturing wounds [3]. Aside from the interesting histological and physiological comparisons between the proliferative retinopathies and soft tissue wound repair, further direct comparisons of these two systems have not been provided. Such comparisons might yield useful basic insights into new directions of research in the biochemistry and cell biology of proliferative retinal disease based on the body of similar work in soft tissue wound repair as a conceptual model.

The purpose of the review presented here is the examination of just one facet of the fundamental biochemistry of both proliferative disease of the retina and wound repair. Growth factors play a central role in the wound repair response as soluble mediators of the directed migration and proliferation of connective tissue and endothelial cells. A growing body of evidence also suggests that growth factors play a central role in the formation and growth of cellular membranes in the proliferative retinopathies. Other fields of research into the biochemistry and cell biology of fibrotic diseases, such as idiopathic pulmonary fibrosis and atherosclerosis, have also demonstrated important roles for growth factors.

This review first briefly considers the cellular events of wound repair, with a special emphasis on cells that produce growth factors or respond to these same macromolecules. In the second section, the biochemistry of cellular growth factors is examined. The third section then presents findings concerning the role of growth factors in pulmonary fibrosis, to illustrate the impact of growth factor research in the field of fibrosis. The fourth section

Birth Defects: Original Article Series, Volume 24, Number 1, pages 87–102
© **1988 March of Dimes Birth Defects Foundation**

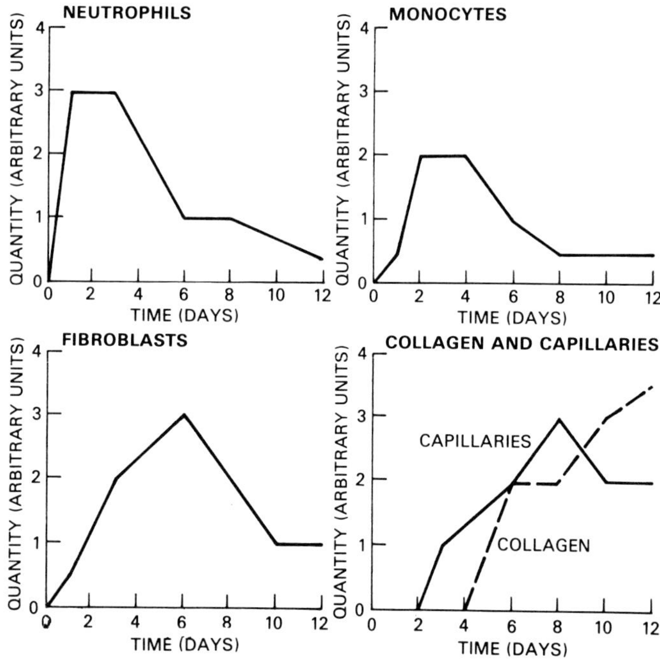

Fig. 1. Cell populations that occupy the wound at different times can be divided into three groups, each with its own special task to perform. The stages tend to overlap one another and may well be interdependent, since suppression of one can delay the start of the next. (Figure and legend taken from Ross R. "Wound Healing." Sci Am 220:40–50, 1969.)

reviews results concerning the role of ocular growth factors in pathology of the retina and vitreous body.

THE PHYSIOLOGY OF WOUND REPAIR: CELLULAR EVENTS

The precise time course of the many cellular events that cooperate to yield the healing wound has been well studied. A schematic representation of the temporal sequence of cellular events in soft tissue wound repair is given in Figure 1. After the initial traumatic event, a thrombus or clot forms at the site of injury. Aggregated platelets and fibrin form the essential constituents of the thrombus, and the presence of platelets is especially important in that these cells contain several important growth factors that initiate the migration and proliferation of fibroblastic cells in the wound space. During the first 24 hours, the wound is invaded by polymorphonuclear leukocytes, which function primarily to phagocytize bacteria that may be present. During the second 24-hour period, the wound is invaded by monocytes from the circulatory system, which then mature into tissue macrophages. These cells play an essential role in the healing of wounds via their role both as phagocytic cell functioning to debride the wound and also as sources of cellular growth factors that stimulate the growth and migration of both connective tissue cells and endothelial cells. Studies by Ross [4] have demonstrated that platelets and macrophages are the essential sources of cellular growth factors in repairing wounds and that polymorphonuclear leukocytes play no role in stimulating growth. During days 3–7, fibroblastic cells and endothelial cells migrate to the center of the wound space and proliferate to form capillaries and granulation tissue. After one week, extracellular matrix is deposited by these cells, and later cellular contraction occurs, which functions to close the wound.

Many similarities exist between wound repair and fibrotic disease. The cellular bases of both fibrotic lesions and wounds have all been compared. In general, it is believed that fibrosis is a problem of hypercellularity, with resultant excessive deposition of otherwise normal extracellular matrix by what appear to be normal cells. Figure 2 presents a conceptual model of the pathogenesis of generalized fibrotic disease. After initial tissue damage, which may occur from any of a variety of insults, chronic inflammation leads to the recruitment of excessive numbers of fibroblasts, which then deposit excessive amounts of extracellular matrix. The role of inflammatory cells thus is clearly central to this process via their production of growth factors, the soluble mediators of fibroblast recruitment and proliferation. Contrasting opinions do exist, notably the published reports that proliferated smooth muscle found in atherosclerotic plaques may be phenotypically different from normal smooth muscle found in the medial layers of large vessels [5]. Nonetheless, fibroblastic cells, elements of the vasculature, and phagocytic cells are found in fibrotic lesions as well as in repairing wounds. These results suggest the general conclusion that many fibrotic diseases are the result of inadequate biological controls on cellular proliferation. Since growth factors are the major soluble mediators of cellular proliferation, this fact suggests that growth factors may play a central role in the development of fibrotic disease.

Besides the similarities noted, however, many differences also exist between wound repair and fibrosis. Quite obviously the etiology of fibrotic diseases is varied and is unrelated to simple traumatic events. In addition, the time course of the cellular events in the two cases is different. As stated above, cellular proliferation in wound repair occupies approximately a 2-week period, whereas the time courses of many fibrotic diseases vary and occupy many months. Again, perhaps the most crucial difference is the relative hypercellularity of the fibrotic lesion and the resultant excessive deposition of extracellular matrix.

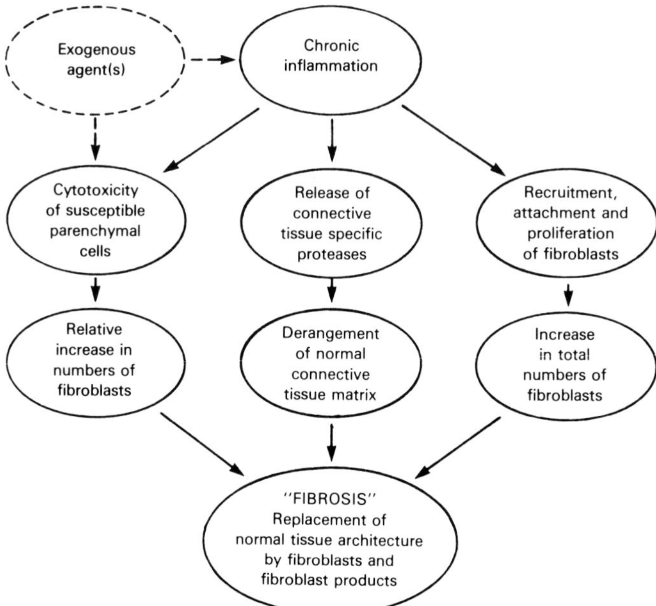

Fig. 2. Injury caused by exogenous agents, or by the inflammation induced by such agents, leads to fibrosis through a variety of processes. There are cytotoxic effects, with loss of susceptible normal parenchymal cells, frequently resulting in a relative increase in fibroblast numbers. Simultaneously, there is a release of connective tissue-specific proteases, which cause derangement of normal tissue matrix components, disrupting normal tissue architecture. In addition, recruitment, attachment, and proliferation of fibroblasts are stimulated, further increasing fibroblast numbers. The end result is fibrosis, ie, the replacement of normal tissue architecture by fibroblasts and fibroblast products. (Reproduced from Rennard SI, Bitterman PB, Crystal RG: Current concepts of the pathogenesis of fibrosis: Lessons from pulmonary fibrosis. In Berk PD, Castro-Malaspina H, Wasserman LR (eds): "Myelofibrosis and the Biology of Connective Tissue." New York: Alan R. Liss, Inc., 1984, pp 359–377, with permission of the authors.)

GROWTH FACTORS

Growth factors that function in the wound repair response and thus are suspect as important factors in fibrotic disease can be conveniently classified on the basis of the major cell types responsible for their production. Platelets, wound macrophages, and endothelial cells are all known to produce chemotactic and mitogenic activities for a variety of cell types, and now the clear distinctions among many of the previously named growth factors from each of these cell types are dissolving, as more precise biochemical information concerning these species becomes available.

TABLE I. Cellular Sources of Growth Factors Involved in Wound Repair

Platelets	Wound macrophages	Endothelial cells
Platelet-derived growth factor	Interleukin-1	Platelet-derived growth factor
Epidermal growth factor	Basic fibroblast growth factor	Unidentified endothelial mitogens
Transforming growth factor-β	Platelet-derived growth factor	
Fibronectin		
Unidentified endothelial mitogens		

Platelets have long been recognized as the major source of mitogenic activity in clotted serum. This activity has been purified to homogeneity from human platelets and named the platelet-derived growth factor (PDGF). PDGF has a wide spectrum of chemotactic and mitogenic activities for mesenchymal and glial cells [6–9]. Platelets are also known to contain transforming growth factor-β [10]. Although the specific role of this growth factor is currently not understood, a possible role in wound repair has been proposed [10]. Platelets also contain fibronectin, epidermal growth factor, and as yet unpurified endothelial mitogens [11]. The growth factor content of platelets, wound macrophages, and endothelial cells is summarized in Table I.

Although wound macrophages were originally considered to be important primarily in stimulating the immune response via production of interleukin-1, it is now clear that these cells play a major role in maintaining cellular proliferation at the wound site after initiation of these events by platelets. Studies by Ross [4] in which animals were made devoid of either neutrophils or peripheral monocytes, the precursor cells of the wound macrophage, demonstrated that neutrophils play essentially no role in cellular proliferation, whereas wound macrophages had a substantial role.

Macrophages have recently been shown to secrete the basic fibroblast growth factor, a potent stimulator of endothelial and connective tissue proliferation [12]. An even more curious finding suggests that wound macrophages synthesize and secrete PDGF [13,14].

Endothelial cells that are proliferating also secrete a connective tissue mitogen, which has recently been demonstrated to be identical with PDGF [15]. Other reports indicate that these cells make an endothelial mitogen as well, which is currently not well characterized [16].

Finally, plasma contains several growth factors that play an essential role in connective tissue proliferation. Insulin, the insulin-like growth factors 1 and 2, and epidermal growth factor have all been variously determined as essential requirements for traversal of the eukaryotic cell cycle [17].

The ways in which all of these growth factors function together to cause

$$G_0 \xrightarrow{\quad 1 \quad} G_1 \xrightarrow{\quad 2 \quad} S$$

1. Competence Factors:
   Platelet Derived Growth Factor
   Acidic Fibroblast Growth Factor
   Basic Fibroblast Growth Factor

2. Progression Factors:
   Epidermal Growth Factor
   Insulin-like Growth Factor — I
   Transforming Growth Factors

Fig. 3. Control of the eukaryotic cell cycle by competence and progression factors. Competence factors induce cells that are in a growth-arrested state (or G_0) to enter G_1, after which the progression factors act sequentially to cause the cell to enter S phase and therefore to initiate DNA synthesis.

cellular proliferation have been the subject of intensive research efforts. The most important model divides the action of growth factors on resting cells into two broad classes, competence and progression [17]. The competence factors act to render resting cells in G_0 capable of division, whereas progression factors cause traversal of G_0/G_1 and entrance into S phase, where DNA synthesis begins. Figure 3 is a schematic representation of the cell cycle, indicating the action of competence and progression factors. Generally speaking, competence factors are contained within special cells and are released according to specific stimuli. Thus platelets, macrophages, and endothelial cells are all capable of secreting competence factors, but only when necessary. Progression factors, on the other hand, appear to be generally available constituents of plasma. In this fashion, the two classes of factors act in concert to produce the intermittent proliferation of cells that is the hallmark of well functioning wound repair. The biological effects of growth factors on cells include proliferation, chemotaxis, and stimulation of extracellular matrix production. Curiously, it is the competence factors that appear to be responsible for chemotaxis, the directed migration of cells. PDGF has been shown to be chemotactic for connective tissue cells [6,7], glia [8], and pigmented epithelium [18]. Fibronectin is likewise chemotactic for connective tissue cells [19], glia [8], and pigmented epithelium [20]. The basic fibroblast growth factor is a chemotactic factor for transformed glia and embryonic connective tissue cells [21], and the acidic fibroblast growth factor is chemotactic for endothelial cells [22]. Table II lists growth factors with chemotactic properties and their target cells.

TABLE II. Chemotactic Growth Factors and Their Target Cells

Platelet-derived growth factor	Basic fibroblast growth factor	Acidic fibroblast growth factor
Fibroblasts Smooth muscle cells Rat brain astrocytes Rat retinal glia Pigment epithelium C_6 glioma Leukocytes (?)	Fibroblasts Rat brain astrocytes C_6 glioma	Human umbilical vein endothelial cells

THE ROLE OF GROWTH FACTORS IN FIBROSIS

Having thus had a brief introduction to cellular growth factors and their function in normal wound repair, it is instructive to consider a field of research in fibrosis in which these two elements, growth factors and wound repair, have been brought together and integrated into the pathogenesis. Recent efforts by Crystal, Renard, Bitterman, and Martinet, have delineated the role of the alveolar macrophage in producing mitogenic substances that are likely to play a major role in causing pulmonary fibrosis. Studies by this group have shown that these cells are responsible for producing PDGF [14], alveolar macrophage-derived growth factor (an activity similar to that of insulin-like growth factor 1) [23,24], and fibronectin [25], all of which apparently stimulate fibroblastic cells in the alveolar wall to divide.

Figures 4 and 5 present data concerning the production of fibronectin and the alveolar macrophage-derived growth factor by macrophages obtained by pulmonary lavage from patients with a variety of fibrotic lung diseases. The data clearly demonstrate that, for both of these important mediators of connective tissue growth, patients with fibrotic disease have resident macrophages that are producing dramatically increased levels compared to normal controls. These findings again illustrate the importance of chronically activated inflammatory cells in fibrotic disease, in this case the alveolar wall.

OCULAR GROWTH FACTORS

With the advent of research on angiogenesis in tumors, basic research in the eye became directed at growth-promoting substances as well. A great number of papers concerning the production of mitogenic or chemotactic substances in vitro have appeared without the benefit of further characterization of these substances. These papers will not be reviewed here. A smaller number of groups have gone on to purify these macromolecules partially or completely, and their results are easily summarized. Table III

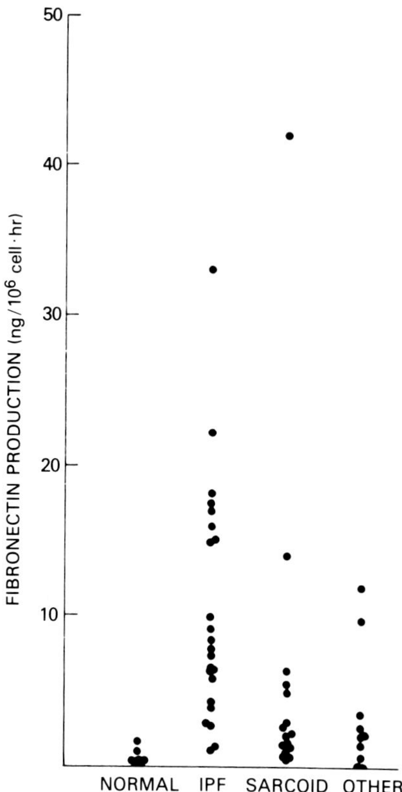

Fig. 4. Production of fibronectin by alveolar cells of normal controls and patients with interstitial lung disease. Cells were cultured for 24 hours in RPMI-1640 medium without serum at a density of 106 cells/ml. Four groups were evaluated: normal adults, patients with idiopathic pulmonary fibrosis (IPF), patients with pulmonary sarcoidosis (sarcoid), and patients with other interstitial lung diseases (other). All values represent the mean of four determinations. (Reproduced from Rennard et al [25], with permission of the publisher.)

presents essential information concerning ocular growth factors and their relationships. As we shall see, many factors with differing names are identical, and these relationships are presented in Table III as well.

Research on ocular growth factors began in the 1970s with the efforts of groups in the United States and in France. Studies by Courtois, Barritault, and colleagues focused on the biochemical and biological properties of a retina-derived mitogenic factor, which they termed eye-derived growth factor [26]. This activity was also found in vitreous, pigmented epithelium, and iris [27]. Most recently, this group has expanded the definition to include

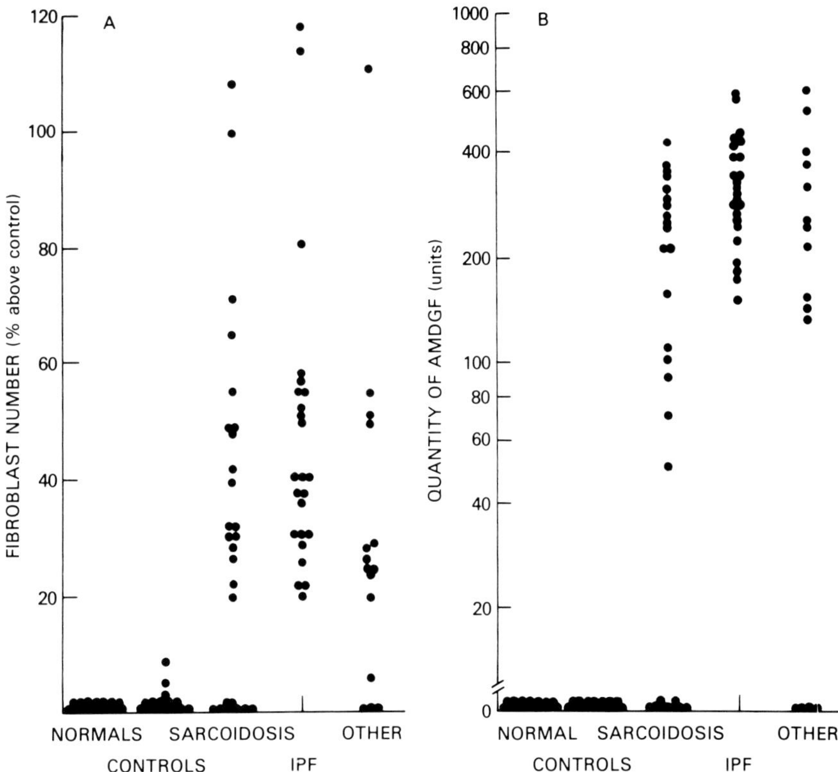

Fig. 5. Spontaneous release of alveolar macrophage-derived growth factor (AMDGF) by alveolar macrophages from patients with interstitial lung disease. A: Growth of fibroblasts in response to macrophage supernates. Noncycling fibroblasts were cultured with undiluted supernates from alveolar macrophages (2 days at 37°C), and the resultant increase in fibroblast number was determined. Shown is the percent increase in fibroblast number above control (medium alone) caused by macrophage supernates from the different patient groups. B: Quantity of AMDGF released spontaneously by macrophages from the different patient groups shown in A. The quantity of growth factor was defined as the reciprocal of the dilution resulting in 50% of the maximum growth response. (Reproduced from Bitterman et al [24], with permission of the publisher.)

eye-derived growth factors (Table III) [28]. The three activities are discrete in terms of both biochemical and biological properties, and EDGF I and II represent the basic and acidic fibroblast growth factors, respectively.

At approximately the same time, efforts of d'Amore, Fenselau, Mello, Lutty, Glaser, and Patz were focused on both stimulators and inhibitors of vascular endothelial cell proliferation found in the retina and vitreous body

TABLE III. Ocular Growth Factors

Growth factor	Source	Distribution	Target cells	High-affinity binding to heparin
Basic fibroblast growth factors				
Eye-derived growth factor I	Bovine retina	Retina Vitreous Choroid/PE Iris	Lens epithelium Connective tissue Vascular endothelium	Yes
Fibroblast growth factor	Bovine retina	Retina Pituitary Brain	Vascular endothelium 3T3 fibroblasts	Yes
Retinal chemotactic protein	Bovine retina	Retina	C_6 glioma Astrocytes Retinal glia	Yes
Acidic fibroblast growth factors				
Retina-derived growth factor	Bovine retina	Retina Hypothalamus	Vascular endothelium 3T3 fibroblasts	Yes
Eye-derived growth factor II	Bovine retina	Retina Vitreous Choroid/PE Iris	Lens epithelium Connective tissue Vascular endothelium	Yes
Other				
Retinoblastoma-derived growth factor	Y79 retinoblastoma	Retinoblastoma	Lens epithelium Retinoblastoma	No
Eye-derived growth factor III	Bovine retina	Retina Vitreous Choroid/PE Iris	—	No

TABLE IV. Eyes With Vasoproliferation

No.	Diagnosis	Endothelial cell migration (cells/20 OIF*)
8	PDR [+]	65 ± 11
9	PDR	50 ± 8
10	PDR	30 ± 3
11	PDR	29 ± 3
12	PDR	33 ± 5
13	PDR	7 ± 3
14	PDR	5 ± 2
15	Rheg. RD[‡] & rubeosis	4 ± 2
16	MPP[§] & rubeosis	5 ± 3

*OIF = oil immersion fields; [+]PDR = proliferative diabetic retinopathy; [‡]Rheg. RD = rhegmatogenous; retinal detachment; [§]MPP = massive periretinal proliferation.
Reproduced from Glaser et al [30], with permission of the publisher.

[29–31]. This work is now being pursued by d'Amore, who has purified a factor termed the retina-derived growth factor, which is apparently equivalent to the eye-derived growth factor II preparation and thus to the acidic fibroblast growth factor [32]. Independent work by Lutty has characterized an inhibitor of vascular endothelial cell proliferation in the vitreous body. [33] Similar studies by Jacobson have also given a characterization of a vitreous inhibitor of endothelial cell proliferation [34].

A group at Yale, led by Reid, has purified a mitogenic factor from retinoblastoma-conditioned medium, which they termed the retinoblastoma-derived growth factor [35]. This material apparently bears no resemblance to any of the other ocular growth factors studied thus far. One chemotactic activity has been substantially purified by Hjelmeland, termed the retinal chemotactic protein, and recently has been shown to be equivalent to the eye-derived growth factor I preparation and thus to the basic fibroblast growth factor (FGF) [36].

Early studies by Glaser, d'Amore, and Michels examined both the mitogenic and chemotactic properties of vitreous aspirates from eyes with proliferative diabetic retinopathy [30]. Tables IV and V are reprinted from this article and demonstrate a significant difference between diabetic samples and control samples with respect to their abilities to stimulate chemotaxis of endothelial cells. More recently, Weiss and collaborators evaluated similar vitreous aspirates for angiogenic activity on the chorioallantoic membrane (CAM) assay [37]. After sample clean-up on diethylaminoethyl (DEAE) chromatography, all samples from diabetic eyes showed major angiogenic activity on the CAM assay, whereas control samples were essentially negative. Although many investigators believe that the retina factor involved

TABLE V. Eyes Without Vasoproliferation

No.	Diagnosis	Endothelial cell migration (cells/20 OIF*)
1	Macular hole	7 ± 2
2	Epiretinal membrane s/p[†] RD	6 ± 1
3	Rheg.[‡] RD[§] s/p excision of membrane behind IOL[‖]	5 ± 1
4	Rheg. RD & MPP**	280 ± 12
5	Rheg. RD s/p vitrectomy	8 ± 3
6	Rheg. RD s/p vitrectomy	4 ± 1
7	Rheg. RD s/p vitrectomy	5 ± 2

*OIF = oil immersion fields; [†]s/p = status post; [‡]Rheg. = rhegmatogenous; [§]RD = retinal detachment; [‖]IOL = intraocular lens; **MPP = massive periretinal proliferation. Reproduced from Glaser et al [30], with permission of the publisher.

TABLE VI. Angiogenic Factor in Human Ocular Fluid

Patient	Age (years)/sex	FGF	
		pmol/ml	ng/ml
1	73, female	1.0, 1.6, 1.0	17, 27.2, 17
2	79, male	0.6	10.2
3	74, male	0.8	13.6
4	57, male	8.9	151.3

Reproduced from Baird et al [38], with permission of the publisher.

in the stimulation of these activities for endothelial cells is the acidic FGF, or equivalently the retina-derived growth factor of d'Amore, recent evidence by Baird, Guillemin, and others has demonstrated the presence of the basic FGF (equivalent to the retinal chemotactic protein and EDGF I) in vitreous [38]. Table VI presents the data reported in that article in terms of directly quantitated concentrations of the basic fibroblast growth factor. It is very significant that the concentrations reported exceed the values determined in vitro for strong mitogenic effects of this protein. Clearly, this brief report gives the first evidence that a specific growth factor plays an important role in abnormal ocular proliferation.

PROLIFERATIVE VITREORETINOPATHY (PVR)

Much less experimental effort has been directed toward establishing the role of growth factors in cellular migration and proliferation associated with periretinal proliferation. In the early papers by d'Amore, Glaser, and Michels, mention of a case of massive PVR was made. Table V gives the

TABLE VII. Chemotaxis, and Proliferation-Stimulating Activities in Human Vitrectomy Specimens; Correlation With Proliferative Vitreoretinopathy Severity[†]

Source of vitreous aspirate	No.	High chemotactic activity or high mitogenic activity	High chemotactic activity and high mitogenic activity
High pathology	66	58	26
Low pathology	76	48	7

[†]PVR grade C1 or greater is classified as high pathology and macular pucker or simple-epiretinal membranes are classified as low pathology. Chemotaxis and mitogenesis assays were performed with rabbit dermal fibroblasts and rabbit or human retinal pigment epithelium. Reproduced from Burke et al [39], with permission of the publisher.

TABLE VIII. Vitreous Aspirates From Eyes With Proliferative Vitreoretinopathy Stimulate Retinal Pigment Epithelium Migration

Source of vitreous aspirate	Chemotactic activity for retinal pigment epithelium	Relative concentration of fibronectin
Proliferative vitreoretinopathy	+	7
Uncomplicated retinal detachment	−	1
Macular pucker	−	1

Reproduced from Jerdan et al [40], with permission of the publisher.

data concerning this case and presence of chemotactic activity for endothelial cells is very evident. Curiously, the assay employed in this study utilizes endothelial cells, but no vascular proliferation is associated with PVR on a routine basis. This fact suggests that the presence of individual growth factors does not uniquely determine the extent or nature of cellular proliferation in pathologies of the retina and that other elements of the pathophysiology play a major role in determining these events.

More recently, Burke has examined the presence of chemotactic and mitogenic activity for fibroblasts in vitreous aspirates from eyes with PVR [39]. A very good correlation between the presence of chemotactic and mitogenic activity and the severity of PVR was noted, and these results are presented in Table VII.

Finally, Jerdan et al have also presented data on the presence of chemotactic activity for pigment epithelium in vitreous aspirates from patients with PVR. The activity in these samples was attributed to both fibronectin and other growth factors, one of which may be PDGF [40]. Table VIII presents these data and comparisons with control patients.

CONCLUSIONS

Quite clearly, several groups have presented evidence for the presence of elevated levels of both chemotactic and mitogenic substances in intraocular fluids of patients with vitreoretinal proliferations. Although the data are currently limited to diabetic vitreoretinopathy and proliferative retinopathy, it is to be expected that further examination of other classes of vitreoretinal proliferation will yield similar results. As was mentioned above, it is also becoming clear that the presence of any particular mitogenic or chemotactic substance does not uniquely determine the nature or extent of the pathology. This is undoubtedly related not only to the complex nature of the pathogenesis of the proliferative disorders of the retina and vitreous body but also to the fact that clinical samples are available only at certain times in the overall progress of these diseases. Nonetheless, growth factors obviously do play a significant role in these processes via their modulation of the directed migration and proliferation of connective tissue, vascular, and glial cells of the retina.

With the advent of homogeneous preparations of the major growth factors found in the eye, more accurate determination of the concentrations of these substances in both experimental and clinical proliferations can be expected. Significant biological investigations of these proteins can then be expected to follow, which will reveal the cellular origins of these proteins in the pigmented epithelium, retina, and vitreous body. Such examinations will then undoubtedly lead to a better understanding of the pathogenesis of this damaging class of ocular diseases.

REFERENCES

1. Wallow IHL, Stevens TS, Greaser ML, Bindley C, Wilson R: Actin filaments in contracting preretinal membranes. Arch Ophthalmol 102:1370–1375, 1984.
2. Hiscott PS, Grierson I, Hitchins CA, Rahi AHS, McLeod D: Epiretinal membranes in vitro. Trans Ophthalmol Soc UK 103:89–102, 1983.
3. Silver IA: The physiology of wound healing. In Hunt TK (ed): "Wound Healing and Wound Infection: Theory and Surgical Practice." New York: Appleton-Century-Crofts, 1980.
4. Ross R: Inflammation, cell proliferation, and connective tissue formation in wound repair. In Hunt TK (ed): "Wound Healing and Wound Infection: Theory and Surgical Practice." New York: Appleton-Century-Crofts, 1980.
5. Benditt EP: Evidence for a monoclonal origin of human atherosclerotic plaques and some implications. Circulation 50:650–652, 1974.
6. Seppa H, Grotendorst GR, Seppa S, Schiffmann E, Martin GR: Platelet-derived growth factor is chemotactic for fibroblasts. J Cell Biol 92:584–588, 1982.
7. Grotendorst GR, Chang T, Seppa HE, Kleinman HK, Martin GR: Platelet-derived growth factor is a chemoattractant for vascular smooth muscle cells. J Cell Physiol 113:261–266, 1982.
8. Bressler JP, Grotendorst GR, Levitov C, Hjelmeland LM: Chemotaxis of rat brain astrocytes to platelet-derived growth factor. Brain Res 344:249–254, 1985.
9. Heldin CH, Westermark B, Wasteson A: Specific receptors for platelet-derived growth factor on cells derived from connective tissue and glia. Proc Natl Acad Sci USA 78:3664–3668, 1981.

10. Assoian RK, Grotendorst GR, Miller DM, Sporn MB: Cellular transformation by coordinated action of three peptide growth factors from human platelets. Nature 309:804–806, 1984.
11. King GL, Buchwald S: Characterization and partial purification of an endothelial cell growth factor from human platelets. J Clin Invest 73:392–396, 1984.
12. Baird A, Mormede P, Bohlen P: Immunoreactive fibroblast growth factor in cells of peritoneal exudate suggests its identity with macrophage-derived growth factor. Biochem Biophys Res Commun 126:358–364, 1985.
13. Ross R, Raines EW, Bowen Pope DF: The biology of platelet-derived growth factor. Cell 46:155–169, 1986.
14. Martinet Y, Bitterman PB, Mornex JF, Grotendorst GR, Martin GR, Crystal RG: Activated human monocytes express the C-SIS proto-oncogene and release a mediator showing PDGF-like activity. Nature 319:158–160, 1986.
15. Barrett TB, Gajdusek CM, Schwartz SM, McDougall JK, Benditt EP: Expression of the sis gene by endothelial cells in culture and in vivo. Proc Natl Acad Sci USA 81:6772–6774, 1984.
16. Gajdusek CM, Schwartz SM: Ability of endothelial cells to condition culture medium. J Cell Physiol 110:35–42, 1982.
17. Stiles CD, Capone GT, Scher CD, Antoniades HN, Van Wyk JJ, Pledger WJ: Dual control of cell growth by somatomedins and platelet-derived growth factor. Proc Natl Acad Sci USA 76:1279–1283, 1979.
18. Campochiaro PA, Glaser BM: Platelet-derived growth factor is chemotactic for human retinal pigment epithelial cells. Arch Ophthalmol 103:576–579, 1985.
19. Gauss-Muller V, Kleinman HK, Martin GR, Schiffmann E: Role of attachment factors and attractants in fibroblast chemotaxis. J Lab Clin Med 96:1071–1080, 1980.
20. Campochiaro PA, Jerdan JA, Glaser BM: Serum contains chemoattractants for human retinal pigment epithelial cells. Arch Ophthalmol 102:1830–1833, 1984.
21. Harvey AK, Aotoki-Keen A, Hjelmeland LM: Manuscript in preparation, 1987.
22. Terranova VP, Aumailley M, Sultan LH, Martin GR, Kleinman HK: Regulation of cell attachment and cell number by fibronectin and laminin. J Cell Physiol 127:473–479, 1986.
23. Bitterman PB, Rennard SI, Hunninghake GW, Crystal RG: Human alveolar macrophage growth factor for fibroblasts: Regulation and partial characterization. J Clin Invest 70:806–822, 1982.
24. Bitterman PB, Adelberg S, Crystal RG: Mechanisms of pulmonary fibrosis: Spontaneous release of the alveolar macrophage-derived growth factor in the interstitial lung disorders. J Clin Invest 72:1801–1813, 1983.
25. Rennard SI, Hunninghake GW, Bitterman PB, Crystal RG: Production of fibronectin by the human alveolar macrophage: Mechanism for the recruitment of fibroblasts to sites of tissue injury in interstitial lung diseases. Proc Natl Acad Sci USA 78:7147–7151, 1981.
26. Barritault D, Plouet J, Courty J, Courtois Y: Purification, characterization, and biological properties of the eye-derived growth factor from retina: Analogies with brain-derived growth factor. J Neurosci Res 8:477–490, 1982.
27. Barritault D, Arruti C, Courtois Y: Is there a ubiquitous growth factor in the eye? Proliferation induced in different cell types by eye-derived growth factors. Differentiation 18:29–42, 1981.
28. Courty J, Loret C, Moenner M, Chevallier B, Lagent O, Courtois Y, Barritault D: Bovine retina contains three growth factor activities with different affinity to heparin: Eye-derived growth factor I, II, III. Biochimie 67:265–269, 1985.
29. Glaser BM, D'Amore PA, Michels RG, Brunson SK, Fenselau AH, Rice T, Patz A: The

demonstration of angiogenic activity from ocular tissues: Preliminary report. Ophthalmology 87:440–446, 1980.

30. Glaser BM, D'Amore PA, Michels RG: The effect of human intraocular fluid vascular endothelial cell migration. Ophthalmology 88:986–991, 1981.

31. Lutty GA, Thompson DC, Gallup JY, Mello RJ, Patz A, Fenselau A: Vitreous: An inhibitor of retinal extract-induced neovascularization. Invest Ophthalmol Vis Sci 24:52–56, 1983.

32. D'Amore PA, Klagsbrun M: Endothelial cell mitogens derived from retina and hypothalamus: Biochemical and biological similarities. J Cell Biol 99:1545–1549, 1984.

33. Lutty GA, Chandler C, Bennett A, Fait C, Patz A: Presence of endothelial cell growth factor activity in normal and diabetic eyes. Curr Eye Res 5:9–17, 1986.

34. Jacobson B, Basu PK, Hasany SM: Vascular endothelial cell growth inhibitor of normal and pathologic human vitreous. Arch Ophthalmol 102:1543–1545, 1984.

35. Tarsio JF, Rubin NA, Russell P, Gregerson DS, Reid TW: Growth stimulatory effects of retinoblastoma-derived growth factors and other mitogens on Nakano mouse lens epithelial cells. Exp Cell Res 146:71–78, 1983.

36. Hjelmeland LM, Harvey AK: Partial purification and biological properties of a chemotactic protein from bovine retina. Invest Ophthalmol Vis Sci 26 [suppl]:335, 1985.

37. Elstow SF, Schor AM, Weiss JB: Bovine retinal angiogenesis factor is a small molecule (molecular mass less than 600). Invest Ophthalmol Vis Sci 26:74–79, 1985.

38. Baird A, Culler F, Jones KL, Guillemin R: Angiogenic factor in human ocular fluid. Lancet 2:563, 1985.

39. Burke J, Abrams G, Aaberg T, Williams G: Chemotaxis and proliferation-stimulating activities in human vitrectomy specimens: Correlation with PVR severity. Invest Ophthalmol Vis Sci 26 [suppl]:283, 1985.

40. Jerdan JA, Campochiaro PA, Glaser BM: Vitreous aspirates from eyes with proliferative vitreoretinopathy stimulate RPE migration. Invest Ophthalmol Vis Sci 26 [suppl]:283, 1985.

Role of Light Toxicity in the Developing Retinal Vasculature

Penny Glass, PhD

Division of Neonatology, Childrens Hospital, National Medical Center, Washington, DC 20010

Advances in medical care and technology have dramatically increased the survival rate of very low-birthweight infants. At the same time, retinopathy of prematurity (ROP) appears to be increasing. Retinal immaturity and oxygen are generally accepted as the principal factors associated with ROP; however, other factors are thought to contribute. One such factor may be precocious exposure of the immature retina to light. The purpose of this chapter is to describe the light exposure by preterm infants in today's intensive care nurseries, to summarize the evidence for light toxicity on the retina, and to suggest some possible mechanisms for the role of light in the pathogenesis of oxygen-induced ROP.

LIGHT EXPOSURE OF PRETERM INFANTS

The preterm infant is exposed to a considerable amount of light from both ambient and supplementary sources (Fig. 1A). The level of ambient illumination in the hospital nursery is bright, having increased five- to tenfold over the last 20 years. Compared to current recommended levels of office lighting (40–50 ftc), the average levels recently reported for hospital nurseries were 50–90 ftc, with peak levels frequently over 220 ftc [1–4]. The exposure of any particular infant depends on the proximity of the infant's incubator to overhead lights or windows. When the sun was entering the windows of one nursery, peak measurements were over 1,000 ftc. In most high-risk nurseries, the lights are on 24 hours per day. Exposure time is a function of length of hospital stay. In general, the smaller the infant, the longer the period of hospitalization. The average length of stay is 40–50 days for infants weighing 1,000–1,500 gm and 100 days for infants weighing less than 1,000 gm at birth [2].

In addition to ambient light, the preterm infant may be exposed to

Birth Defects: Original Article Series, Volume 24, Number 1, pages 103–117

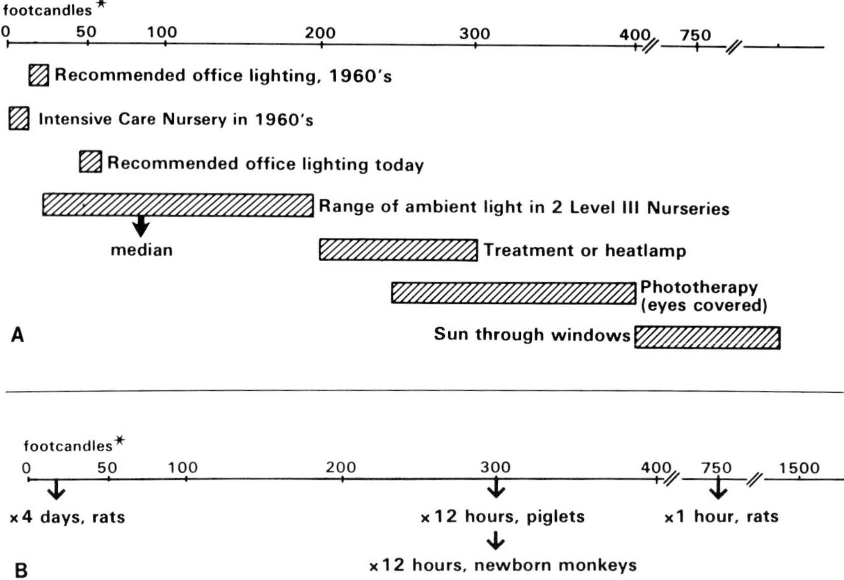

Fig. 1. A: Levels of light exposure in the intensive care nursery. B: Fig. 1b. Light exposure and retinal damage in animals.

supplementary sources of light, such as the bililights, the heat lamp (treatment lamp), and the indirect ophthalmoscope. The bililight is the most frequent treatment for a form of jaundice particularly common among preterm infants, which if untreated can cause brain damage or even death. The phototherapy unit typically consists of a bank of eight to ten fluorescent tubes placed over the infant's incubator, which produce 300–400 ftc of illumination. The duration of the treatment usually ranges from 1 to 5 days but may last longer. The eyes of the treated infants are routinely covered, but the infants adjacent to the phototherapy unit are unprotected. In some cases, the eye pads for the treated infants are inadequate or may slip off.

The second supplementary source of light is the heat lamp. This lamp is dual-purpose, providing the medical personnel caring for the infant with additional light that may be needed to perform delicate medical procedures and helping to maintain the infant's body temperature. Both the necessity for medical procedures and the difficulty in maintaining normal body temperature are more likely to occur with the youngest and smallest preterm infants. The heat lamp may consist of one or two 150–250 watt bulbs. The intensity produced at the infant's face is approximately 250 ftc. Exposure time varies, but it may be prolonged. The infant's eyes are not routinely protected.

Finally, preterm infants are at increased risk for ROP and therefore have at least one ophthalmic examination prior to discharge. Thus they are also routinely exposed to the light of an indirect ophthalmoscope. It has been estimated that exposure to an indirect ophthalmoscope for 2 minutes delivers the same amount of light as 2,000 ftc for 3 hours [5]. Furthermore, the infant's eyes are fully dilated for the examination. Extra precautions for protecting the infant's dilated eyes from ambient or supplementary sources of light prior to and following the eye exam are not routine. The necessity for adequate illumination in the hospital nursery is unquestionable, but there is mounting concern that both the high level and the continuous nature of the exposure may be hazardous [6–10].

LIGHT TOXICITY IN ANIMALS

Retinal damage in animals exposed to excess light is widely recognized [10–16,18–20]. Evidence of phototoxicity is typically demonstrated by electron or light microscopy. Nearly ten times the microscopically visible damage is necessary before a lesion is visible by ophthalmoscope. The lesion is primarily photochemical rather than thermal. The most effective light in producing damage is that which produces maximum bleaching of rhodopsin. Retinal damage is facilitated by maintaining the animal in constant dark prior to light exposure and by an increase in body temperature, hyperoxia, hypoxia, and retinal disease. In general, increasing the length of exposure time lowers the threshold for light damage (Fig. 1B).

Of particular relevance to the light exposure that preterm infants experience in the hospital nursery are the studies finding retinal damage in animals such as the rat [12,13], piglet [10], and newborn monkey [14]. The rat studies are important because they demonstrate the damaging effects of continuous compared to cyclic illumination, using even the low-to-moderate light levels that were standard for the animals in the laboratory. For example, retinal damage was found after 4 days of continuous low-intensity light (18 ftc) [13] and after 1 hour of exposure to high-intensity light (750 ftc) [12]. This suggests that even the levels of illumination that are thought to be safe are still potentially hazardous if the lighting is continuous rather than cyclic.

Perhaps the most appropriate human analog for the effect of high levels of illumination would be the studies with the piglets and monkeys. Unlike the rat, both of these animals are diurnal, and their eyes more closely resemble those of human infants, although not necessarily those of preterm infants. Sisson and his associates [10] exposed piglets to 300 ftc for 12–72 hours. Histology revealed photoreceptor damage after as little as 12 hours of exposure. Messner et al [14] reported similar findings with newborn monkeys. Both studies emphasized that a normal ophthalmic exam was not sufficient to rule out retinal damage. Although extrapolation from animal studies to human infants can be problematic, the evidence raises serious questions regarding the safety of current levels and durations of exposure for immature infants.

The phototoxic effects reported in animals include retinal disorganization, with damage to photorecepter cells, pigment epithelium, and the choroid [12,15–17]. The early effects are usually in the outer segments of the photoreceptors. The outer segments become swollen, lose their lamellar structure, and break away from the inner segments. The inner segments shrink and the nuclei become pyknotic. First the outer segments and then the inner segments may disappear.

The pigment epithelium has an important role in phagocytosis. When the photoreceptors are degenerating, the pigment epithelium may become overburdened; or portions of the pigment epithelial layer may be destroyed, leading to an accumulation of extralamellar matter. Glial cells around the blood vessels fill with cell debris.

As further effects of light exposure, microvilli of the pigment epithelium increase in size and number, and invade into the photoreceptor layer. Damage to the photoreceptor layer or the pigment epithelial layer may disrupt the normal adhesion of these two layers, leading to a localized retinal detachment. Finally, the choroid may be damaged by exposure to excess light. Fluorescein angiography reveals early filling defects in the choroid. The choroidal capillaries can form buds, which can grow through the spaces in the Bruch membrane and into the vitreous.

In summary, the evidence suggests that excess light exposure can lead to retinal damage, disorganization, or alteration of normal retinal metabolism. Furthermore, certain factors may increase retinal sensitivity to light damage, which is particularly relevant for preterm infants. Research with animals has shown that hyperoxia lowers the threshold for light damage in animals [18,19]. In addition, ischemic conditions during light exposure lead to more retinal damage than either ischemia or light alone [20]. It should be noted that ischemia is very different from hypoxia in its effect. Commensurate with their immaturity, preterm infants frequently require supplementary oxygen in the nursery and often fluctuate between relative hypoxia and hyperoxia. In fact, one issue for students of retinopathy is whether the culprit is hyperoxia or hypoxia at the retina. In view of these findings of phototoxicity in animals, it is somewhat surprising that only a limited amount of research has been conducted with human infants.

HUMAN DATA

Until recently, human studies of the effect of exposure of neonates to bright hospital nursery light have been limited to small samples of otherwise healthy preterm and full-term infants. For example, 4–5-year-old children who had been exposed to 90 ftc of nursery illumination for 6 days as newborns showed no effect on dark adaptation rate on a visual acuity screening [7]. Likewise, Hamer and his associates [21] found no difference between healthy preterm and full-term infants on a behavioral measure of absolute threshold to light or on an acuity screening when infants were tested at term. Although gross retinal damage from the nursery light was not demonstrated in these studies, the results are inconclusive regarding the safety of current levels of light and lengths of exposure for very low-birthweight infants and infants receiving supplementary oxygen, because these infants have never been studied previously. Furthermore, the question of light and ROP was not addressed.

LIGHT AND ROP
Previous Studies

With his first clinical reports of retrolental fibroplasia in the 1940s, Terry [22] suggested early light exposure as a leading cause. Subsequent studies reported that patching the eyes of preterm infants from birth until discharge did not reduce the incidence of ROP [23,24], leading to the conclusion that light was not a factor. However, the nursery conditions at that time were quite different from today's. Oxygen was still in liberal use even in the absence of clinical indications, and the ambient illumination level, as described earlier, was quite dim (Fig. 1A).

During the 1950s, clinical and laboratory studies demonstrated a relation between prolonged administration of supplementary oxygen and the development of ROP. Research into other possible factors essentially ceased [25]. Following the advent of the modern intensive care nursery in the early 1960s, higher levels of lighting (100–200 ftc) began to be recommended, initially as prophylaxis for neonatal jaundice [26] and ultimately for better visualization of sick infants [27]. At the same time, concern was repeatedly expressed over the possible consequences to the visual system of prolonged exposure of the preterm infant to this bright light [7,10,21,28,29]. No studies demonstrated the safety to exposure to bright nursery light, especially for the very low-birthweight infant or the infant receiving supplementary oxygen.

Current Investigation

In 1982, a prospective study was undertaken to examine once again the question of a relationship between light and ROP [2]. All infants included in the study had been admitted by the second day after birth for a minimum of 7 days to the intensive care nursery at either Children's Hospital National Medical Center or Georgetown University Medical Center in Washington,

TABLE I. Distribution of Sample by Birthweight

	Weight (gm)				
	<1,000	1,001–1,250	1,251–1,500	1,501–1,750	1,751–2,000
Control (n = 74) (%)	21 (28)	17 (23)	13 (18)	14 (19)	9 (12)
Light-protected (n = 154) (%)	45 (29)	31 (20)	33 (21)	23 (15)	22 (14)

DC. The infants weighed less than 2,001 gm and had a gestational age of less than 35 weeks at birth. Infants who weighed between 1,500 and 2,000 gm were included in the study only if they required supplementary oxygen in the nursery. The final sample consisted of 74 infants in the control group and 154 infants in the treatment or light-protected group (Table I).

Experimental treatment. The treatment was designed to attenuate the level of light in the face of each preterm infant in the light-protected group. It consisted of the application of a neutral density filter to the top and rear surface of the incubator as soon after birth as the infant was medically stable. The filter, a grey, transparent material similar to sunglasses, remained for the duration of the hospital stay. The level of light was monitored twice weekly for all infants. Median light level for the control infants was 60 ftc and for the light-protected infants was 25 ftc.

Group assignment. Assignment to the control or light-protected group was accomplished sequentially. That is, during the 6-month control period, all the infants were exposed to the customary level of illumination in each hospital nursery. During the following 12 months, the treatment condition was instituted for all infants within each hospital. Thus control and treatment were not simultaneous. The purpose of this design was to prevent control group contamination that might occur once the parents became familiar with the treatment. The treatment condition was likely to be preferred, and it was impossible to apply the treatment blindly. No attempt was made to increase the use of lighting for the control infants. In fact, precautions regarding the use of eye protection for infants under heat lamps were instituted at the beginning of the study.

Procedure. Infants in these high-risk nurseries were routinely examined for ROP by pediatric ophthalmologists near the time of discharge. Classification of retinopathy was similar to McCormick's method. Grade I was a sharp demarcation line between the vascular and avascular zone, or shunt formation; grades II and III were defined by a raised shunt and/or intravitreal neovascularization; grades IV and V were defined by partial or complete retinal detachment. For the purpose of this study, the highest grade of ROP was used if the two eyes differed or if more than one eye examination was conducted.

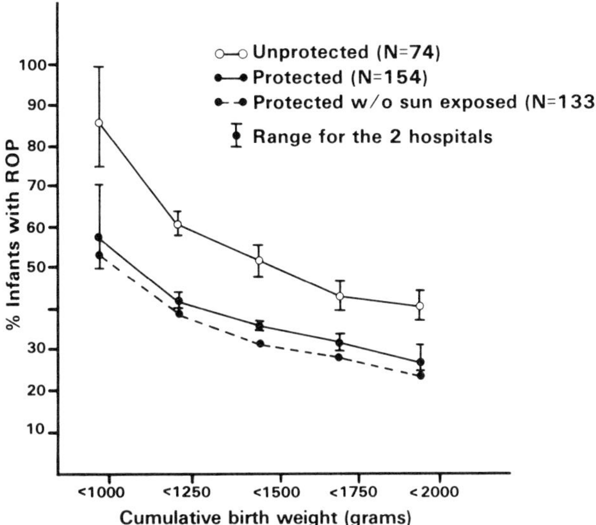

Fig. 2. Effect of light intensity on the incidence of ROP in two intensive care nurseries (cumulative birthweight function). (Reproduced from Glass et al [2], with permission of the publisher.)

Results. The results indicated a significant relation between the intensity of ambient nursery light and the incidence of ROP, with a higher incidence of ROP among unprotected infants exposed to the brighter ambient light (Fig. 2).

An association between light level and ROP was also found for a subgroup of infants. During the treatment period, nursery renovations in one hospital resulted in the intermediate nursery having a southern exposure. On occasion, infants in the light-protected group whose beds were next to the window were observed with the sun in their faces. Since the neutral density filter had been placed over the top and back of the incubator, and not the front, this meant periodic exposure to intensities in excess of 400 ftc. Of the 14 infants who had ROP in the treatment group in that hospital, 11 (79%) had been in a bed next to the window (chance was 25%). Ten of these infants could be matched for birthweight with non-ROP infants within the same treatment group. In contrast to the infants with ROP, only one (10%) of these non-ROP infants had been in a bed next to the window. Based on this empirical relationship between probable sun exposure and ROP (Fisher's exact test, P = 0.005), subsequent analyses excluded from the light-protected group the 21 babies whose beds had been next to the window in that intermediate nursery, whether or not they developed ROP. As can be seen in Figure 2, removal of this subgroup further enhanced the treatment effect.

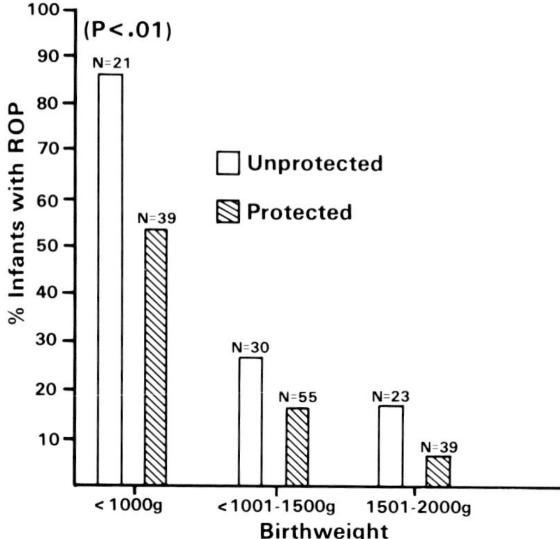

Fig. 3. Effect of light intensity in the hospital nurseries on the incidence of ROP. (Reproduced from Glass et al [2], with permission of the publisher.)

The data were then classified into separate birthweight categories, 500–1,000 gm, 1,001–1,500 gm, and 1,501–2,000 gm. As is shown in Figure 3, exposure to bright nursery light increased the probability of ROP in each birthweight category. Furthermore, the effect of light exposure was consistent within each hospital (Fig. 4).

To determine if the relationship between light exposure and ROP for the infants weighing less than 1,000 gm at birth might be accounted for by some other variable, light-protected and control infants in this birthweight category were compared on a number of factors. As is outlined in Table II, the increased incidence in ROP among the control infants cannot be attributed to their being sicker or smaller than the light-protected infants. Furthermore, a similar proportion of infants in the two groups received oxygen for less than 2 weeks (4/21 controls and 7/39 light-protected infants). It is interesting to note that all four of the infants in the control group who were exposed to oxygen for less than 2 weeks developed ROP, whereas only one of the seven infants in the light-protected group who had been exposed to oxygen less than 2 weeks developed ROP.

Finally, the infants were classified according to the severity of ROP (Fig. 5). Two infants had bilateral retinal detachments (ROP IV–V) and blindness. Both were in the control group. Given the overall incidence of cicatricial ROP, the sample size in this study is too small to draw any meaningful conclusions regarding the effect of light on the severity of ROP.

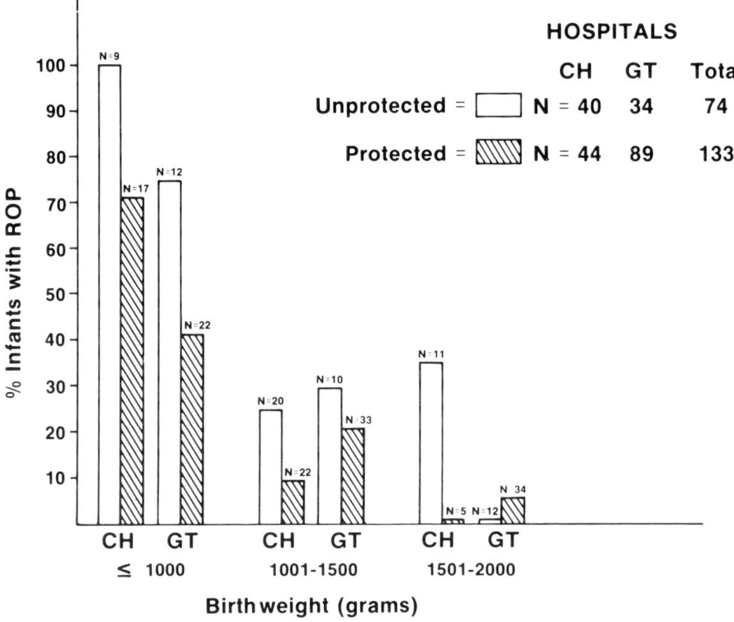

**Effect of bright light in two hospital nurseries on
the incidence of retinopathy of prematurity (ROP).**

Fig. 4. Effect of light intensity in two different hospital nurseries on the incidence of ROP.

In summary, this study suggests that the bright level of light customarily found in intensive care nurseries may be one factor contributing to oxygen-induced ROP. Given the problems of a nonrandomized design, the results must be considered preliminary; however, the findings are substantiated by parallel results in the two hospitals and by an effect of exposure to light within the treatment group.

SPECULATION REGARDING MECHANISMS OF LIGHT AND ROP

The early clinical signs for diagnosing ROP are vascular changes in the periphery of the retina with more severe vascular changes involving the region of the posterior pole. However, as illustrated by Phelps and Rosenbaum [30], ROP need not be a purely vascular disease. The retinal cross section of a kitten exposed to supplementary oxygen shows considerable swelling of the inner retinal layers and an apparent loss of the inner limiting membrane as compared to a control retina (Fig. 6). The mechanism of light

TABLE II. Characteristics of Infants Weighing Less Than 1,000 Grams

	Control (n = 21) (%)	Light-protected (n = 39) (%)
ROP	18/21 (86)	21/39 (54)
No. of males	8/21 (38)	13/39 (33)
Mean birthweight (gm)	910	830
No. less than 750 gm	0/21	7/39
Mean gestational age (weeks)	27.7	26.9
No. less than 26 weeks	0/21	5/39
Mean 1-minute Apgar[†]	3.2	3.4
1-Minute Apgar less than 4	10/18 (56)	21/36 (58)
Mean 5-minute Apgar[†]	5.7	6.1
5-Minute Apgar less than 7	11/18 (61)	18/36 (50)
Duration of ventilator therapy		
Less than 1 week	4 (19)	8 (21)
1–2 Weeks	1 (5)	4 (10)
2–4 Weeks	3 (14)	3 (8)
More than 4 weeks	13 (62)	24 (62)
Duration of oxygen therapy		
Less than 1 week	3 (14)	6 (15)
1–2 Weeks	1 (5)	1 (3)
2–4 Weeks	1 (5)	3 (8)
More than 4 weeks	16 (76)	29 (74)
CNS manifestations		
None	4 (19)	9 (23)
Minor (IVH[‡] grades I–II)	8 (38)	18 (46)
Major (IVH grades III–IV), periventricular leukomalacia, seizures, or confirmed meningitis)	9 (43)	12 (31)
Requiring exchange transfusions	5 (24)	5 (13)

[†]Apgar scores not recorded for some infants.
[‡]IVH, intraventricular hemorrhage.

in ROP may parallel oxygen toxicity. Vascular pathology may be accompanied by, or be secondary to, underlying retinal changes. With this premise, speculations regarding some possible basis for light as one of the factors contributing to ROP include alteration of normal retinal metabolism, damage to retinal structures, and generation of free radicals.

Local oxygen concentration in the retina is determined by the rate of oxygen diffusing from the choroid and retinal vessels and by the level of oxygen consumption in the intermediate retinal layers. Located between these two vascular systems is the major oxygen consumer in the retina, the photoreceptor/retinal pigment epithelial (RPE) complex. Oxygen tension at the retina affects the development of retinal vasculature. Retinal vessels do not grow in high PO_2. Therefore, any factor that could lead to increased

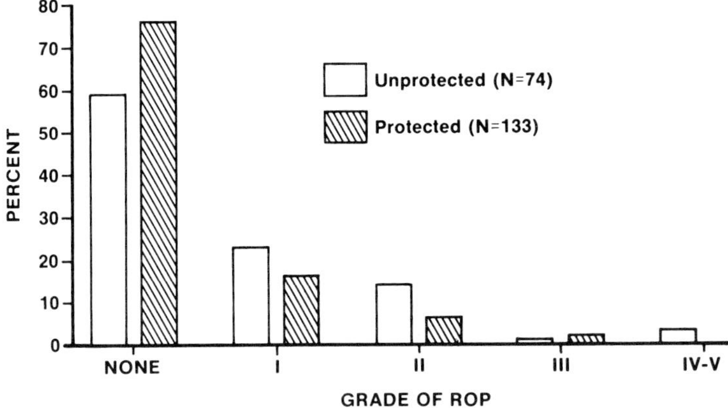

Fig. 5. Effect of light intensity on the severity of ROP.

retinal PO_2 could contribute to ROP. During light exposure, oxygen consumption by the retina decreases [31–33]. Thus light exposure could lead to hyperoxic conditions in the region of developing retinal vasculature whether or not an infant was receiving supplementary oxygen.

Light exposure can lead to considerable retinal disorganization or damage to nonvascular retinal structures, which could contribute to ROP. For example, damage to the photoreceptor/RPE complex would also alter oxygen consumption and probably disrupt the gating function of the complex in controlling the level of oxygen in the inner retina. The effect would be to increase oxygen concentration in the inner retina [34]. In addition, damage to the pigment epithelium could disturb its important phagocytic role, which in turn could result in an accumulation of extralamellar matter [35]. The presence of this matter could lead to abnormal patterns of vascularization.

Structural damage to the Mueller cells could also contribute to ROP. The Mueller cells form cystic spaces in the retina, which are thought to provide an organizing structure for the advancing mesenchyme [36]. Following localized photoreceptor damage, the Mueller cells may grow and close off the damaged from the undamaged portion of the retina. Alteration of this matrix could contribute to anomalous vascularization.

Light exposure changes the retinal biochemistry [37]. For example, the retina shifts from aerobic to more anerobic metabolism during light exposure [38]. Lactic acid is a normal byproduct of anerobic metabolism, and its accumulation has been proposed as one possible angiogenic factor in ROP [39].

Finally, oxygen radicals are widely recognized agents of oxygen toxicity

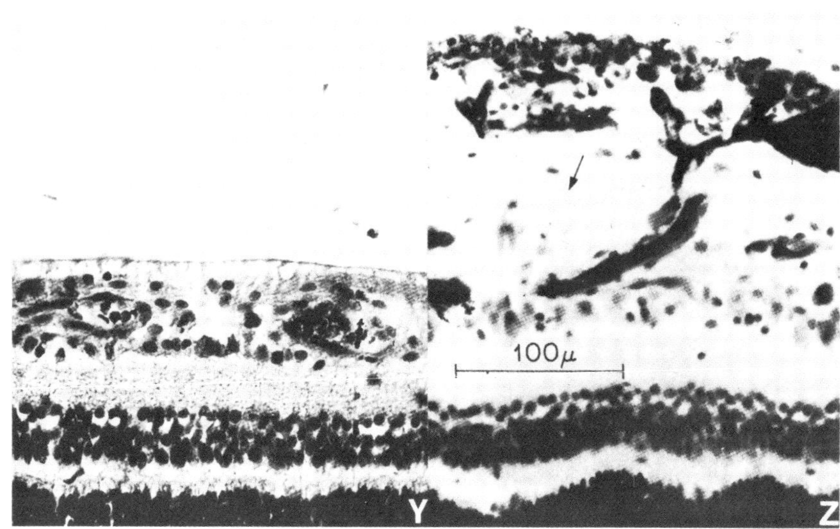

Fig. 6. Photomicrograph of retinal cross section showing normal kitten architecture (Y), and the thickened retina with extra-retinal neovascularization (Z) as seen in an 80-hour oxygen exposure. Both micrographs are taken at the same magnification and the arrow points out the poorly defined retinal surface in the abnormal section (H & E). (Reproduced from Phelps and Rosenbaum [30], with permission of the publisher.)

[18,40,41]. The reduction of a molecule of oxygen is a sequential process requiring the transfer of four electrons. The products of oxygen reduction include the superoxide radical (O_2-), hydrogen peroxide (H_2O_2), and the very active hydroxyl radical (OH). Damage by free radicals to retinal cells or vascular precursors has been proposed by a number of researchers as a mechanism underlying oxygen induced ROP [41–44].

It follows that factors that increase free radical formation would increase the potential for tissue damage [44]. Free radicals are also generated during light exposure [18,41] and more expediently under bright light. Thus the combination of light and oxygen could increase the formation of free radicals and the potential for tissue damage. Research with animals has shown that exposure to oxygen lowers the threshold for light damage [18,19,29]. In the immature human retina, light and oxygen may act synergistically to increase the probability of ROP.

CONCLUSIONS

The proposed mechanisms are speculative, but they provide a theoretical framework for our empirical finding of a relationship between the level of light in the intensive care nursery and the incidence of ROP. The mechanisms are readily compatible with other theories regarding the pathogenesis of ROP. Light exposure is probably not necessary for ROP to occur, but it may increase the risk [41,45].

FUTURE DIRECTIONS

Although reducing the intensity of light exposure may reduce the risk of ROP, low levels of continuous light may not be the optimal environment for the preterm infant. Furthermore, the extensive literature on the effects of visual deprivation would advise against maintaining a preterm infant in continuous darkness. Some evidence indicates that cycled lighting (light/dark) may even be protective against light damage [46]. Also, following light damage, considerable recovery occurs once the animals are returned to normal cycled lighting. No study has looked at the effect of cycled lighting (dark/dim or dark/light) on ROP. Theoretically, cycled lighting could reduce the risk of ROP. It may be useful to pursue this line of research in the future. Until sufficient evidence makes it clear that current levels of light exposure are safe for the preterm infant, a prudent approach might be to shade the infants' eyes from exposure to excess levels of light [47].

REFERENCES

1. Gaiter J, Avery G, Temple C, Johnson A, White N: Stimulation characteristics of nursery environments for critically ill preterm infants and infant behavior. In Stern D (ed): ''Intensive Care in the Newborn, 3rd Ed.'' New York, Masson Publishing Co., 1981, pp 389–410.
2. Glass P, Avery GB, Subramanian KN, Keys MP, Sostek AM, Friendly DS: Effect of bright light in the hospital nursery on the incidence of retinopathy of prematurity. N Engl J Med 313:401–404, 1985.
3. Gottfried AW, Wallace-Lande P, Sherman-Brown S, King J, Coen C: Physical and social environment of newborn infants in special care units. Science 214:673–675, 1981.
4. Lawson K: Environmental characteristics of a neonatal intensive-care unit. Child Dev 48:1633–1639, 1977.
5. Lanum J: The damaging effects of light on the retina: Empirical findings, theoretical and practical implications. Surv Ophthalmol 22:221–249, 1978.
6. Abramov I, Hainline L, Lemerise E, Brown AK: Changes in visual functions of children exposed as infants to prolonged illumination. J Am Optometry Assoc 56:614–619, 1985.
7. Dobson V, Riggs LA, Siqueland ER: Electroretinographic determination of dark adaptation functions of children exposed to phototherapy as infants. J Pediatr 85:25–29, 1974.
8. Dobson V, Cowett RM, Riggs LA: Long-term effect of phototherapy on visual function. J Pediatr 86:555–559, 1975.
9. Dubowitz LM, Dubowitz V, Morante A, Verghote M: Visual function in the preterm and fullterm newborn infant. Dev Med Child Neurol 22:465–475, 1980.

10. Sisson TR, Glauser SC, Glauser EM et al: Retinal changes produced by phototherapy. J Pediatr 77:221–227, 1970.

11. Williams T, Baker B (eds): "Symposium on Effects of Constant Light on Visual Processes." New York: Plenum Press, 1980.

12. Kuwabara T, Gorn RA: Retinal damage by visible light. Arch Ophthalmol 79:69–78, 1968.

13. O'Steen WK: Retinal and optic nerve serotonin and retinal degeneration as influenced by photoperiod. Exp Neurol 27:194–205, 1970.

14. Messner K, Maisels M, Leure-duPree A: Phototoxicity in the newborn primate retina. Invest Ophthalmol Vis Sci 17:178–182, 1978.

15. Lawwill T: Three major pathologic processes caused by light in the primate retina: A search for mechanisms. Trans Am Ophthalmol Soc 80:517–579, 1982.

16. Noell WK: Possible mechanism of photoreceptor damage by light in mammalian eyes. Vis Res 20:1163–1171, 1980.

17. Young RW: A theory of central retinal disease. In Sears ML (ed): "New Directions in Ophthalmic Research." New Haven, CT: Yale University Press, 1981, pp 237–270.

18. Ham WT, Mueller HA, Ruffolo JJ et al: Mechanisms underlying the production of photochemical lesions in the mammalian retina. Curr Eye Res 3:165–174, 1984.

19. Ruffolo JJ, Ham WT, Mueller HA, Millen JE: Photochemical lesions in the primate retina under conditions of elevated blood oxygen. Invest Ophthalmol Vis Sci 25:893–898, 1984.

20. McKechnie NM, Johnson NF, Foulds WS: The combined effects of light and acute ischemia on the structure of the rabbit retina: A light and electron microscopic study. Invest Ophthalmol Vis Sci 22:449–459, 1982.

21. Hamer RD, Dobson V, Mayer MJ: Absolute thresholds in human infants exposed to continuous illumination. Invest Ophthalmol Vis Sci 25:381–388, 1984.

22. Terry TL: Retrolental fibroplasia. J Pediatr 29:770–773, 1946.

23. Hepner WR, Krause AC, Davis ME: Retrolental fibroplasia and light. Pediatrics 3:824–828, 1949.

24. Locke JC, Reese AB: Retrolental fibroplasia. Arch Ophthalmol 48:44–47, 1952.

25. Silverman WA, Flynn JT: Overview: A "developmental" retinopathy reconsidered. In Silverman WA, Flynn JT (eds): "Contemporary Issues in Fetal and Neonatal Medicine. Vol. II: Retinopathy of Prematurity." Boston: Blackwell Scientific Publications, 1985, pp 11–23.

26. Lucey JF: Nursery illumination as a factor in neonatal hyperbilirubinemia. Pediatrics 44:155–157, 1969.

27. Korones S: Physical structure and functional organization of neonatal intensive care units. In Gottfried AW, Gaiter JL (eds): "Infant Stress Under Intensive Care." Baltimore: University Park Press, 1985.

28. Fulton A, Abromov I, Allen J, Gwiazda J, Hainline L, O'Neill JF, Raymond P, Varner D: Optical radiation effects on visual development. In Waxler M, Hitchins VM (eds): "Optical Radiation and Visual Health." Boca Raton, FL: CRC Press, Inc, 1986, pp 137–146.

29. Sisson T: The effect of light and various light concentrations of oxygen on the retina of the newborn pig. In: "Retinopathy of Prematurity Conference Syllabus." Washington, DC: 1981, pp 581–599.

30. Phelps DL, Rosenbaum AL: The role of tocopherol in oxygen-induced retinopathy: Kitten model. Pediatrics 59 [suppl]:998–1005, 1977.

31. Feke GT, Zuckerman R, Green GJ, Weiter JJ: Response of human retinal blood flow to light and dark. Invest Ophthalmol Vis Sci 24:136–141, 1983.

32. Stefansson E, Wolbarsht ML, Landers MB III: In vivo O_2 consumption in rhesus monkeys in light and dark. Exp Eye Res 37:251–256, 1983.
33. Zuckerman R, Weiter JJ: Oxygen transport in the bullfrog retina. Exp Eye Res 30:117–127, 1980.
34. Weiter JJ, Zuckerman R: The influence of the photoreceptor-RPE complex on the inner retina. Ophthalmology 87:1133–1139, 1980.
35. Kaitz M, Auerbach E: Light damage in dystrophic and normal rats. In Williams TP, Baker BN (eds): "The Effects of Constant Light on Visual Processes." New York: Plenum Press, 1980.
36. Flower RW, McLeod DS, Lutty GA, Goldberg B, Wajer SD: Postnatal retinal vascular development of the puppy. Invest Ophthalmol Vis Sci 26:957–968, 1985.
37. Hansson H-A: A histochemical study of cellular reactions in rat retina transiently damaged by visible light. Exp Eye Res 12:270–274, 1971.
38. Howell WL, Rapp LM, Williams TP: Distribution of melanosomes across the retinal pigment epithelium of a hooded rat: Implications for light damage. Invest Ophthalmol Vis Sci 22:139–144, 1982.
39. Imre G: Studies on the mechanism of retinal neovascularization: Role of lactic acid. Br J Ophthalmol 48:75–82, 1964.
40. Fridovich I: The biology of oxygen radicals. Science 201:875–880, 1978.
41. Riley PA, Slater TF: Pathogenesis of retrolental fibroplasia. Lancet 2:265, 1969.
42. Hittner HM, Kretzer FL: Efficacy of vitamin E in retinopathy of prematurity. In McPherson AR, Hittner HM, Kretzer FL (eds): "Retinopathy of Prematurity: Current Concepts and Controversies." Toronto: B.C. Decker, Inc, 1986, pp 89–103.
43. Katz ML, Robison WG: Autoxidative damage to the retina: Potential role in retinopathy of prematurity. This volume.
44. Crowe J, Rea PA, Rolfe P: Retinopathy of prematurity, intraventricular hemorrhage, and oxidative damage (letter). Pediatrics 77:129–130, 1986.
45. Slater TF, Riley PA: Free radical damage in retrolental fibroplasia. Lancet 2:467, 1970.
46. Noell W, Albrecht R: Irreversible effects on visible light on the retina: Role of vitamin A. Science 172:76–79, 1971.
47. Avery GB, Glass P: Light and retinopathy of prematurity: What's prudent for 1986? Pediatrics 78:519–520, 1986.

IV. BASIC VASCULAR RESEARCH

Retinal Pigment Epithelial Cells Release an Inhibitor of Neovascularization

Bert M. Glaser, MD, Peter A. Campochiaro, MD, John L. Davis, Jr., MAS, and Misao Sato, MD

Department of Ophthalmology, Johns Hopkins University, Baltimore, Maryland 21205 (B.M.G., J.L.D.); Department of Ophthalmology, University of Virginia Medical School, Charlottesville, Virginia 22908 (P.A.C.); Department of Ophthalmology, Nippon University, Tokyo, Japan (M.S.)

The possibility that controlling neovascularization will aid in the treatment of a variety of ocular disorders has prompted an extensive search for inhibitors of new blood vessel formation [1]. Most inhibitors of neovascularization so far identified have been extracted from avascular tissues [2–8]. Unfortunately, the study of these inhibitors is severely limited by the fact that only small quantities of active material can be extracted from these sources [9].

It has been suggested that diabetic intraocular neovascularization is less likely to occur in eyes with chorioretinal scars [10]. This has led to the widespread use of photocoagulation to induce chorioretinal scar formation. The production of these scars often results in the rapid regression of intraocular neovascularization in eyes with proliferative diabetic retinopathy [10,11]. Regression occurs even when photocoagulation and resultant chorioretinal scarring take place in areas remote from the new blood vessels [10–15]. Retinal pigment epithelial (RPE) cells are one component of these scars. We report herein our findings that human RPE cells in culture release a substance (or substances) that causes the regression of new blood vessels on the chick embryonic yolk sac.

MATERIALS AND METHODS
Cell Cultures

RPE cells were harvested from human eyes obtained from the Medical Eye Bank of Maryland, as previously described [16]. The cells were grown in 75 cm^2 flasks containing Eagle's minimal essential medium with 20% fetal bovine serum (MEM/20), in 5% CO_2 at 37°C, and they were subcultured

Birth Defects: Original Article Series, Volume 24, Number 1, pages 121–127

once per week. Second- to sixth-passage cultures were used for all experiments. All experiments were repeated with RPE cells from four different donor eyes, with identical results.

Astrocytes were cultured from neonatal rat brain cortex, as described by McCarthy and de Vellis [17]. More than 90% of the cells in culture stained with antibodies to glial fibrillary acidic protein using indirect immunofluorescence [18,19]. The astrocytes were grown in 75 cm^2 flasks containing Eagle's minimal essential medium with 10% fetal bovine serum (MEM/10), in 5% CO_2 at 37°C. Cells were subcultured once per week. Third- to tenth-passage cultures were used for all experiments. All experiments were repeated with astrocytes from two different preparations, with identical results.

Bovine corneal fibroblasts were cultured as previously described [20]. Cells were grown in 75 cm^2 flasks containing MEM/10 in 5% CO_2 at 37°C. Cells were subcultured twice per week, and third- to twelfth-passage cultures were used for all experiments.

Fetal bovine aortic endothelial (FBAE) cells were grown as previously described [20] in 75 cm^2 flasks (Falcon) containing MEM/10 in 5% CO_2 at 37°C. Cells were subcultured twice per week, and fourth- to thirteenth-passage cultures were used for all experiments. All experiments were repeated with endothelial cells from three different preparations, with identical results.

At confluence, RPE cells, astrocytes, and fibroblasts reached a density of $3.5-4.0 \times 10^6$ cells per 75 cm^2 flask. The FBAE at confluence reached a density of $8-9 \times 10^6$ cells per 75 cm^2 flask.

Conditioned Media

RPE cell-conditioned medium (RPE-CM), astrocyte-conditioned medium (astro-CM), and fibroblast-conditioned medium (fibro-CM) were prepared by plating each cell type in 75 cm^2 tissue culture flasks at a density of 6.6×10^5 cells in 20 ml of either MEM/20 for RPE cells or MEM/10 for astrocytes and fibroblasts. Media were changed every 3 days. After 6 days, all cultures had reached confluence. The media were then removed and replaced with 10 ml of Eagle's minimal essential medium without serum (MEM/0). Forty-eight hours later, the conditioned media were removed and centrifuged, and the supernatant was stored at -20°C for later use. The RPE cells were also grown in MEM/10 prior to transfer to MEM/0, with identical results.

Inhibition of New Blood Vessels

The effect of conditioned media on the vasculature of the chick embryonic yolk sac was evaluated using a modification of the technique described by Taylor and Folkman [21]. Three-day-old fertilized white leghorn chicken eggs were opened and their contents carefully placed in a hammock of plastic wrap suspended in a small plastic drinking cup so that the chick embryo and vascularized yolk sac were fully exposed. The eggs were incubated at 37°C for 6 hours. The various conditioned media were concentrated fivefold by ultrafiltration using an Amicon YM10 filter (molecular weight cut-off 10,000 daltons). The filter disks (13 mm diameter; HATF 01300; Millipore, Bedford, MA) had 4 mm circles punched out of their centers and were soaked for 1 hour in the various concentrated conditioned media. The filter disks were placed on the vascularized yolk sacs. Twenty-four hours later, the yolk sac vasculature within the central cut-out of the filter disk was observed for signs of regression using an operating microscope (Zeiss; ×260). The effects of conditioned media on the yolk sac vasculature within the central cut-out of the filter disk were rated for whether there was regression of blood vessels. Regression was considered present if at least 75% of the area within the central cut-out of the filter had become avascular [22,23].

The chick embryonic yolk sacs were fixed for 1 hour in quarter-strength Karnovsky's 1% paraformaldehyde–1.2% glutaraldehyde fixative at 4°C and washed with 10% sucrose–0.05 N sodium cacodylate (pH, 7.5) for 1 hour. After dehydration in alcohol, they were stained en bloc with 1% uranyl acetate in 100% alcohol for 30 minutes in the dark. After a 100% alcohol rinse, the specimens were embedded in epoxy resin (Epon 812). Sections were cut perpendicular to the culture surface on an ultramicrotome (Sorvall MT2-B) and studied by light and electron microscopy.

RESULTS

Disks of filter paper soaked in RPE-CM media and placed on the surface of the vascularized yolk sac caused regression of adjacent capillaries, resulting in a localized avascular zone (Table I). Histologic examination of yolk sac vessels adjacent to RPE-CM soaked filters showed vessels occluded by packed red blood cells within 24 hours. This is similar to the appearance of regressing vessels in the cornea [24]. In contrast, astro-CM or fibro-CM did not affect the adjacent vasculature (Table I). Before testing, the conditioned media were concentrated fivefold using ultrafiltration membranes with a 10,000-dalton molecular weight cut-off. To determine whether concentrated RPE-CM is toxic to vascular endothelial cells, we grew FBAE cells in concentrated RPE-CM for 24 hours. At the concentrations used on the chick vasculature, RPE-CM showed no toxicity for FBAE cells as determined by trypan blue exclusion. The ability of RPE-CM to cause regression of vessels is lost after boiling for 15 minutes and after trypsin treatment (Table I).

TABLE I. Regression of New Blood Vessels[†]

	No change	Regression[‡]
RPE-CM		
Untreated	16	41*
Boiled for 15 minutes	15	0
Trypsinized	13	0
MEM/0	33	0
Astro-CM	16	0
Fibro-CM	37	0

[†]RPE-CM indicates retinal epithelial cell-conditioned medium; MEM/0, Eagle's minimal essential medium without serum; astro-CM, astrocyte-conditioned medium; fibro-CM, fibroblast-conditioned medium.

[‡]Regression was considered present if at least 75% of the area within the central cut-out of the filter had become avascular.

*$P < .001$ by χ^2 test in comparison with effects of other conditioned media.

DISCUSSION

Chorioretinal scars are composed mainly of astrocytes, RPE cells, and possibly fibroblasts [25–27]. In our experiments, human RPE cells in culture, but not astrocytes or corneal fibroblasts, released a substance (or substances) that caused the regression of new blood vessels on the chick embryonic yolk sac. Vessels appear in the chick embryonic yolk sac at 48 hours and grow rapidly over the next 6–8 days [21]. Therefore, the vasculature of the 4–5-day-old embryos used in our studies was at an actively developing or "neovascular" stage.

Unlike human RPE cells, rat brain astrocytes and bovine corneal fibroblasts are unable to release detectable levels of substances that cause regression of new blood vessels. This finding does not indicate, however, that other cell types or cells under other conditions might not release similar substances. These possibilities are currently being investigated in our laboratory.

Cell–cell interactions play an important role in a large number of biologic processes, including those occurring during development, wound healing, and tumor growth and spread. The establishment and control of an adequate blood supply has a role in all these processes. Therefore, cell–cell interactions are also likely to be involved in controlling new blood vessel formation and regression during these processes. The ability of RPE cells to induce the regression of new blood vessels may be important during ocular development, when the RPE lies between the extremely vascular choroid and the avascular outer retina. In a laser-induced chorioretinal scar, RPE cells may release the same substance into the vitreous cavity and cause regression of intraocular new blood vessels. Previous studies [20] have shown that retina, under certain conditions, can release a stimulator of neovascularization. It is therefore notable that RPE cells, although derived from the same neuroectoderm as the remainder of the retina, release inhibitors of neovascularization.

The release of the RPE-derived inhibitor is dependent on RPE cell density [33]. Inhibitor release by RPE cells in confluent cultures is less than in subconfluent cultures. Several days after RPE cell cultures reach confluence, the release of inhibitor once again increases. Corresponding to the increase in inhibitor release, the RPE cells begin to overgrow the monolayer, forming localized regions with multiple cell layers. The effect of cell density on inhibitor release possibly depends on the cell–cell relationships and associated cellular morphology. The RPE cells in subconfluent and superconfluent cultures do not maintain the highly ordered cell–cell relationships present within the RPE monolayer in the normal eye. Alterations in the highly ordered RPE monolayer that occur in chorioretinal scars and that are possibly mimicked in superconfluent and subconfluent RPE cultures may result in the enhancement of inhibitor release. This may occur in spite of the fact that some RPE cells are destroyed by the photocoagulation, since it is the remaining cells that can then undergo morphologic alterations. The resultant enhancement in the release of inhibitor into the adjacent retina and vitreous may play a role in the effect of photocoagulation-induced chorioretinal scarring on the regression and prevention of neovascularization in diabetic retinopathy. Further studies of the relationship between inhibitor release and RPE cell morphology and environment are underway in our laboratory.

In summary, we have described an RPE-derived substance (or substances) that stimulates the regression of new blood vessels on the chick embryonic yolk sac. This discovery raises several interesting possibilities that require further investigation. Under normal conditions, the RPE and Bruch's membrane are positioned as a barrier between the highly vascular choriocapillaris and the avascular outer retina. The ability of RPE cells to release an inhibitor of vascular endothelial cell proliferation may be the biochemical mechanism by which the barrier functions. Since cell–cell relationships seem to alter inhibitor release by RPE cells, photocoagulation and subsequent chorioretinal scarring may function by altering the local architecture and morphology of the RPE cells so that increased levels of the inhibitor may be achieved in the surrounding retina and vitreous, thereby inhibiting vessel formation in proliferative diabetic retinopathy. Most importantly, further study of the interaction between RPE cells and vasculature is likely to improve our understanding of neovascularization and suggest new approaches to its management.

REFERENCES

1. Folkman J: Tumor angiogenesis: Therapeutic implications. N Engl J Med 285:1182–1186, 1971.
2. Eisenstein R, Sorgente N, Soble LW et al: The resistance of certain tissues to invasion: Penetrability of explanted tissues by vascular mesenchyme. Am J Pathol 73:765–774, 1973.
3. Sorgente N, Kuettner KE, Soble LW, et al: The resistance of certain tissues to invasion: II. Evidence for extractable factors in cartilage which inhibit invasion by vascularized mesenchyme. Lab Invest 32:217–222, 1975.
4. Brem H, Folkman J: Inhibition of tumor angiogenesis mediated by cartilage. J Exp Med 141:427–439, 1975.
5. Langer R, Brem H, Falterman K et al: Isolation of a cartilage factor that inhibits tumor neovascularization. Science 193:70–72, 1976.
6. Brem S, Preis I, Langer R et al: Inhibition of neovascularization by an extract derived from vitreous. Am J Ophthalmol 84:323–328, 1977.
7. Lutty GA, Thompson DC, Gallup JY et al: Vitreous: An inhibitor of retinal extract-induced neovascularization. Invest Ophthalmol Vis Sci 24:52–56, 1983.
8. Williams GA, Eisenstein R, Schumacher B et al: Inhibitor of vascular endothelial cell growth in the lens. Am J Ophthalmol 97:366–371, 1984.
9. Lee A, Langer R: Shark cartilage contains inhibitors of tumor angiogenesis. Science 221:1185–1187, 1983.
10. Beetham WP, Aiello LM, Balodimos MC et al: Ruby-laser photocoagulation of early diabetic neovascular retinopathy: Preliminary report of a long-term controlled study. Trans Am Ophthalmol Soc 67:39–67, 1969.
11. Doft BH, Blankenship G: Retinopathy risk factor regression after laser panretinal photo-coagulation for proliferative diabetic retinopathy. Ophthalmology 91:1453–1457, 1984.
12. Diabetic Retinopathy Study Research Group: Photocoagulation treatment of proliferative diabetic retinopathy: The second report of diabetic retinopathy study findings. Ophthalmology 85:82–106, 1978.
13. Weiter JJ, Zuckerman R: The influence of the photoreceptor-RPE complex on the inner retina: An explanation for the beneficial effects of photocoagulation. Ophthalmology 87:1133–1139, 1980.
14. Foulds WS: The role of photocoagulation in the treatment of retinal disease. Trans Ophthalmol Soc NZ 32:82–90, 1980.
15. Stefansson E, Landers MB, Wolbarsht ML: Oxygenation and vasodilatation in relation to diabetic and other proliferative retinopathies. Ophthalmic Surg 14:190–226, 1983.
16. Vidaurri-Leal J, Hohman R, Glaser BM: Effect of vitreous on morphologic characteristics of retinal pigment epithelial cells: A new approach to the study of proliferative vitreoretinopathy. Arch Ophthalmol 102:1220–1223, 1984.
17. McCarthy KD, de Vellis J: Preparation of separate astroglial and oligodendroglial cell cultures from rat cerebral tissue. J Cell Biol 85:890–902, 1980.
18. Raff MC, Fields KL, Hakamori SI et al: Cell-type-specific markers for distinguishing and studying neurons and the major classes of glial cells in culture. Brain Res 174:283–308, 1979.
19. Parks DR, Bryan VM, Oi VT et al: Antigen-specific identification and cloning of hybridomas with a fluorescence-activated cell sorter. Proc Natl Acad Sci USA 76:1962–1966, 1979.
20. Glaser BM, D'Amore PA, Michels RG et al: Demonstration of vasoproliferative activity from mammalian retina. J Cell Biol 84:298–304, 1980.

21. Taylor S, Folkman J: Protamine is an inhibitor of angiogenesis. Nature 297:307–312, 1982.
22. Lowry OH, Rosebrough NJ, Farr AL et al: Protein measurement with the Folin phenol reagent. J Biol Chem 193:265–275, 1951.
23. Eckel RH, Fujimoto WY: Quantification of cell death in human fibroblasts by measuring the loss of [^{14}C]thymidine from prelabeled cell monolayers. Anal Biochem 114:118–124, 1981.
24. Ausprunk DH, Falterman K, Folkman J: The sequence of events in the regression of corneal capillaries. Lab Invest 38:284–294, 1978.
25. Wallow IHL, Tso MOM, Fine BS: Retinal repair after experimental xenon arc photocoagulation: I. A comparison between rhesus monkey and rabbit. Am J Ophthalmol 75:32–52, 1973.
26. Wallow IHL, Tso MOM: Repair after xenon arc photocoagulation: III. An electron microscopic study of the evolution of retinal lesions in rhesus monkeys. Am J Ophthalmol 75:957–972, 1973.
27. Wallow IHL, Davis MD: Clinicopathologic correlation of xenon arc and argon laser photocoagulation: Procedure in human diabetic eyes. Arch Ophthalmol 97:2308–2315, 1979.
28. Eisenstein R, Kuettner KE, Neopolitan C et al: The resistance of certain tissues to invasion: III. Cartilage extracts inhibit the growth of fibroblasts and endothelial cells in culture. Am J Pathol 81:337–347, 1975.
29. Goren SB, Eisenstein R, Choromokos E: The inhibition of corneal vascularization in rabbits. Am J Ophthalmol 84:305–309, 1977.
30. Rifkin DB, Gross JL, Moscatelli E et al: Proteases and angiogenesis: Production of plasminogen activator and collagenase by endothelial cells. In Nossel HL, Voge JH (eds): "Pathobiology of the Endothelial Cell." New York, Academic Press, Inc., 1982, pp 191–197.
31. Glaser BM, Kalebic T, Garbisa S et al: In Nugent J, O'Connor M (eds): "Development of the Vascular System: Ciba Foundation Symposium 100." London: Pitman Medical Books, Ltd., 1983, pp 150–162.
32. Kalebic T, Garbisa S, Glaser B et al: Basement membrane collagen: Degradation of migrating endothelial cells. Science 221:281–283, 1983.
33. Glaser BM, Campochiaro PA, Davis JL, Sato M: Retinal pigment epithelial cells release an inhibitor of neovascularization. Arch Ophthalmol 103:1870–1875, 1985.

Physiology of the Developing Ocular Vasculature

Robert W. Flower

Applied Physics Laboratory and Wilmer Ophthalmological Institute, Johns Hopkins University, Baltimore, Maryland 21205

As long as cell physiology per se is excluded, as it will be in this discussion, the physiology of the developing retinal vasculature is covered by a very small body of data. Although a good deal is known about the adult retina, to apply those data to the immature eye, as is sometimes done, is to ignore the significant morphologic and physiologic changes that occur during the perinatal period. These include significant changes in arterial PO_2, PCO_2, and blood pressure.

During the past 40 years, concern over the pathogenesis of retinopathy of prematurity (ROP) has focused primarily on the effects of induced hyperoxia, seemingly ignoring that normoxia in a premature infant is quite abnormal in comparison to the intrauterine oxygen tension. Relatively little attention has been given to other physiologic factors, yet today ROP remains a concern, one that appears to become greater as infants of increasing prematurity survive. Consequently, it has become my belief that it is necessary to back away a little from studying ROP per se until a far better understanding of the physiology as well as the morphology of the immature retinal vasculature is developed. It seems unlikely that abnormal developmental processes like those leading to ROP can be recognized, much less understood, without first thoroughly understanding the normal ones.

Investigating physiology of the immature retinal vasculature goes hand in hand with investigating its morphology. Whereas, with the adult retina, investigators typically ignore the adjacent choroidal circulation, the adjacent choroidal and hyaloid circulations cannot be ignored in the case of the immature retina. Clearly, there is a dynamically changing relationship between these two circulations and the developing retinal vasculature that must be taken into account; in fact, the atrophic hyaloid system is hydrostatically coupled directly to the developing retinal vasculature at the optic disk.

There is one final difficulty. The scarcity of both human diseased and

Birth Defects: Original Article Series, Volume 24, Number 1, pages 129–146
© **1988 March of Dimes Birth Defects Foundation**

normal ocular tissues for examination and the enormous obstacles to direct study of the immature human ocular vasculatures make it necessary to turn to experimental animal models. Unfortunately, the validity of such models remains a subject of controversy, and, since the brief overview to be presented is of data principally derived from animal studies, we must first say a word on this subject.

THE BEAGLE PUPPY MODEL

The main criterion by which a model is judged is the faithfulness with which it mimics the human disease, but an animal model used for studying physiology of a vasculature *must* also meet the requirement that its morphologic development is similar to that in the human. Given the acknowledged shortcomings of the well known kitten ROP model, we began using the beagle puppy in hope of achieving a more faithful model. Our recently completed morphologic study [1] demonstrated the similarities between development of the canine and human retinal vasculatures; that is, the method of vasculogenesis observed to occur in the puppy is strikingly similar to that noted by Ashton [2] in human fetal retinas. The process is summarized in Figure 1. Vascular precursors, or angioblasts, were found in the puppy avascular retina. These angioblasts were observed to organize subsequently into a vascular network essentially by the same sequence of steps described by Ashton, but the whole process could be observed in much greater detail in the puppy.

Müller cells processes appear to provide a structural matrix throughout the avascular retina on which differentiated angioblasts organize into a vascular network. Arteries develop in beds of primordial capillaries lying near the edge of the developing vasculature. This precedes vein formation, which occurs through a process involving coalesence of embryonic capillaries that themselves were derived from primordial capillaries. Then, through a gradual process of reorganization, the mature vasculature emerges. These events occur in a wavelike progression that moves radially across the avascular retina from the optic disk. Throughout this process, the important structures are the so-called embryonic and primordial capillaries that lie at the leading edge of vascularization. These thin-walled, structurally immature vessels carry whole blood; therefore, they are very much subject to the effects of pressure and blood gas content.

Perhaps the most significant observation is that the angioblasts throughout the avascular puppy retina were observed to differentiate in situ. The maturation of angioblasts is demonstrated in Figure 2. Ashton [2] observed only differentiated angioblasts (ie, so-called spindle cells) in the human retina and concluded that they represent an invasion of primitive

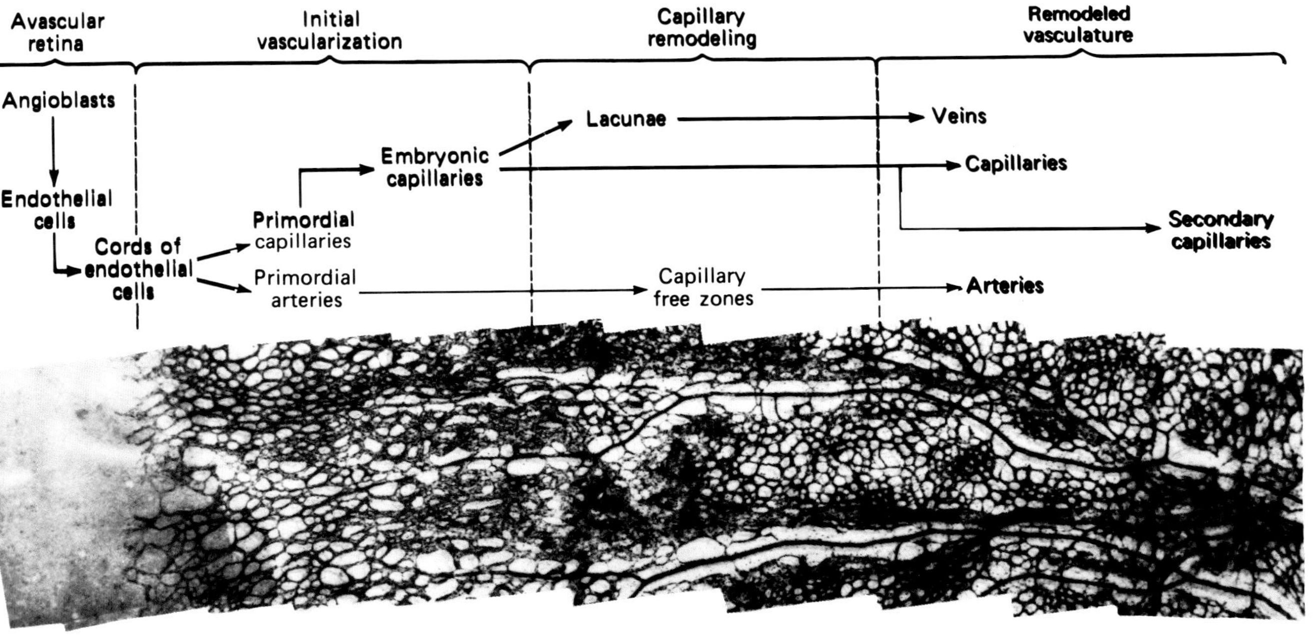

Fig. 1.   Summary of vasculogenesis in an ATPase flat-mounted retina from a 14-day-old puppy. (original magnification, ×60). Reproduced from Flower RW et al [1], with permission of the publisher.

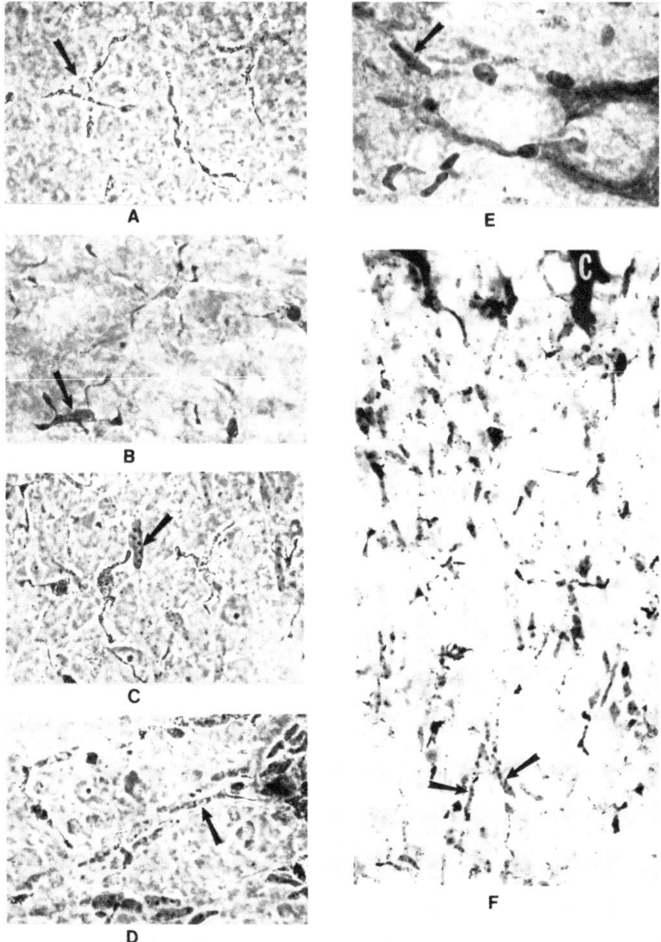

Fig. 2. Appearance of angioblasts in ATPase-reacted puppy retinas at 2 (A), 4 (B), 6 (C,D), and 14 (E) days postnatal. A: At two days of age, angioblasts in peripheral retina have spherical, ATPase-negative nuclei, and ATPase-positive mitochondria in their cytoplasmic processes (arrow). B: In avascular peripheral retina at four days of age, angioblast nuclear envelope and nucleoli are ATPase-positive and less spherical, and mitochondrial ATPase activity is still present. C: By six days of age, some angioblasts have completely differentiated and appear spindle-shaped (arrow). Differentiated angioblasts have no mitochondrial ATPase activity, but nucleolar and nuclear envelope activity is prominent. D: At the edge of established vasculature at six days of age, angioblasts are found organizing into endothelial cell cords (arrow). E: By 14 days of age, all angioblasts at the edge of the vasculature are spindle-shaped with prominent nucleolar and nuclear envelope reaction product (arrow), bearing the appearance of endothelial cells in established vasculature (A–E, ×845). F: Lower magnification view of peripheral retina adjacent to established vasculature (at the top) showing a population of angioblasts at various stages in differentiation. Note that angioblasts appear to be organizing (arrows) even distant from established endothelial cell cords (C, at top of figure). (×630). Reproduced from Flower RW et al [1], with permission of the publisher.

mesenchymal precursors, but we were able to employ methods permitting visualization of less differentiated angioblast precursors in the puppy. As a result, we concluded that the so-called spindle cells differentiate from angioblast precursors and mature in place. Thus primordial vessels form by organization of differentiating angioblasts that exist in peripheral retinal cystic spaces at birth or by addition of fully differentiated endothelium. They form *unlike* neovascularization.

Eventually, we produced cicatricial ROP in the puppy eye [3], thereby answering a major criticism of the animal model. All this strengthens the confidence with which results from such animal studies might be extrapolated ultimately to the clinical situation.

It is interesting to note at this point that preliminary examination of mongrel kitten retinas, using the same techniques, indicates that the puppy retina is much more completely vascularized at birth than that of the newborn kitten, as shown in Figure 3. The kitten retina is on top; yet, by postnatal day 14, vascularization reaches the retinal periphery in both kitten and puppy. This observation might explain why more severe ROP has not been produced in kittens. During oxygen exposure, the more rapid cellular differentiation that occurs in the kitten retina might permit it to cope more effectively with whatever vascular damage is induced by oxygen, whereas the less rapidly differentiating puppy vasculature cannot.

The puppy, therefore, appears to be a good choice as a model for investigation of physiologic factors affecting the developing ocular vasculatures. Nevertheless, since this chapter discusses chiefly animal data, and with most of that coming from my own laboratory, it would be presumptuous to suppose that this chapter contains the last words on the subject. To underscore that fact, the subtitle of the rest of this discussion will be ''Work in Progress.'' Also, even though the body of data on immature retina physiology is small, it is large enough that a chapter this short can touch only on some main points.

From experimental observations, the effects of hyperoxia can be divided into two stages [4]. The first consists of vasoconstriction and possibly vaso-obliteration of the retinal blood vessels. So long as vasoconstriction persists, further forward growth of vessels toward the periphery of the retina is halted. The second stage occurs when breathing of room air resumes. Those vessels not permanently obliterated can recannulate, and new vessel growth can commence again. However, the vessels no longer necessarily develop along normal pathways. Whether the damage done is a result of ischemia or of direct oxygen cytotoxicity has long been a question of great interest, and it is one to which the experimental animal model might be applied.

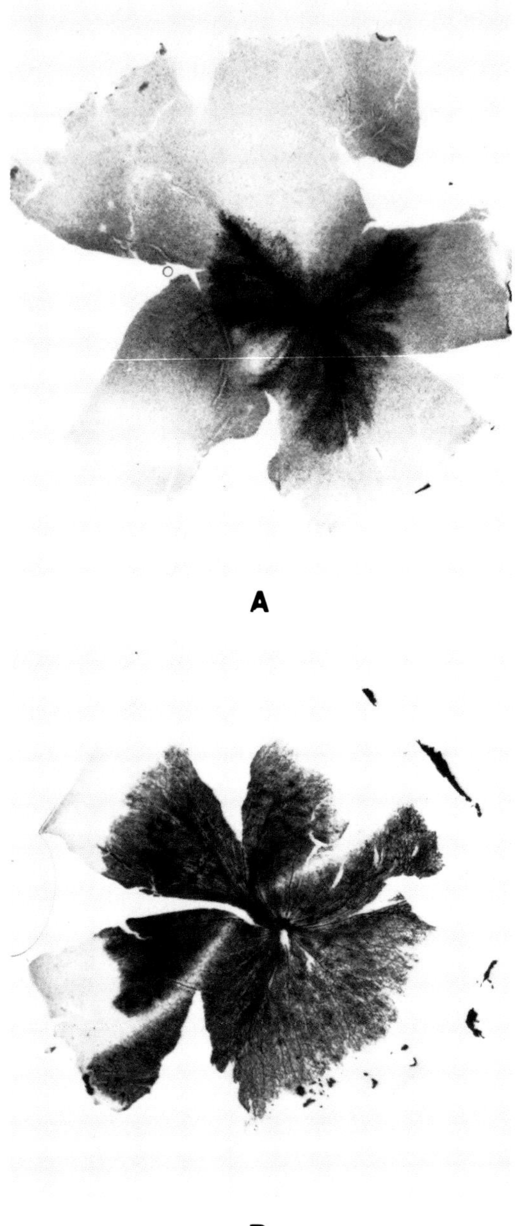

A

B

Fig. 3. Flat-mounted retinas prepared by the ATPase method from the right eyes of a 2-day-old kitten (A, top) and a 2-day-old puppy (B, bottom). ($\times 3.7$.) Reproduced from Flower RW et al [1], with permission of the publisher.

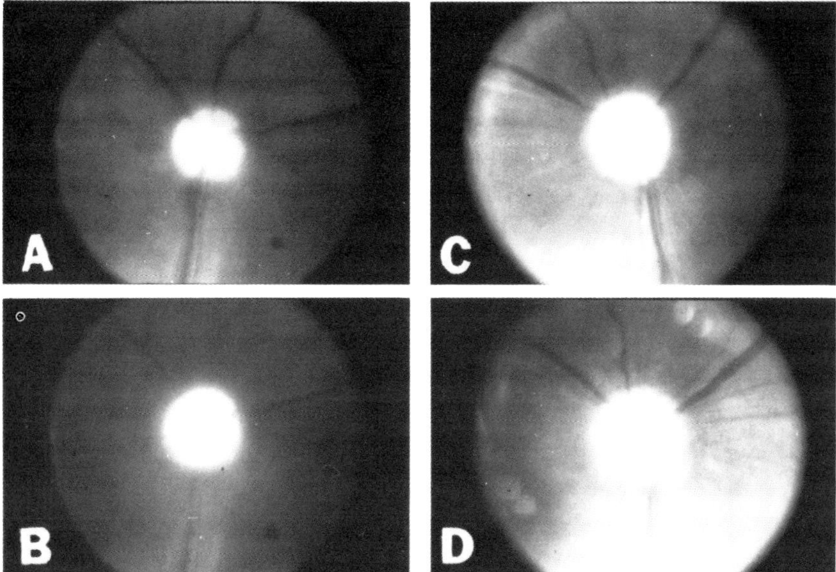

Fig. 4. Comparison of fundus photographs from a pair of beagle puppy littermates. The puppy on the left (A and B) was unmedicated, and the puppy on the right (C and D) was aspirin-treated. The top photographs were taken while both animals were breathing ambient air, and those on the bottom were taken after two hours of breathing 100% oxygen. Reproduced from Flower RW et al [3], with permission of the publisher.

PROSTAGLANDIN SUPPRESSORS

In the late 1970s, evidence appeared linking manipulation of the prostaglandin system to oxygen-dependent changes in the ductus arteriosus [5,6]. This suggested looking for a similar link between the prostaglandin system and the well recognized oxygen-induced changes in the immature retina. Eventually, one was found by which retinal vasotonia could be manipulated independently of PO_2.

Aspirin, administered at dosages producing plasma levels within the human therapeutic range, was demonstrated to inhibit oxygen-induced retinal vasconstriction in puppies [3]. Figures 4-A and C are of the funduses of two air-breathing littermates. B and D are of the same puppies after 2 hours of breathing oxygen. The puppy on the right was aspirin-treated at the start of the experiment; note the absence of vasoconstriction. It was also found that the aspirin-treated puppies developed significantly more severe retinopathy than their simultaneously oxygen-exposed littermates. In fact, a number of the aspirin-treated, oxygen-exposed puppies developed cicatricial changes of ROP.

We postulated from these results that the more severe retinopathy developed by the aspirin-treated puppies resulted from prostaglandin-mediated inhibition of retinal vasoconstriction and that vasoconstriction may be a normal physiologic mechanism to protect the immature retina from excessive oxygen. That is, retinal vasoconstriction may in fact be a protective rather than a pathologic process in response to hyperoxia. The vasoconstriction observed in oxygen-exposed premature infants may be only the extreme of a normal physiologic response by which retinal blood flow is modulated during in utero development. During that period, retinal tissue gradually ceases to be totally dependent for maintenance on the adjacent choroidal and hyaloid blood flows. This same mechanism may also be active throughout the perinatal period.

It is possible then that susceptibility of an eye to oxygen-induced retinopathy depends on the extent to which the protective vasoconstriction response is functional at birth as well as on the degree of retinal maturity attained. From this point of view, it may be argued that cases of spontaneous ROP reported in premature infants never administered oxygen [7], or in full-term infants who were [8], are simply examples of inadequate retinal vasotonia at birth to protect structurally immature vessels. We also speculated that the apparently strong vasoconstriction response normally present in both the kitten and puppy contribute to the fact that cicatricial retinopathy was never produced in these animals until vasoconstriction was inhibited by aspirin administration.

On the assumption that retinal vasotonia is a predisposing factor in development of ROP, the greater vascular damage to the dilated retinal blood vessels of the aspirin-treated puppies could be attributed simply to a greater than usual flow of oxygenated blood through the immature vessels, those farthest from the optic nerve. This explanation supports the suggestion of Ashton and Pedler [9] that retinal vessel damage can result from direct cytotoxic effects of oxygen on endothelial cells.

A second possible explanation, however, takes into account occurrence of a presumed normal degree of vasoconstriction at birth concomitantly with the normally occurring rise in arterial blood pressure, as shown at left in Figure 5. (Vasoconstriction would not, however, be uniform throughout the vasculature as shown. This schematic simplification is used here only to make a point about the peripheral capillary transmural pressure.) Vasoconstriction, nevertheless, could add resistance to blood flow throughout the retinal vasculature in such a way that the most peripheral, and hence the most structurally immature, vessels would experience the smallest increase in transmural pressure. However, failure of such vasoconstriction to occur at

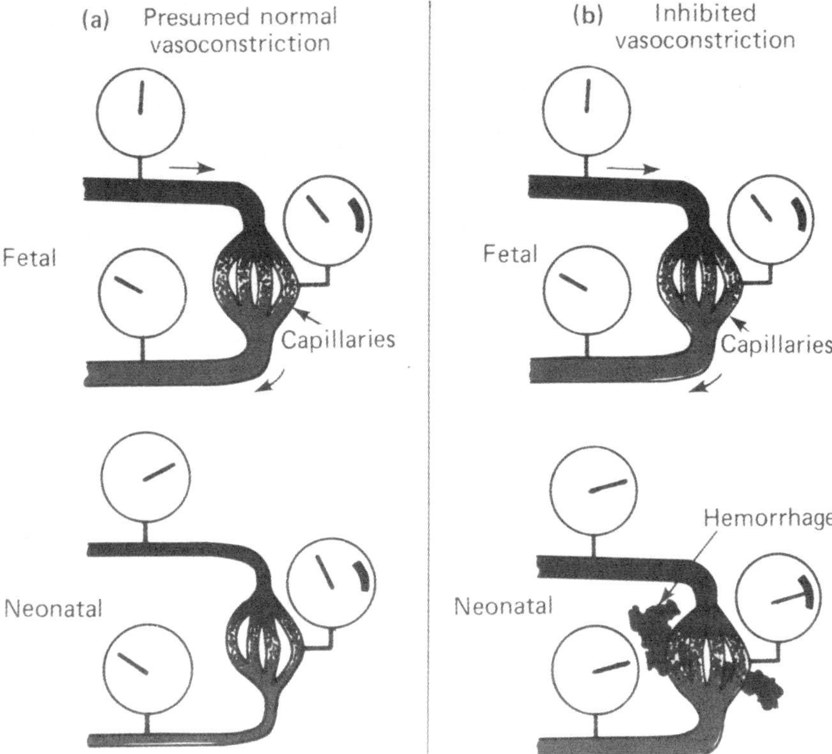

Fig. 5. Schematic representation of the changes in transmural pressure that might occur in the retinal vasculatures of fetal and neonatal eyes. A: Pressure relationships resulting from a presumed normal degree of vasoconstriction: B: Pressure relationships resulting from inhibited vasoconstriction. Under such circumstances it is possible for hemorrhage to occur. Reproduced with permission from Flower RW: "A mechanism for oxygen damage to the immature retinal vasculature." In: Lubbers DW, Acker H, Leniger-Follart E et al (eds): "Oxygen Transport to Tissue." New York: Plenum Press, Vol. 5, 1984.

birth (as indicated on the right) could result in excessively high transmural pressures, possibly producing retinal capillary hemorrhage. This mechanism could conceivably work independently of, or concomitantly with, direct oxygen cytotoxic effects.

At this point, it seemed desirable to pursue the effects of inhibited vasoconstriction by a method besides aspirin treatment. Regulation of arterial PCO_2 came to mind, since up to that time only passing attention had been given to it by earlier investigators. However, they looked only at the effects produced by breathing 5% CO_2 in conjunction with oxygen exposure of kittens and reported that CO_2 had no significant effect on the severity of retinopathy [10,11].

STUDIES WITH HYPERCARBIA

Our own investigation of the acute effects of CO_2 breathing was carried out in puppies under conditions in which arterial PCO_2 could be monitored and independently varied while blood pressure was maintained constant. We found that immature retinal vessels, in fact, respond dramatically to CO_2 breathing. The tendency of the retinal vessels to dilate in response to elevated PCO_2 is greater than their tendency to constrict in response to elevated PO_2, so much so that, when PCO_2 was elevated while PO_2 was maintained as high as 460 mm Hg, the vessels became more dilated than they were during normal air breathing [12] (see Fig. 6).

In keeping with the hypothesis that vasoconstriction plays an important role in modulating blood flow through the developing retinal vasculature, the changes that can be induced in puppy retinal vessels by manipulating arterial PCO_2 can be thought of as analogous to various changes in retinal vascular status during the perinatal period. When PCO_2 is relatively high and arterial blood pressure is low in utero, the retinal blood vessels are maximally dilated (as in the fundus at top in Fig. 6). At birth, when PCO_2 drops and blood pressure rises, the retinal blood vessels constrict to a degree recognized as clinically normal retinal vasotonia (as in the fundus in the middle). Of course, as long as the PCO_2 remains within the normal air breathing range, elevation of PO_2 will result in retinal vasoconstriction (as in the fundus at bottom).

Inspiration of 10% CO_2 was used, therefore, as an alternative to aspirin administration to induce retinal vasodilation. Litters of newborn puppies were randomly divided; half the puppies were reared for 3 days in humidified 10% CO_2/90% O_2, and half were reared in 10% N_2/90% O_2. They then matured to 20 days of age in air, at which time their retinas were examined [13].

The vascular patterns in both groups of littermates were abnormal, but the CO_2/O_2-reared groups had vascular anomalies distinctly different from those of the N_2/O_2-reared groups. The major retinal vessels of the CO_2/O_2 puppies were significantly dilated in comparison to those of the N_2/O_2 littermates, even though the animals had been removed from the high CO_2 environment for more than 2 weeks before euthanasia. Whereas vascularization to the periphery was halted in the N_2/O_2 retinas, it was not in the CO_2/O_2 retinas.

At the microscopic level, the retinas of the N_2/O_2 puppies showed characteristic oxygen-induced vascular changes. These included a ''brush-border'' configuration of peripheral capillaries and persistence of large areas

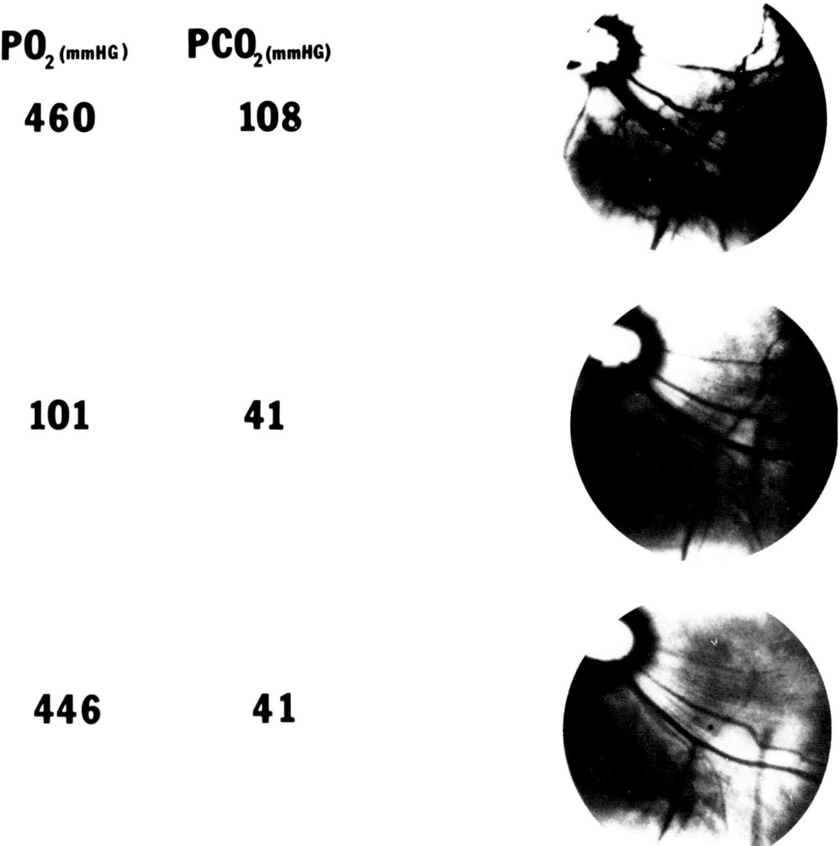

Fig. 6. Response of the immature retinal vasculature to manipulation of arterial PCO$_2$ level while holding systemic blood pressure constant. The middle fundus photograph shows the condition of the retinal vessels of an anesthetized puppy that was breathing room air. The bottom fundus photograph shows the constricted state of the same retinal vessels after the puppy breathed oxygen, which raised the arterial PO$_2$ but did not affect arterial PCO$_2$. The top fundus photograph shows retinal vessels, both arteries and veins, more dilated than during either air-breathing or oxygen-breathing states as a result of simultaneously breathing a high oxygen and high CO$_2$ concentration gas mixture. Reproduced from Flower RW et al [12], with permission of the publisher.

of avascular peripheral retina. Segments of peripheral retinal capillaries in some of the CO$_2$/O$_2$ puppies, on the other hand, were of such large caliber that they resembled the sinusoid-like embryonic capillaries; this is consistent with capillary blood pressures having risen to the point that the capillaries dilated beyond the elastic limits of their walls, resulting in a ballooned-out appearance.

In animals exposed for 3 days to 10% CO_2/90%O_2 and then returned for one day to air, focal hemorrhages have been found. What appeared to be microaneurysms were also found. All these effects can be explained, at least in part, on the basis of excessively high transmural pressures having been placed across structurally immature blood vessels.

To separate the presumed oxygen toxic effect from that presumably associated with excessive transmural capillary pressure, randomly selected puppy littermates were reared for 3 days in an environment of humidified 10% CO_2/90% air. At approximately 3 weeks of age, these puppies' retinas were compared to those of their littermates reared in air. In terms of vessel diameters, the same kinds of differences existed as were found between the CO_2/O_2- and N_2/O_2-reared puppies; that is, compared to the vascular periphery of a normal air-breathing puppy, the vascular diameters of a puppy of the same age killed in a 10% CO_2/90% air environment after breathing that mixture for 3 days, especially those of the capillaries, were significantly greater. Again, the effects of excessively high transmural pressures can explain these vascular changes. In some animals exposed to CO_2 and then returned to air, exaggerated avascular zones were seen.

In several of the CO_2/air-reared littermates whose ocular media were sufficiently clear to permit ophthalmic examination prior to euthanasia, lesions resembling those found in clinical ROP were observed and photographed. These lesions were also found to leak intravenously injected sodium fluorescein dye as observed clinically in ROP.

On the basis of results suggesting that PCO_2 is a risk factor in ROP pathogenesis, Bauer and Widmayer [14] reevaluated their data by discriminant analysis on a group of 74 surviving infants whose birthweights were under 1,000 gm. Of these, 37 had been diagnosed to have ROP. Of 28 independent variables evaluated by discriminant analysis to determine their roles in occurrence of ROP in this patient population, nine variables were found to correlate. The total function, consisting of the nine variables, correctly predicted infants with ROP 84% of the time. It is interesting that the most significant prediction of ROP was the highest PCO_2 measured, followed by the number of PCO_2 measurements greater than 50 torr that occurred simultaneously with an elevated PO_2 (greater than 100 torr).

Some consideration also must be given to the hyaloid and choroidal vasculatures.

A review of the color fundus photographs made prior to euthanasia of 62 puppies reared in either 90% or 100% O_2 indicated that, in 31 (ie, 50%), hemorrhage had occurred at the base of the hyaloid artery. However,

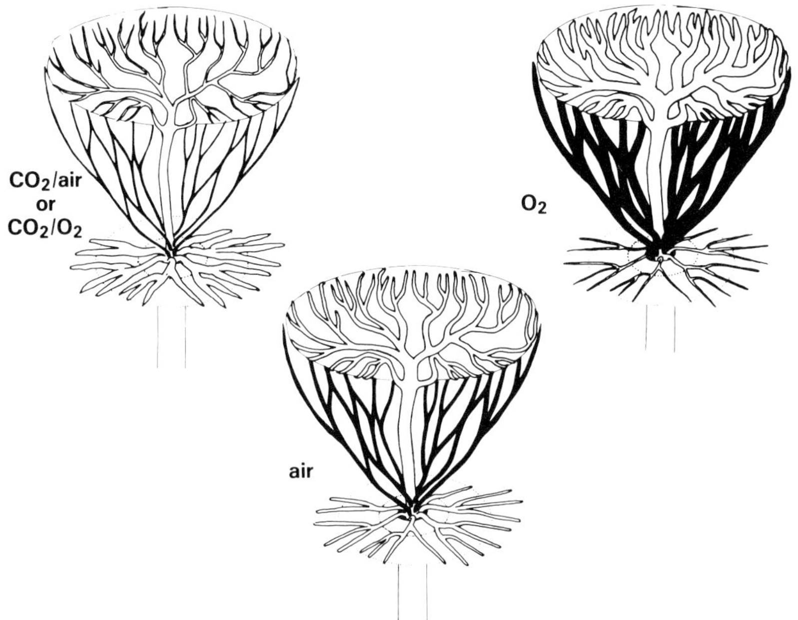

Fig. 7. Schematic representations of hypothetic relationships between retinal and hyaloid vessels during gas exposure. Reproduced from Bischoff PM et al [15], with permission of the publisher.

hemorrhage occurred in only one of 24 puppies (ie, 4%) reared in 10% CO_2/90% O_2 [13]. These data were interpreted as further evidence that administration of 10% CO_2, even concomitantly with oxygen, can reduce resistance to blood flow through the retinal vasculature.

In a puppy breathing oxygen continuously for 3 days, severe constriction of the retinal vasculatures must reduce blood flow and result in an elevation of the pressure head in retinal arteries near the disk as indicated at the top right in Figure 7. Since the retinal and hyaloid vasculatures share a common arterial supply at the optic nerve and are therefore hydrostatically coupled, of the two, the atrophic hyaloid artery is most likely to "leak" if intraarterial blood pressure rises sufficiently. The same puppy breathing 10% CO_2 /90% O_2 would be spared such a blood pressure rise in vessels near the disk if elevated PCO_2 inhibited downstream retinal vasoconstriction (this is indicated at the top left in Fig. 7).

The hyaloid vessels appear to be genetically programmed to atrophy concomitantly with retina vessel development. Compared to the retina, the hyaloid is relatively resistant to blood flow under normal circumstances. The hydrostatic coupling between the passive, yet flow-resistant, hyaloid and the active retinal vasculatures may tie the rate of atrophy of the former to the rate of development of the latter. The common rate-limiting factor is the magnitude of the pressure gradient that produces blood flow. Thus an inverse relationship may exist between hyaloid artery pressure and rate of hyaloid atrophy. During O_2 exposure, retinal vasoconstriction conceivably results in elevation of pressure in the hyaloid vessels and inhibits the normal process of atrophy. Assuming vasodilation of the retinal vessels during CO_2 exposure, hydrostatic pressure in the hyaloid artery would drop, producing passive vasoconstriction of the hyaloid vessels compared to their state during air breathing.

Since the newborn puppy hyaloid vasculature is usually in an advanced state of atrophy, a preliminary study of O_2 and CO_2 exposure on the hyaloid was undertaken using the newborn mouse eye, where it is still relatively patent. We used a scanning electron microscopy technique to study its response in mice exposed to various humidified gas mixtures [15].

For example, compared to the rate of hyaloid atrophy in air-reared mice, the rate of atrophy in O_2-exposed mice was retarded, and the hyaloid vessels of the O_2-exposed mice were of slightly greater caliber than those of air-reared mice of identical age. At the top left in Figure 8, the tunica vasculosis lentis of a 3-day-old, air-reared mouse is compared to that of a 3-day-old mouse reared in O_2; a similar comparison is made of two 10-day-old mice on the right side. Notice also the more prominently visible vaso hyaloidea propria in the O_2-exposed mice.

In the case of CO_2 exposure, the rate of atrophy *increased* significantly, and the hyaloid vessel calibers were less than those of air-reared mice. These observations were also in agreement with the inverse relationship postulated to exist between hyaloid artery pressure and atrophy.

CHOROIDAL STUDIES

Finally, we come to the choroidal vasculature. Various studies have suggested that, under some conditions, the entire oxygen needs of the retina can be met by the choroidal circulation [16,17]. Other studies demonstrated that a significantly attenuated choroidal circulation alone (less than 10% intact) could supply the necessary retinal oxygen when the animal was breathing 100% oxygen at an elevated ambient pressure. Several investigators have hypothesized the choroidal vasculature of the mature eye to be capable of autoregulating its blood flow, but choroidal autoregulation has not been rigorously demonstrated. In the specific case of the immature eye, it has been suggested more than once that the choroidal circulation is unaffected by oxygen exposure. At best, the choroidal circulation remains a bit of a mystery.

Fluorescein dye studies have shown that, in kittens whose arterial O_2

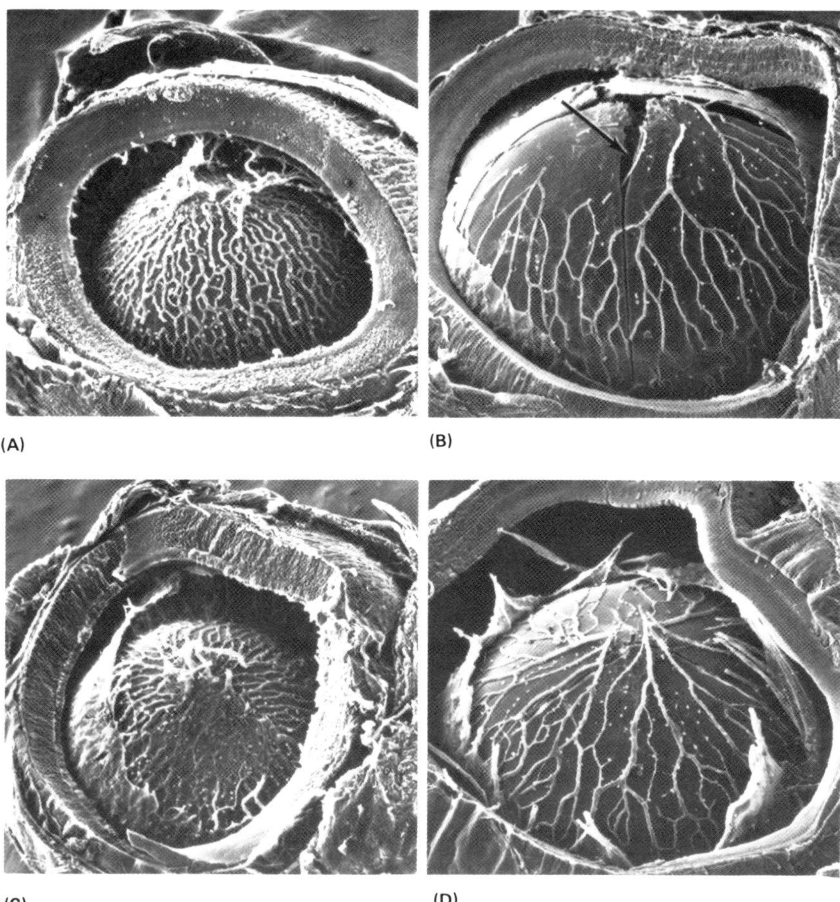

Fig. 8. A-D. Scanning electron micrographs of the hyaloid vascular system (magnification ×75). A: Three-day-old mouse reared in air. The vessels of the tunica vasculosis lentis (TVL) form a complex vascular network with numerous interconnections. B: Ten-day-old mouse reared in air. The vessels of the TVL are further separated than those of the 3-day-old, have fewer interconnections, and have narrower diameters. Some vessels are reduced to threadlike strands. The vaso hyaloidea propria (VHP) vessels are barely visible on the peripheral lens surface. Fixation artifact in lens (arrow). C: Three-day-old mouse reared in oxygen since the first day of life. The hyaloid vessels are not constricted but are similar to those in the air controls. D: Ten-day-old mouse reared in oxygen continuously since the first day of life. Compared to B, there is marked vascular distention in the VHP and slight dilation in the TVL. Reproduced from Bischoff PM et al [15], with permission of the publisher.

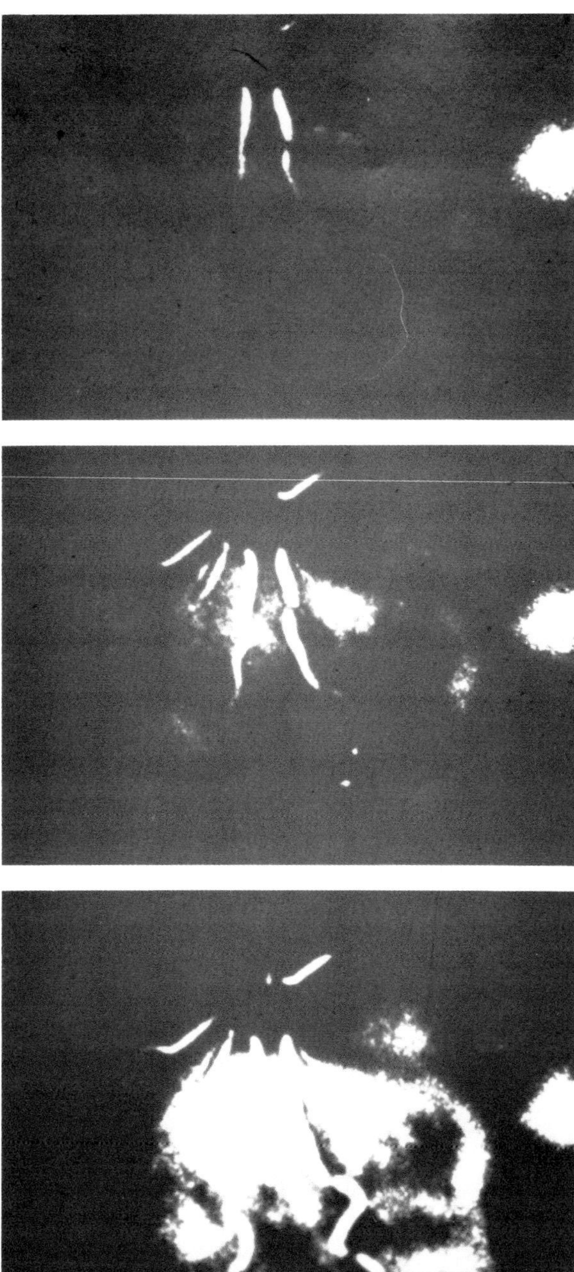

Fig. 9. Three selected frames from a 16-mm motion picture fluorescein angiogram. Top, fluorescein dye wave front shortly after entering retinal artery. Center, 0.016 seconds later. Bottom, 0.047 seconds later. Reproduced from Flower RW, Patz A [19], with permission of the publisher.

levels were maintained above 400 torr for a period of 4 hours, virtually all the retinal vessels became threadlike, leaving only the highly reflective disk as a landmark in the fundus [18]. More importantly, however, the dye studies also showed that the background choroidal flush was extremely sluggish compared to the extremely rapid choroidal flush seen in the same kitten breathing room air [19]; its blood velocity was reduced by as much as sixfold.

An example of sluggish choroidal circulation in an oxygen-exposed kitten is demonstrated in Figure 9. Three frames of an angiogram are shown of an oxygen-breathing kitten in which the choroidal flush greatly lags behind dye-filling of the retinal circulation, indicating that the choroidal circulation can be affected by sustained oxygen breathing.

Existing data on the choroid of the immature eye obviously leave much to be desired, but the choroid clearly has the potential to play a major role in maintaining the retina until the retinal vasculature develops fully. It seems reasonable that its role in controlling tissue oxygenation in the immature retina even exceeds the role it plays in the adult eye; therefore, its role in the etiology of ROP deserves extensive investigation.

SUMMARY

A conservative view of some of the data discussed here would be that they are anecdotal, but the possibility that factors other than oxygen alone contribute to genesis of ROP is compelling, as is the possibility that clinically observed ROP is only a narrow range of a broad spectrum of retinopathies that could be produced in the immature retina were appropriate physiologic parameters varied outside the current clinically acceptable range. In this context, the significance of such preliminary investigations as these is that they should alert investigators and clinicians to look for correlations between incidence of ROP and factors other than oxygen alone.

REFERENCES

1. Flower RW, McLeod DS, Lutty GA, Goldberg B, Wager SD: Postnatal retinal vascular development of the puppy. Invest Ophthal Vis Sci 26:957–968, 1985.
2. Ashton N: Retinal angiogenesis in the human embryo. Br Med Bull 26:103–106, 1970.
3. Flower RW, Blake DA, Wajer SD, Egner PG, McLeod DS, Pitts SM: Retrolental fibroplasia: Evidence for a role of the prostaglandin cascade in the pathogenesis of oxygen-induced retinopathy in the newborn beagle. Pediatr Res 15:1293–1302, 1981.
4. Patz A: Retrolental fibroplasia. Surv Ophthalmol 14:1–29, 1969.
5. Clyman RI, Mauray F, Heymann MA, Rudolph AM: Ductus arteriosus: Developmental response to oxygen and indomethacin. Prostaglandin 15:993–998, 1978.
6. Friedman WF, Hirschklau MJ, Printz MP, Pitlick PT, Kirkpatrick SE: Pharmacologic

closure of patent ductus arteriosus in the premature infant. N Engl J Med 295:526–529, 1976.

7. Foos RY: Acute retrolental fibroplasia. Albrecht von Graefes Arch Klin Exp Ophthalmol 195:87–100, 1975.

8. Brockhurst RJ, Chishti MI: Cicatricial retrolental fibroplasia: Its occurrence without oxygen administration and in full term infants. Albrecht von Graefes Arch Klin Exp Ophthalmol 195:113–128, 1975.

9. Ashton N, Pedler C: Studies on developing retinal vessels: IX. Reaction of endothelial cells to oxygen. Br J Ophthalmol 46:257–276, 1962.

10. Ashton N, Cook C: Direct observation of the effect of oxygen on developing vessels: Preliminary report. Br J Ophthalmol 38:433–440, 1954.

11. Patz A: Clinical and experimental studies on role of oxygen in retrolental fibroplasia. Trans Am Acad Ophthalmol Otolaryngol 58:45–50, 1954.

12. Flower RW, McLeod DS, Wajer SD, Sendi GS, Egner PG, Dubin NH: Prostaglandins as mediators of vasotonia in the immature retina. Pediatrics 73:440–444, 1984.

13. Flower RW: A mechanism for oxygen damage to the immature retinal vasculature. In Lubbers DW, Acker H, Leniger-Follart E, Goldstick TK (eds): "Oxygen Transport to Tissue." New York: Plenum Press, Vol 5, 1984.

14. Bauer CR, Widmayer SM: A relationship between $PaCO_2$ and retrolental fibroplasia. Pediatr Res 15:1236A, 1981.

15. Bischoff PM, Wajer SD, Flower RW: Scanning electron microscopic studies of the hyaloid vascular system in newborn mice exposed to O_2 and CO_2. Albrecht von Graefes Arch Clin Exp Ophthalmol 220:257–263, 1983.

16. Bietti G: Effects of experimentally decreased or increased oxygen supply in some ophthalmic diseases. Arch Ophthalmol 49:491–513, 1953.

17. Dollery CT, Bulpitt CJ, Kohner EM: Oxygen supply to the retina from the retinal and choroidal circulations at normal and increased arterial oxygen tensions. Invest Ophthalmol 8:588–594, 1969.

18. Patz A: The role of oxygen in retrolental fibroplasia. Trans Am Ophthal Soc 66:940–985, 1968.

19. Flower RW, Patz A: Oxygen studies in retrolental fibroplasia: IX. The effects of elevated arterial oxygen tension on retinal vascular dynamics in the kitten. Arch Ophthal 85:197–203, 1971.

Spindle Cells and Retinopathy of Prematurity: Interpretations and Predictions

Frank L. Kretzer, PhD, and Helen M. Hittner, MD

Cullen Eye Institute (F.L.K., H.M.H.); and Departments of Pediatrics (H.M.H.) and Cell Biology (F.L.K.), Baylor College of Medicine, Houston, Texas 77030

Spindle cells in the hyperoxygenated, avascular, vanguard retina are proposed to be the peripheral inducers of the neovascularization associated with retinopathy of prematurity (ROP) [1–3]. The induction of ROP is conceptualized in terms of three basic events. 1) Activation of spindle cells results initially in the increase in gap junctions between adjacent spindle cells, secondarily in the increase in cytoplasmic volume of rough endoplasmic reticulum, and ultimately in the synthesis and secretion of angiogenic factors. 2) Maturation of spindle cells is associated with a decrease in gap junctions, a diminished cytoplasmic volume of rough endoplasmic reticulum, and a cessation of synthesis and secretion of angiogenic factors from spindle cells. 3) Myofibroblasts, which differentiate from the shunt, invade the vitreous concomitantly with spindle cell maturation and provide the tractional force that can produce retinal separation.

Data obtained by studying preterm infant postmortem retinas have led us to eight conclusions that we see as pieces fitting into the larger puzzle that is ROP. These increase our understanding of ROP and can assist in focusing future research so that potential prophylactic and therapeutic medical and surgical interventions can be understood, predicted, and tested.

PUZZLE PIECE 1: SPINDLE CELLS MIGRATE THROUGH CYSTOID SPACES

Whole eye donations were obtained within 1–5 hours postmortem from 73 liveborn, anomaly-free, ≤ 1,500 gm-birthweight infants who were enrolled in one of three clinical trials performed at Texas Children's Hopsital [4–6]. These 73 infants were from 20 to 32 weeks of gestational age and survived

This research was supported by grants from the Retina Research Foundation, Research to Prevent Blindness, Cullen Foundation, and Hoffmann-LaRoche, Inc.

Birth Defects: Original Article Series, Volume 24, Number 1, pages 147–168
© 1988 March of Dimes Birth Defects Foundation

from 30 minutes to 23 weeks on continuous oxygen. Along the optic disk-ora serrata axis of these 73 eyes, light and electron microscopy revealed the following observations about spindle cells.

The process of spindle cell migration through the nerve fiber layer occurs in the low-oxygen environment of the intrauterine fetus. The migration starts around the optic disk before 20 weeks of gestational age and reaches the temporal ora serrata at 29 weeks of gestational age [1–3]. Spindle cells arise from the adventitia of the hyaloid artery. Migrating spindle cells in the human appear to be postmitotic because of the absence of mitotic figures. The peripheral edge of the migrating spindle cell apron follows the formation of the outer plexiform layer. Migrating spindle cells are fusiform in shape, form a meshwork apron that occupies a minimal volume of the nerve fiber layer, and possess minimal gap junctions. Spindle cells have extensive surface contacts with each other and with the lateral processes of transretinal Müller cells.

Posterior to the migrating apron, spindle cells form solid cords and eventually metamorphose into endothelium by canalization. The process of normal inner retinal vasoformation lags far behind the advancing apron of spindle cells and does not reach the temporal ora serrata until term. Thus the preterm infant is born with a circumferential zone of avascular, peripheral, vanguard retina that is laden with spindle cells [7,8]. The vanguard retina is proportionately larger in infants of lower gestational age.

The process of vasoformation from spindle cell precursors is not universal in mammals and does not occur in the term kitten, term beagle puppy, or preterm baboon [9]. Thus, in these animal models, the mechanism of inner retinal vasoformation is different from that of the preterm infant. Furthermore, in the kitten, there is vasoobliteration but no mesenchymal shunt formation nor any terminal retinal separation [10]. In the kitten, antioxidant (vitamin E) megadose therapy designed to halt vitreal neovascularization [11] or oxygen weaning designed to open gradually vasoobliterated vessels [12] cannot be extrapolated to the preterm infant because the vasoformative process is so different. We believe that the rat model, which does contain spindle cells [13,14], is the most appropriate animal model currently available to probe the molecular basis of human ROP. However, the rat retina is very immature at birth. The animals are difficult to keep alive on vitamin E-free formula to allow experimentation to start 5 days postnatally, when extensive spindle cells have invaded the nerve fiber layer.

PUZZLE PIECE 2: SPINDLE CELLS ARE TRANSRETINAL TO IMMATURE PHOTORECEPTORS

In the preterm retina, there is a continuum of photoreceptor maturation along the optic disk-ora serrata axis. With increasing gestational age,

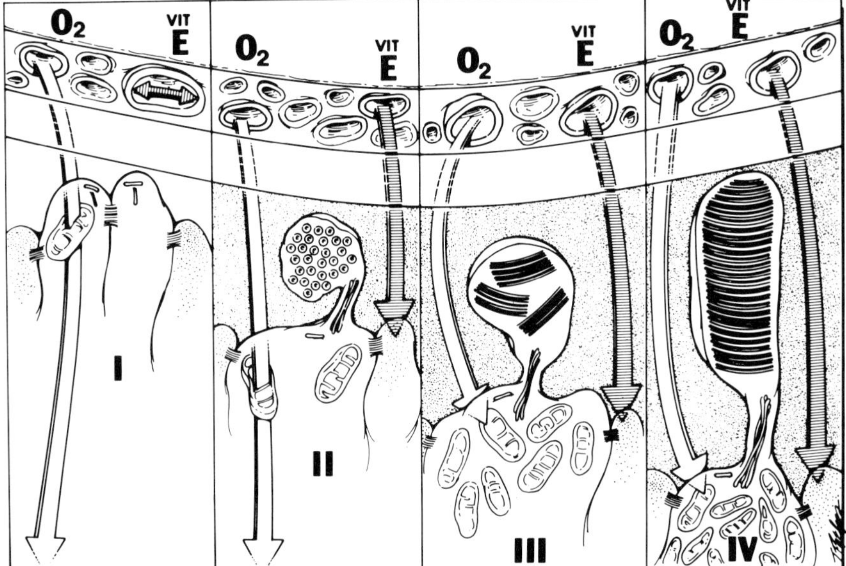

Fig. 1. Cartoon showing stage I, II, III, and IV photoreceptors. The stippled material represents interstitial retinol binding protein (IRBP) in the subretinal space. Note the increasing mitochondrial aggregation within the maturing inner segment. Hypothetical oxygen flux from the nonconstricting choroidal vessels across the retinal pigment epithelium is designated as an open arrow. There is no oxygen sink created by the low metabolic requirements of stage I and II photoreceptors. There is a formidable barrier created by stage III and IV photoreceptors, as indicated morphologically by the dense packing of mitochondria. IRBP is not secreted by stage I photoreceptors. IRBP is secreted by stage II, III, and IV photoreceptors. The potential transport of vitamin E into Müller cells by IRBP is designated by the shaded arrow.

photoreceptors mature slowly around the optic disk and gradually radiate toward the ora serrata as defined by Johnson and colleagues [15,16]. The maturation process is incomplete even at term birth. The stages of photoreceptor maturation are schematized in Figure 1. This cartoon is based on 73 pairs of whole eye donations in which the following parameters were studied along the optic disk-ora serrata axis: development of the subretinal space and photoreceptors, photoreceptor maturation as related to inner retinal vasoformation, location of the spindle cell apron as related to retinal maturation, and percentage volume of the nerve fiber layer occupied by spindle cells. The development of photoreceptor inner and outer segments was studied by transmission electron microscopy in 11 eyes.

Immature stage I photoreceptors contain only precursor inner segments, with few mitochondria, and reach the temporal ora serrata by about 27 weeks

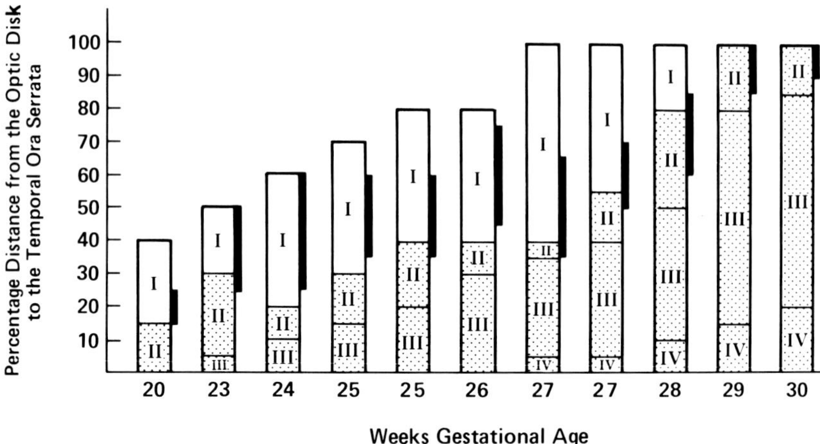

Fig. 2. This bar graph shows photoreceptor maturation along the optic disk-ora serrata axis in continuous montages of the horizontal meridian in the retinas of 11 preterm infants of 20–30 weeks of gestational age who survived for <4 hours. The Roman numerals indicate the stage of photoreceptor development; the stippled area represents the distribution of IRBP in the subretinal space; the solid black bars mark the location of the spindle cell apron.

of gestational age. With maturation, stage II photoreceptors develop balloon-shaped primitive outer segments with random tubular disks, have primitive inner segments with scarce mitochondria, and reach the temporal ora serrata by 29 weeks of gestational age. With continued maturation, stage III photoreceptors appear with outer segments containing stacked profiles of randomly oriented disks, possess inner segments with a dense aggregation of mitochondria, and reach the temporal ora serrata near term. Ultimately, stage IV photoreceptors have elongate outer segments with organized and stacked disks, possess inner segments with a denser aggregation of mitochondria, and reach the temporal ora serrata postterm.

In the developing human retina, there is a tight geometric relationship between photoreceptor maturation and the composition of the nerve fiber layer. The higher metabolic rate of stage III and IV photoreceptors [17–20] (as inferred from the mitochondrial accumulation in the inner segment) is counterbalanced by the transretinal development of small inner retinal capillaries and larger inner retinal vessels, respectively. The majority of spindle cells are transretinal initially to stage I photoreceptors and later to stage II photoreceptors (Fig. 2). Both have low metabolic rates, as deduced from the scarce mitochondria in their inner segments. Such immature photoreceptors create no barrier to oxygen diffusing from the nonvasoconstricted choroid. Thus, in the preterm human retina, it appears that spindle cells and the interface between the vanguard and rear guard retina are in a hyperoxic environment with or without oxygen administration. In infants ≤27 weeks of gestational age, the majority of the spindle cell apron is transretinal to stage I photoreceptors (Fig. 2). In contrast, stage II photoreceptors are transretinal to the majority of the spindle cell apron in infants ≥28 weeks of gestational age (Fig. 2).

PUZZLE PIECE 3: INTERSTITIAL RETINOL BINDING PROTEIN (IRBP) SECRETION BY MATURING PHOTORECEPTORS DETERMINES VITAMIN E UPTAKE INTO THE VANGUARD RETINA

Twenty-four additional eyes (obtained within 3 hours postmortem from infants 20–33 weeks of gestational age who survived <4 hours) were appraised for the length of the IRBP fluorescent band in the subretinal space from the optic disk to the temporal ora serrata in the horizontal meridian [3,15,16]. Spindle cells are far removed from inner retinal vessels, and potentially, therefore, only minimal amounts of vitamin E could reach the peripheral spindle cells from these centrally located vessels. IRBP in the hydrophilic subretinal space likely plays a critical role in the delivery of vitamin E to the vanguard neural retina in the preterm infant. IRBP is a major constituent of the adult interphotoreceptor matrix [21–23]. IRBP is a sialated glycoprotein [24] that binds retinol [22,24,25] and vitamin E [24,26,27] and is probably identical to the 7S retinol receptor of retina and brain described by Wiggert et al [28,29]. IRBP, with an approximate Stokes' radius of 55 Å, is contained within the subretinal space by the tight junctions between photoreceptors and Müller cells that form the outer limiting membrane. These tight junctions have a Stokes' radius pore size of 30–36 Å [30].

Vitamin E uptake into vanguard retinal membranes therefore seems dependent on retinal maturation (photoreceptor development to stage II and secretion of IRBP; Fig. 1). The correlation between IRBP production and outer segment disk formation is consistent with the hypothesis that photoreceptors synthesize and secrete IRBP [31–33]. Thus, IRBP appears in the subretinal space at a time when the exchange of retinol between the retinal pigment epithelium and photoreceptors begins. Likewise IRBP may be involved in delivering vitamin E to the retina at a time when antioxidant protection is first needed for the highly unsaturated disk membranes [34].

We propose that Müller cells are the connecting link between vitamin E transport across the subretinal space and spindle cells located transretinally within the nerve fiber layer. Müller cells have extensive apical microvilli, which protrude beyond the outer limiting membrane into the subretinal space. They also have lateral processes that enshroud retinal neurons as well as spindle cells. Vitamin E may be shuttled across the subretinal space by IRBP, be absorbed by Müller cell microvilli, be transported transretinally, and provide antioxidant protection to spindle cells within the nerve fiber layer [3,15,16]. This function of Müller cells would be important only in the premature, peripheral retina, which is devoid of inner retinal vessels. Since a given area of IRBP exists at any given gestational age, efficacy of vitamin E in suppressing the development of severe ROP is dependent on filling a threshold level of IRBP with vitamin E by creating a state of plasma sufficiency in the normally vitamin E-deficient preterm infant [35].

The complex relationship between the area of IRBP and the location of spindle cells (Fig. 2) explains why clinical efficacy of vitamin E supplementation may have a breakpoint at 28 weeks of gestational age. In those infants ≤27 weeks of gestational age, most spindle cells may not be protected by vitamin E.

If secretion of IRBP into the subretinal space (stage II photoreceptors) occurred prior to the peripheral migration of spindle cells toward the ora serrata, or if spindle cells were restricted to regions around the last-formed inner retinal blood vessels, vitamin E supplementation would eliminate ROP. It would be possible to transport sufficient levels of the fat-soluble vitamin E from the plasma to retinal membranes and protect spindle cells from oxidative insults in infants of all gestational ages. Unfortunately, vitamin E uptake into peripheral retinal membranes is dependent on retinal maturation. Thus, vitamin E is not a panacea for the suppression of severe ROP. Perhaps supplementation with selenium (a water-soluble antioxidant) can circumvent this maturation dependency and offer antioxidant protection to spindle cells in the youngest viable preterm infants (24–27 weeks of gestational age).

Currently, infants of ≤1,000 gm birthweight are still at high risk for development of severe ROP despite continuous oral, intramuscular, or slow intravenous infusion vitamin E supplementation from the first hours postpartum. However, even in these infants, vitamin E may cause a delay in the clinical development of severe ROP [36].

PUZZLE PIECE 4: NO ENDOTHELIAL NECROSIS OCCURS CENTRALLY AND NO HYPOXIA OCCURS PERIPHERALLY

In all 73 eyes studied morphologically, there is no indication of inner retinal vasoobliteration, endothelial cell destruction, or phagocytosis of nascent vessels despite clinically evident, physiologic oxygen-induced vasoconstriction. Although there are reports that hyperoxia uniquely induces a cessation of endothelial cell proliferation in vitro [37,38], there is no indication in the preterm human retina of parallel lysosomal alterations, mitochondrial fragmentation and nuclear aggregation, or increased size of the endothelium in the retinal vessels of the preterm infant on continuous oxygen supplementation. The absence of ganglion cell swelling, bloated mitochondria, or enlarged extracellular spaces negates the idea that peripheral inner retinal hypoxia or ischemia is the physiologic inducer of the neovascularization associated with ROP. ROP is distinctly different from diabetic retinopathy. In ROP, there is no basal lamina thickening, there is no alteration in junctional complexes between adjacent endothelia, and there is no hypoxia. In fact, the neovascularization associated with ROP occurs from immature vessels that have not even acquired pericytes.

PUZZLE PIECE 5: WHEN SPINDLE CELLS ARE STRESSED, GAP JUNCTIONS FORM

When spindle cells are stressed, the first morphologic manifestation is an increase in the extent of gap junctions between adjacent spindle cells (Fig. 3). Gap junctions are sites of electrical coupling between cells that appear ultrastructurally as two adjacent plasma membranes separated by a space of 20 Å that contains a central dense line [39] (Fig. 3B). Biologically, modulations in the total surface area of gap junctions can be triggered by cell damage [40], environmental stress [41], low pH [42], low temperature [43], and lipid peroxidation [44].

When spindle cells are extensively gap junction-linked, normal inner retinal vasoformation ceases, with no further migration. The kinetics of gap junction formation as modulated by vitamin E are summarized in Figure 4 for 22 control infants <32 weeks of gestational age (≤1,500 gm birthweight), 29 treatment infants ≤27 weeks of gestational age (≤1,000 gm birthweight), and 22 treatment infants ≥28 weeks of gestational age (>1,000 gm birthweight). The 22 control infants achieved mean plasma vitamin E levels of 0.3–0.6 mg% with oral supplementation [4]. The 51 treatment infants achieved mean plasma vitamin E levels of 1.2–3.3 mg% with oral (with or without intramuscular) supplementation [4–6].

In control infants, with all risk factors operant (Fig. 4, upper panel), extensive gap junction formation (activation) can occur as early as 4 days of life. Spindle cells can remain gap junction-linked for approximately 8–10 weeks. When spindle cells stack to >42% of the nerve fiber volume at about 8–10 weeks, the level of gap junctions drastically decreases (maturation). In treatment infants of ≤27 weeks of gestational age (Fig. 4, middle panel), gap junction levels remain low for approximately 2 weeks. After this lag, activation occurs to levels commensurate with control infants (delayed activation). Spindle cells remain gap junction-linked for approximately 8–10 weeks, and maturation occurs at about 10–12 weeks (delayed maturation) with stacking to >46% of the nerve fiber volume and a decrease in gap

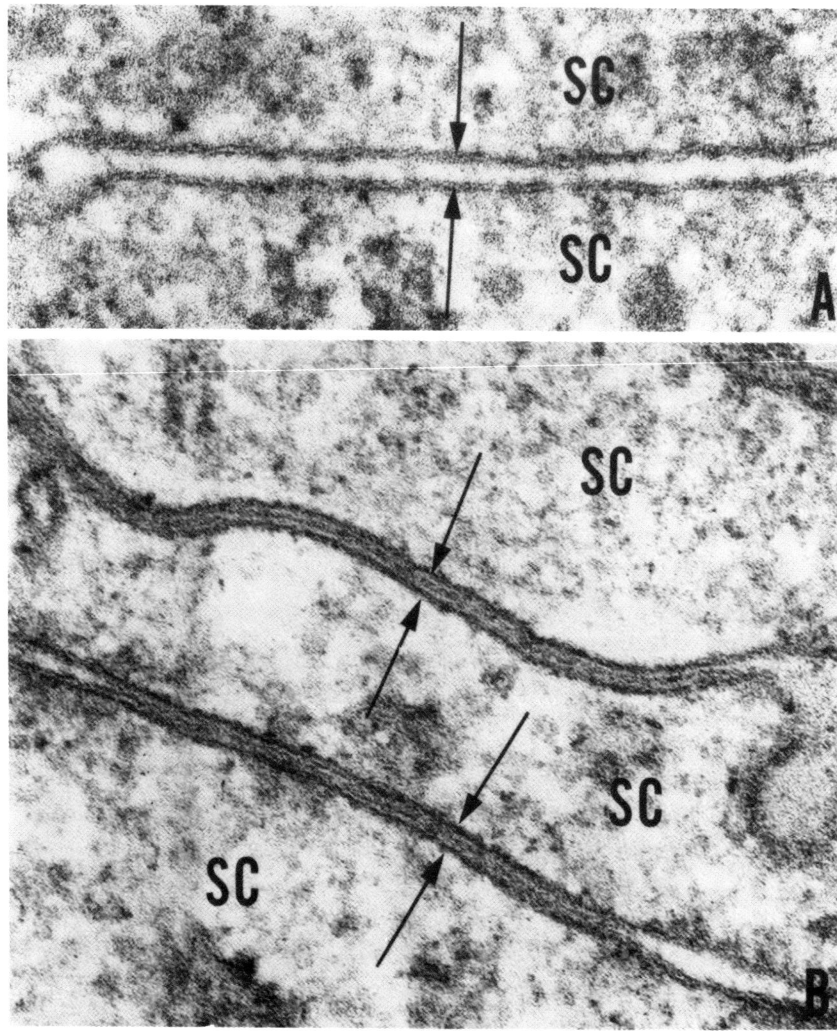

Fig. 3. Transmission electron micrographs (×181,000) demonstrating the absence of gap junctions between the two adjacent plasma membranes (arrows) of nonactivated spindle cells (SC) (A) as contrasted with the extensive gap junctions (arrows) between activated spindle cells (B).

junctions. In treatment infants of ≥28 weeks of gestational age (Fig. 4, lower panel), extensive gap junction formation never occurs, despite significant risk factors (suppressed activation).

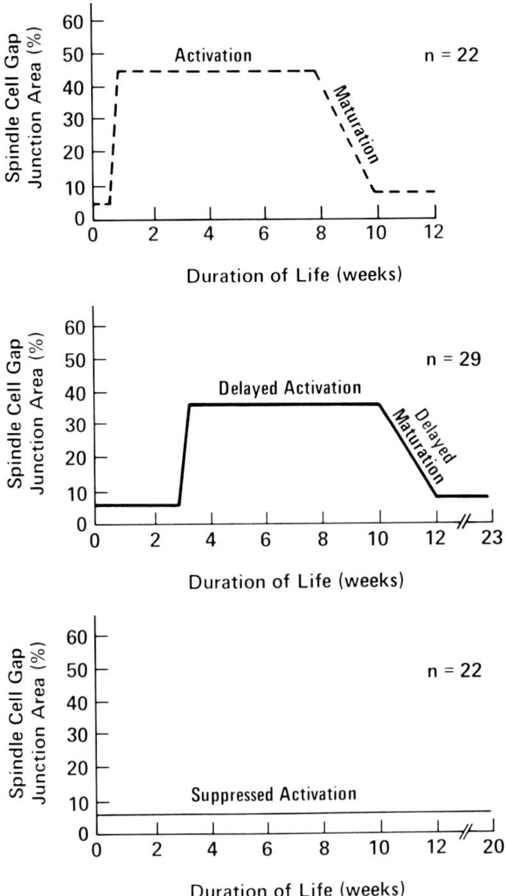

Fig. 4. These diagrams summarize the kinetics of gap junction formation between adjacent spindle cells in 22 control infants of <32 weeks of gestational age (upper panel), 29 treatment infants of ≤27 weeks gestational age (middle panel), and 22 treatment infants of ≥28 weeks of gestational age (lower panel) as a function of duration of life.

Any alteration in oxygen tension (in utero hypoxia, postpartum hyperoxia or hypoxia) may stress spindle cells and initiate the development of ROP. According to our theory, since immature photoreceptors create no metabolic sink to buffer the transretinal flux of oxygen from the nonconstricting choroidal vessels, the preterm vanguard retina is uniquely vulnerable to hyperoxia. Thus spindle cells can be oxidatively stressed when hemoglobin releases additional oxygen. This can occur when adult hemoglobin is transfused to replace lost blood (intraventricular hemorrhage or multiple laboratory tests) or is exchanged when hyperbilirubinemia occurs. Additionally, an oxidative stress can be induced by sepsis when macrophages engulf bacteria and release superoxide radicals [45] or when prolonged high light intensity [46] damages the maturing photoreceptors and diminishes the oxygen barrier between the choroid and spindle cells in the nerve fiber layer [17,18]. All these oxidative stresses on spindle cells can be minimized by a favorable oxidant–antioxidant balance. This is the proposed role of vitamin E prophylaxis in the preterm infant.

If an intrauterine hypoxic insult occurs sometime after 16 weeks of gestational age, when spindle cells first enter the nerve fiber layer but before the temporal spindle cell apron has become very small, ROP can be induced. The infant might be found to have cicatricial retinopathy or severe active ROP at birth [47]. Only early postpartum retinal examinations can identify these cases that occur earlier than 8–10 weeks of life as predicted by the natural history of ROP.

In infants of ≤1,500 gm birthweight experiencing early postpartum severe hypoxia or hypothermia, gap junction formation between adjacent spindle cells may be extensive and irreversible despite subsequent vitamin E supplementation. Pathologically, the kinetics of gap junction formation in these infants parallels that of control infants. This could explain the clinical development of severe ROP despite continuous vitamin E supplementation from the first hours of life in infants who are difficult to stabilize or must be transported.

When fewer ROP risk factors are operant, spontaneous regression occurs clinically. This correlates with an early decrease in gap junctions and no spindle cell stacking. It is not understood what environmental factors trigger this decrease in gap junctions.

The ultrastructural data show that prophylactic, minimal elevation of the deficient plasma vitamin E levels of the premature infant to sufficiency minimizes gap junction formation in infants of 28–32 weeks of gestational age, permitting normal vasoformation and suppressing the development of severe ROP. Infants of >32 weeks of gestational age and >1,500 gm birthweight are not usually at high risk, because the small spindle cell apron has minimal potential to secrete threshold levels of angiogenic factors. This makes vitamin E therapy unnecessary for ROP prevention in this population according to our theory.

In infants ≤27 weeks of gestational age, the restricted central domain of IRBP (Fig. 2) is apparently not sufficient to shuttle an effective level of the antioxidant into peripheral retinal membranes to stabilize the majority of the spindle cell apron against extensive gap junction formation. At around 28 weeks of gestational age, the extent of overlap between IRBP in the subretinal space (stage II photoreceptors) and the majority of the spindle cells in nerve fiber layer increases (Fig. 2). At this gestational age, most spindle cells can be protected against hyperoxic damage by sufficient antioxidant retinal levels.

PUZZLE PIECE 6: THERE IS A RELATIONSHIP BETWEEN GAP JUNCTIONS AND PROLIFERATION OF ROUGH ENDOPLASMIC RETICULUM

A significant increase in the cytoplasmic volume of the rough endoplasmic reticulum within spindle cells (Fig. 5) parallels extensive gap junction formation (Fig. 6). Similarly, when spindle cell maturation occurs with a decrease in gap junctions, there is a diminished cytoplasmic volume of the rough endoplasmic reticulum. These gap junction and rough endoplasmic reticulum changes have been stereologically quantified in 30 eyes ($R = 0.85$, $P \leq 0.0001$) and do not occur in any other retinal cell types [3].

PUZZLE PIECE 7: THERE IS A RELATIONSHIP BETWEEN PROLIFERATION OF THE ROUGH ENDOPLASMIC RETICULUM AND DETECTABLE LEVELS OF ANGIOGENIC FACTORS

The presence of angiogenic factors has been assayed by the induction of loop formation from the chorioallantoic membrane (CAM) of the fertilized chicken egg as per the protocols of Glaser et al [48–50]. The retinas from 12 eyes were isolated. The vanguard retina was dissected from the rear guard, and the 24 coded, masked pieces were homogenized in hypotonic salt solution. The supernate was filtered, freeze-dried, and stored at $-70°C$. The crystals were resuspended in 10 µl salt solution. This saturated a 1 mm pad of glass fiber that was impregnated with 5% acrylamide. Identical control pads were saturated with 10 µl of sterile salt solution. All 27 samples were assayed at the same time. A glass pad was placed over the CAM of 8-day-old fertilized chicken eggs and incubated for 4 days, and the number of new vascular loops was counted. The three blank saline pads induced from zero to three loops as background.

Angiogenic factors can be detected only in extracts of the vanguard retina as early as the fourth day of life in control infants and the third week of life in treatment infants of ≤ 27 weeks of gestational age (16–18 loops). Angiogenic factors are no longer detectable in extracts of the vanguard retina after 8–10 weeks of life in control infants and after 10–12 weeks of life in treatment infants of ≤ 27 weeks of gestational age (zero to three loops). In other words, positive angiogenic stimulation of the CAM occurs only in homogenates of the vanguard retina during a finite period of time when the

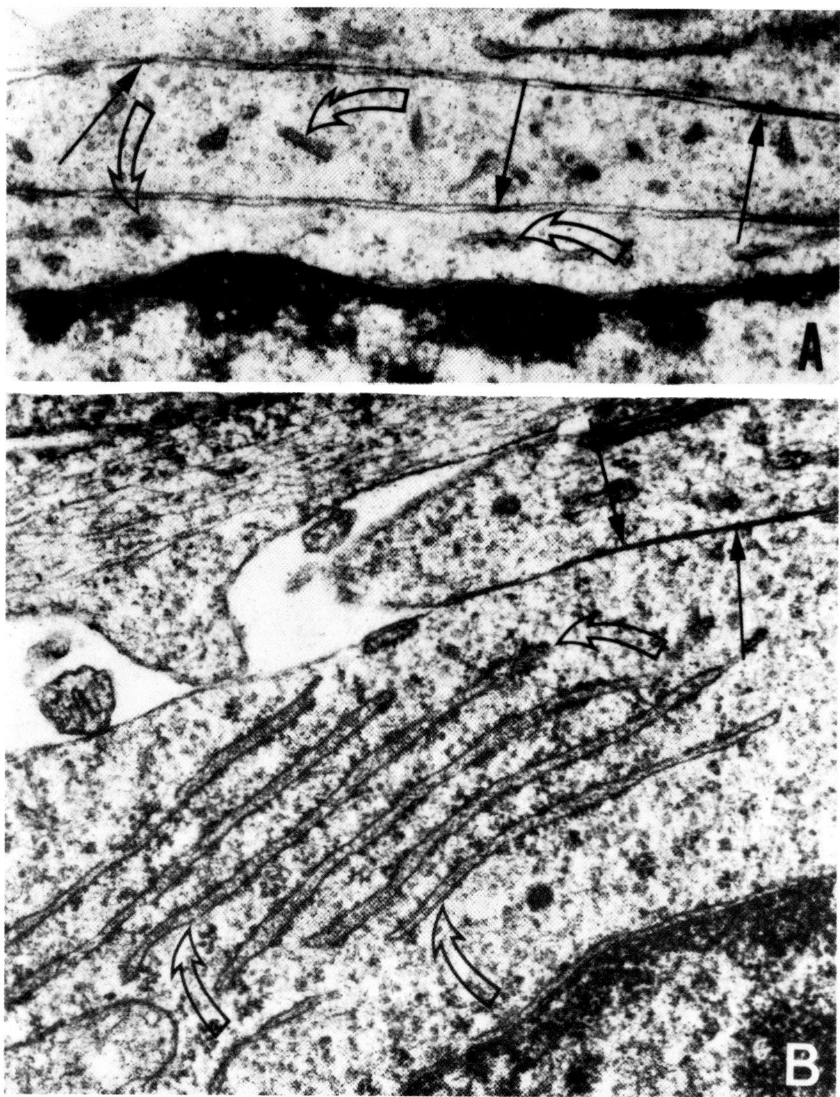

Fig. 5. Transmission electron micrographs ($\times 44,000$) showing the small cytoplasmic volume of rough endoplasmic reticulum (open arrows) associated with scarce gap junctions (solid arrows) in nonactivated spindle cells (A) as contrasted with the large cytoplasmic volume of RER associated with extensive gap junctions in activated spindle cells (B).

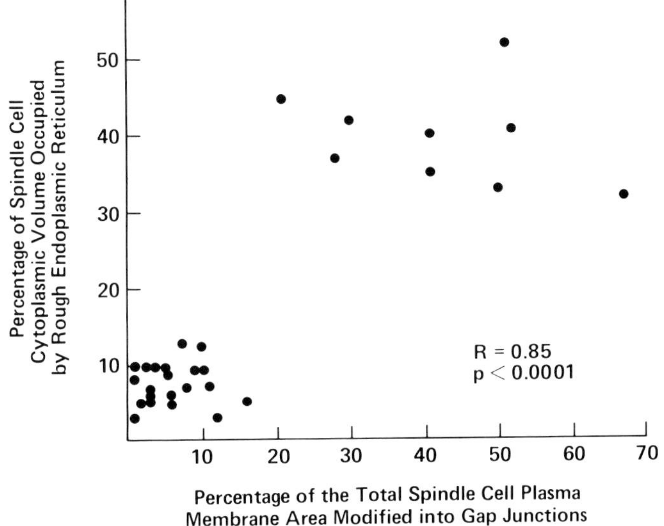

Fig. 6. Relationship between the percentage of spindle cell cytoplasmic volume occupied by rough endoplasmic reticulum and the percentage of the total spindle cell plasma membrane area modified into gap junctions in 30 preterm retinas. The statistic is the Pearson nonparametric coefficient.

vanguard retina contains spindle cells with a large cytoplasmic volume of rough endoplasmic reticulum (R = 0.97, P ≤0.0001, Fig. 7) and follows the time course of spindle cell activation shown in Figure 4 [3,36].

Angiogenic factors may be secreted in vitamin E-treated infants of ≥28 weeks of gestational age, but this probably occurs at much lower levels. Although ROP develops in many of these more mature infants, it spontaneously regresses in most. The cellular explanation proposed is that only a few spindle cells are activated, and a low level of angiogenic factors is secreted, which then induces only mild intraretinal neovascularization from the last-formed inner retinal vessels. Thus, with this scenario, vitamin E supplementation would prevent the development of severe ROP but not the total incidence of all stages of ROP [36].

Extracts of the rear guard retina at all 12 time points during the pathogenesis of ROP contain no assayable levels of angiogenic factors (zero to three loops) [3]. Even when tortuous and dilated vessels are present, this region is not the source of angiogenic factors.

These angiogenic factors have not been isolated, their molecular weights are unknown, and their activity has been detected only in homogenates of the vanguard retina that contain gap junction-linked spindle cells with a large

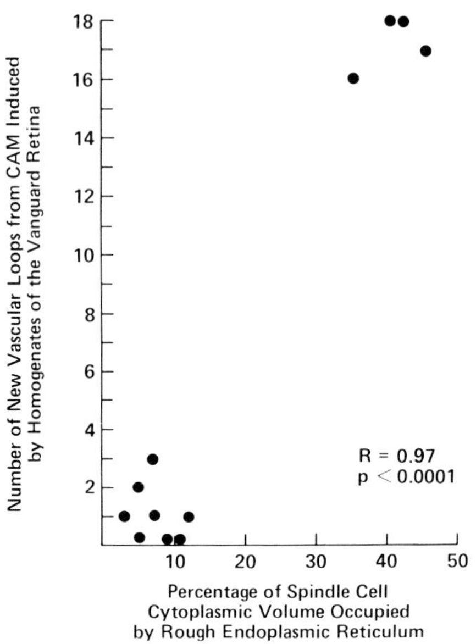

Fig. 7. Relationship between the number of vascular loops growing from the chorioallantoic membrane (CAM) of the 8-day-old fertilized chicken egg by homogenates of the vanguard retina and the percentage of spindle cell cytoplasmic volume occupied by rough endoplasmic reticulum in 12 preterm retinas. In all samples, homogenates of the rear guard retina as well as blank saline pads produced from zero to three loops. The statistic is the Pearson nonparametric coefficient.

cytoplasmic volume of rough endoplasmic reticulum. The peripheral spindle cells are the only retinal cells showing kinetic changes of gap junctions and volumetric increases in rough endoplasmic reticulum that parallel the detection of angiogenic factors in extracts of the vanguard retina. It is therefore concluded that spindle cells are the peripheral inducers of the neovascularization associated with ROP.

There are more sophisticated techniques to establish the presence of angiogenic factors, such as the rabbit corneal micropocket technique [51], proliferation of fetal calf aortic endothelial cell cultures [52], noninflammatory Elvax polymer [53], and implantation of polymer slivers in the chick limb bud [54]. However, the CAM has served in a crude, preliminary effort to focus future research on the angiogenic potential of the vanguard retina in the preterm infant. Numerous angiogenic factors have been suggested, ranging from soluble vitreous proteins in the puppy [55], to plasminogen activators that bind avidly to fibrin [56], to low-molecular weight proteins [57]. To date, it has been impossible to tissue culture isolated human spindle cells to assay directly for angiogenic factors. In the future, the fetal and postnatal rat will be an appropriate animal model in which to study spindle cells. Attempts will be made to isolate the mitotic spindle cell stem line from the adventitia of the rat hyaloid artery and recover angiogenic factors in the incubation medium.

PUZZLE PIECE 8: MYOFIBROBLASTS INVADE THE VITREOUS AND CREATE TRACTIONAL FORCES

Myofibroblasts invade the vitreous simultaneously with the cessation of synthesis and secretion of angiogenic factors from spindle cells. Morphologically, the vitreous invasion of myofibroblasts occurs concomitantly with decreased gap junctions, decreased cytoplasmic volume of rough endoplasmic reticulum, and stacking of spindle cells. Myofibroblasts invade the vitreous from stem cells located at the interface between the vascular and avascular retina (shunt) and form organized sheets. There are no myofibroblasts within the subretinal space, between retinal neurons, or within the cystoid spaces of the nerve fiber layer.

Myofibroblasts are oblong cells that are distinct from spindle cells and Müller cells. Myofibroblasts contain dense cytoplasmic aggregations of actin filaments throughout the cytoplasm (Fig. 8). These filaments are distinct from the GFAP filaments, which are diagnostic for stressed Müller cells [58,59]. The contractile filaments within the cytoplasm of the myofibroblasts provide a tractional force that may result in retinal separation when they are present within the vitreous in sufficient numbers [60].

FOUR RECOMMENDATIONS REGARDING VITAMIN E PROPHYLAXIS BASED ON THE SPINDLE CELL PATHOGENESIS OF ROP

Vitamin E appears to stabilize spindle cells and to minimize the first morphologic event (gap junction formation) in a complex cascade of events that ultimately can result in total retinal detachment. We believe that four recommendations can be generated from the spindle cell hypothesis of the pathogenesis of ROP.

1. *Vitamin E supplementation must begin within the first hours of life.* Oxidative insults impinge on spindle cells at birth from oxygen fluxing across the retina, which results in spindle cell activation as early as 4 days of life (Fig. 4). We believe that these early, subclinical events prime the neovascularization that begins weeks later. Thus antioxidant protection should be given immediately at birth [4–6,36,61].

2. *The initial route of vitamin E administration will affect immediate*

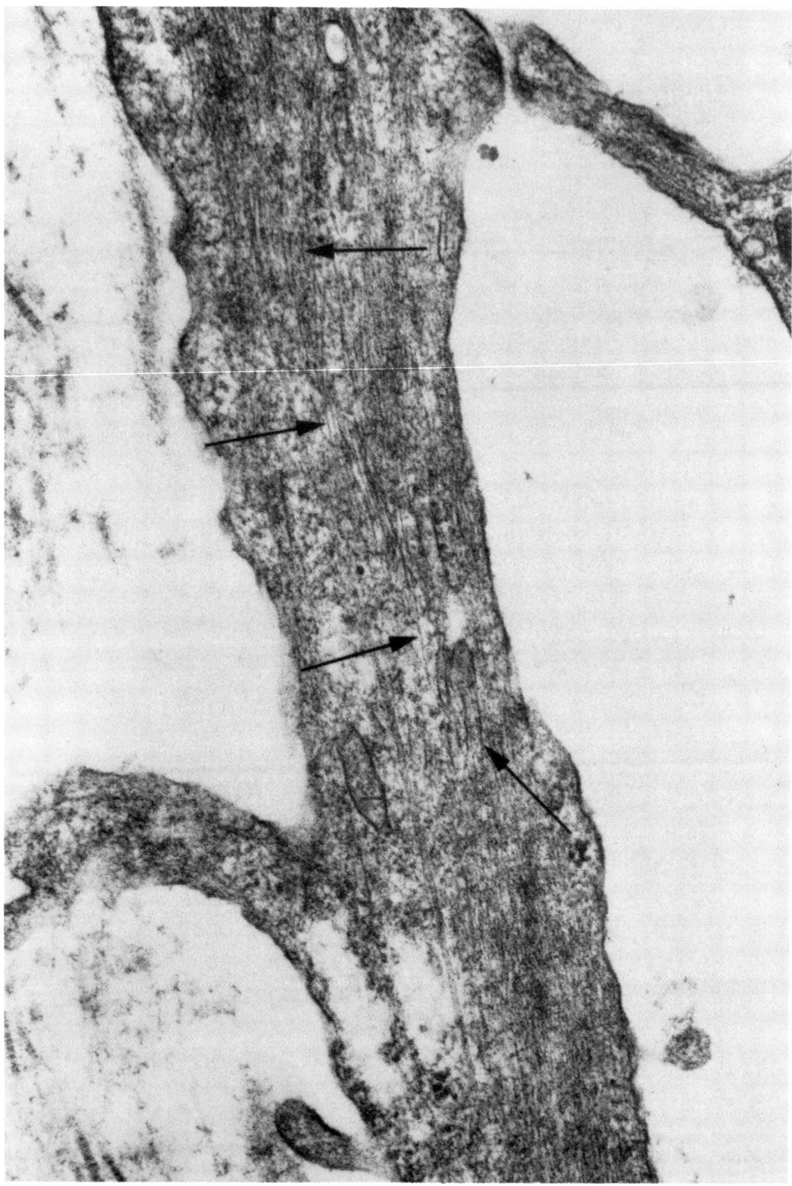

Fig. 8. Transmission electron micrograph ($\times 54,000$) demonstrating the 70 Å actin filaments (arrows) that are the dominant cytoplasmic feature of myofibroblasts that invade the vitreous concomitantly with the maturation of spindle cells and provide the tractional force that can result in retinal detachment.

retinal uptake. Perhaps this explains why the clinical trial of Phelps et al [62], which utilized initial rapid intravenous supplementation, demonstrated no efficacy of vitamin E in suppressing the development of severe ROP. The initial rapid intravenous infusion on days 1 and 2 of life may leave spindle cells vulnerable to early, irreversible oxidative damage and gap junction formation.

3. *Vitamin E supplemention need not electively raise the mean plasma vitamin E level above a threshold level.* If IRBP and stage II photoreceptors overlap the majority of the spindle cell apron (infants of $\geq$28 weeks of gestational age; Fig. 2), retinal vitamin E uptake will occur to some threshold level and protect spindle cells from extensive gap junction formation if minimal plasma sufficiency is obtained (>1.2 mg% but <3.5 mg%). If IRBP is restricted to central regions ($\leq$27 weeks of gestational age; Fig. 2), retinal vitamin E uptake will be minimal, and spindle cells will be prone to gap junction formation even with higher doses that produce toxicity [63].

4. *Vitamin E supplementation should continue until the inner retinal vessels reach the ora serrata.* As long as spindle cells are in the vanguard retina, oxygen diffusing across the retina is sufficient to trigger extensive gap junction formation between spindle cells at any time. Spindle cells are absent from the nerve fiber layer only when the inner retinal vessels reach the ora serrata in both the nasal and temporal hemispheres. Thus vitamin E supplementation should not be interrupted or halted prematurely [36].

THREE PREDICTIONS ABOUT CRYOTHERAPY BASED ON THE HYPOTHESIS OF SPINDLE CELL ACTIVATION/MATURATION AND MYOFIBROBLAST INVASION

Based on the kinetics of spindle cell activation/maturation and the invasion of myofibroblasts into the vitreous, the following three predictions about cryotherapy are made as related to stage III active disease as per the International Classification [64].

1. *When stage III mild ROP is present, 360° contiguous rows of cryomarks should be placed just anterior to the shunt and subsequent rows anterior to the first to decrease the levels of angiogenic factors.* This ablates the area with the highest density of activated spindle cells, which do not reach the temporal ora serrata in utero until the infant is 29 weeks of gestational age. In the smallest infants, cryotherapy adjacent to the ora serrata should be performed subsequently to destroy cystoid spaces in the neuroblastic retina which permit recurrent neovascularization. We believe that cryotherapy is not performed to ablate ischemic retina but to destroy activated spindle cells in the nerve fiber layer prior to extensive myofibroblast invasion and to obliterate cystoid spaces which relate to recurrent

neovascularization. If only the proliferating vessels are destroyed (too posterior), activated spindle cells continue to secrete angiogenic factors, and the correctly timed but misplaced therapy would be nonefficacious.

2. *When stage III moderate or severe ROP is present, the shunt should also be ablated.* This would obliterate not only the activated spindle cells in the vanguard retina that are secreting angiogenic factors but also the apparent site of myofibroblast invasion into the vitreous. We believe that this approach can be useful if traction is minimal; however, cryoablation of the shunt should be the last circumferential row to be done, since hemorrhage may occur and prevent direct visualization for further cryotherapy.

3. *When stage III severe ROP develops, tractional forces at this late stage are great and may induce retinal detachment despite cryotherapy.*

CONCLUSIONS

We have developed a comprehensive hypothesis regarding the role of spindle cells and their interactions with the other elements of the developing retina in ROP. This thesis is consistent with several significant pathologic features of the disease and forms an interesting framework on which to reason out the potential benefits and risks of newly proposed interventions.

ACKNOWLEDGMENTS

Whole eye donations were sensitively encouraged by the Lion's Eyes of Texas Eye Bank. The morphologic analyses included data generated by Rekha S. Mehta, Evelyn S. Brown, and Drs. A. Tim Johnson, David G. Hunter, Donna Goad, C.C. Adams, and Chaula Rana. The IRBP immunocytochemical studies were performed in collaboration with Drs. C.D.B. Bridges and Dominic M.K. Lam with rabbit antibovine IRBP antibody provided by Drs. Shao-Ling Fong and Gregory I. Liou and cryosections produced by Pat A. Glazebrook. The authors acknowledge the photographic expertise of Alexander Kogan and Gilma Miranda, the secretarial talents of Dorothy Carr, the graphic arts assistance of Tim Phelps, and the manuscript critique by Dr. Michael Osato.

REFERENCES

1. Kretzer FL, Mehta RS, Johnson AT, Hunter DG, Brown ES, Hittner HM: Vitamin E protects against retinopathy of prematurity through action on spindle cells. Nature 309:793–795, 1984.
2. Kretzer FL, McPherson AR, Rudolph AJ, Hittner HM: Pathogenic mechanism of retinopathy of prematurity: A controversial explanation for the efficacy of oral and

intramuscular vitamin E supplementation and cryotherapy. Bull NY Acad Med 61:883–900, 1985.

3. Kretzer FL, McPherson AR, Hittner HM: An interpretation of retinopathy of prematurity in terms of spindle cells: Relationship to vitamin E prophylaxis and cryotherapy. Albrecht von Graefes Arch Clin Exp Ophthalmol 224:205–214, 1986.

4. Hittner HM, Godio LB, Rudolph AJ, Adams JM, Garcia-Prats JA, Friedman Z, Kautz JA, Monaco WA: Retrolental fibroplasia: Efficacy of vitamin E in a double-blind clinical study of preterm infants. N Engl J Med 305:1365–1371, 1981.

5. Hittner HM, Godio LB, Speer ME, Rudolph AJ, Taylor MM, Blifeld C, Kretzer FL: Retrolental fibroplasia: further clinical evidence and ultrastructural support for efficacy of vitamin E in the preterm infant. Pediatrics 71:423–432, 1983.

6. Hittner HM, Speer ME, Rudolph AJ, Blifeld C, Chadda P, Holbein MEB, Godio LB, Kretzer FL: Retrolental fibroplasia and vitamin E in the preterm infant: Comparison of oral versus intramuscular:oral administration. Pediatrics 73:238–249, 1984.

7. Foos RY, Kopelow SM: Development of retinal vasculature in paranatal infants. Surv Ophthalmol 18:117–127, 1973.

8. Foos RY: Acute retrolental fibroplasia. Albrecht von Graefes Arch Clin Exp Ophthalmol 195:87–100, 1975.

9. Kretzer FL, Mehta RS, Goad D, Hittner HM: Animal models in research on retinopathy of prematurity. In McPherson AR, Hittner HM, Kretzer FL (eds): ''Retinopathy of Prematurity: Current Concepts and Controversies.'' Toronto: BC Decker, Inc, 1986, pp 79–88.

10. Gole GA, Gannon BJ, Goodger AM: Oxygen induced retinopathy: The kitten model re-examined. Aust J Ophthalmol 10:223–232, 1982.

11. Phelps DL, Rosenbaum A: Vitamin E in kitten oxygen-induced retinopathy. II. blockage of vitreal neovascularization. Arch Ophthalmol 97:1522–1526, 1979.

12. Phelps DL, Rosenbaum AL: Effects of marginal hypoxemia on recovery from oxygen-induced retinopathy in the kitten model. Pediatrics 73:1–6, 1984.

13. Henkind P, deOliveira LF: Development of retinal vessels in the rat. Invest Ophthalmol 6:520–530, 1967.

14. Shakib M, deOliveira LF, Henkind P: Development of retinal vessels II. earliest stages of vessel formation. Invest Ophthalmol 7:689–700, 1968.

15. Johnson AT, Kretzer FL, Hittner HM, Glazebrook PA, Bridges CDB, Lam DMK: Development of the subretinal space in the preterm human eye: Ultrastructural and immunocytochemical studies. J Comp Neurol 233:497–505, 1985.

16. Johnson AT, Kretzer FL: Interstitital retinol binding protein in the developing human retina: A proposed explanation for vitamin E suppression of retinopathy of prematurity. In Bridges CDB, Adler AJ (eds): ''The Interphotoreceptor Matrix in Health and Disease.'' New York: Alan R. Liss, Inc, 1985, pp 251–277.

17. Weiter JJ, Zuckerman R, Schepens CL: A model for the pathogenesis of retrolental fibroplasia based on the metabolic control of blood vessel development. Ophthalmol Surg 13:1013–1017, 1982.

18. Weiter JJ, Zuckerman R: The influence of the photoreceptor-RPE complex on the inner retina: An explanation of the beneficial effects of photocoagulation. Ophthalmology 87:1133–1139, 1980.

19. Adler VA, Cringle SJ, Constable IJ: The retinal oxygen profile in cats. Invest Ophthalmol Vis Sci 24:30–36, 1983.

20. Drujan BD, Svaetichin G: Characterization of different classes of isolated retinal cells. Vision Res 12:1777–1784, 1972.

21. Adler AJ, Martin KJ: Retinol binding proteins in bovine interphotoreceptor matrix. Biochem Biophys Res Commun 108:1601–1608, 1982.

22. Liou GI, Bridges CDB, Fong SL, Alvarez RA, Gonzalez-Fernandez F: Vitamin A transport between retina and pigment epithelium—An interstitial protein carrying endogenous retinol (interstitial retinol-binding protein). Vision Res 22:1457–1467, 1982.
23. Bunt-Milam AH, Sarri JC: Immunocytochemical localization of two retinoid-binding proteins in vertebrate retina. J Cell Biol 97:703–712, 1983.
24. Fong SL, Liou GI, Landers RA, Alvarez RA, Gonzalez-Fernandez F, Glazebrook PA, Lam DMK, Bridges CDB: Characterization, localization, and biosynthesis of an interstitial retinol-binding glycoprotein in the human eye. J Neurochem 42:1667–1676, 1984.
25. Lai YL, Wiggert B, Liu YP, Chader GJ: Interphotoreceptor retinol-binding proteins: Possible transport vehicles between compartments of the retina. Nature 298:848–849, 1982.
26. Bridges CDB, Alvarez RA, Fong SL: Vitamin A storage, esterification and interstitial retinol-binding protein in two cases of retinal degeneration, one with retinitis pigmentosa. Invest Ophthalmol Vis Sci 24 [Suppl]:141, 1983.
27. Liou GI, Bridges CDB, Alvarez RA, Fong SL: Binding specificity of interstitial retinol-binding protein—Possible physiological consequences of competition between vitamins A and E. Invest Ophthalmol Vis Sci 24[Suppl]:42, 1983.
28. Wiggert B, Bergsma DR, Lewis M, Chader GJ: Vitamin A receptors: Retinol binding in neural retina and pigment epithelium. J Neurochem 29:947–954, 1977.
29. Wiggert B, Mizukawa A, Kuwabara T, Chader GJ: Vitamin A receptors: Multiple species in retina and brain and possible compartmentalization in retinal photoreceptors. J Neurochem 30:653–659, 1978.
30. Bunt-Milam AH, Saari JC, Klock IB, Garwin GG: Zonulae adherentes pore size in the external limiting membrane of the rabbit retina. Invest Ophthalmol Vis Sci 26:1377–1380, 1985.
31. Gonzalez-Fernandez F, Landers RA, Glazebrook PA, Fong SL, Liou GI, Lam DMK, Bridges CDB: An extracellular retinol-binding glycoprotein in the eyes of mutant rats with retinal dystrophy—Development, localization, and biosynthesis. J Cell Biol 99:2092–2098, 1984.
32. Hollyfield JG, Fliesler SJ, Rayborn ME, Fong SL, Landers RA, Bridges CDB: Synthesis and secretion of interstitial retinol-binding protein by the human retina. Invest Ophthalmol Vis Sci 26:58–67, 1985.
33. Nir I, Cohen D, Papermaster DS: Immunocytochemical localization of opsin in the cell membrane of developing rat retinal photoreceptors. J Cell Biol 98:1788–1795, 1984.
34. Fliesler SJ, Anderson RE: Chemistry and metabolism of lipids in the vertebrate retina. Prog Lipid Res 22:79–131, 1983.
35. Gutcher GR, Raynor WJ, Farrell PM: An evaluation of vitamin E status in premature infants. Am J Clin Nutr 40:1078–1089, 1984.
36. Hittner HM, Rudolph AJ, Kretzer FL: Suppression of severe retinopathy of prematurity with vitamin E supplementation: Ultrastructural mechanism of clinical efficacy. Ophthalmology 91:1512–1523, 1984.
37. Graeber JE, Glaser BM: Hyperoxia alters endothelial cell proliferation. Invest Ophthalmol Vis Sci 26[Suppl]:284, 1985.
38. Sproul EW, Orlidge A, D'Amore PA: Effects of hyperoxia on the growth and integrity of vascular cells in vitro. Invest Ophthalmol Vis Sci 26[Suppl]:284, 1985.
39. Revel JP, Karnovsky M. Hexagonal array of subunits in intercellular junctions of the mouse heart and liver. J Cell Biol 33:C7–C12, 1967.
40. Yee AG, Revel JP: Loss and reappearance of gap junctions in regenerating liver. J Cell Biol 78:554–564, 1978.

41. Decker RS: Hormonal regulation of gap junction differentiation. J Cell Biol 69:669–685, 1976.

42. Turin L, Warner AE: Intracellular pH in early Xenopus embryos: Its effect on current flow between blastomeres. J Physiol 300:489–504, 1980.

43. Picard-Schneider G, Cartentier JL, Girardier L: Quantitative evaluation of gap junctions in rat brown adipose tissue after cold acclimation. J Membrane Biol 78:85–89, 1984.

44. Halliwell B, Gutteridge JMC: Lipid peroxidation, oxygen radicals, cell damage, and antioxidant therapy. Lancet 1:1396–1397, 1985.

45. Roos D, Weening RS: Defects in the oxidative killing of microorganisms by phagocytic leukocytes. In Fitzsimons DW (ed): "Oxygen Free Radicals and Tissue Damage." New York: Excerpta Medica, 1979, Vol 65, pp 225–262.

46. Glass P, Avery GB, Subramanian KNS, Keys MP, Sostek AM, Friendly DS: Effect of bright light in the hospital nursery on the incidence of retinopathy of prematurity. N Engl J Med 313:401–404, 1985.

47. Hittner HM: Retinal and central nervous system abnormalities: Syndromes which resemble retrolental fibroplasia. Metab Pediatr Syst Ophthalmol 8:5–10, 1985.

48. Glaser BM, D'Amore PA, Seppa H, Seppa S, Schiffmann E: Adult tissues contain chemoattractants for vascular endothelial cells. Nature 288:483–484, 1980.

49. Glaser BM, D'Amore PA, Michels RG, Patz A, Fenselau A: Demonstration of vasoproliferative activity from mammalian retina. J Cell Biol 84:298–304, 1980.

50. Glaser BM, D'Amore PA, Michels RG, Brunson SK, Fenselau AH, Rice T, Patz A: The demonstration of angiogenic activity from ocular tissues. Ophthalmology 87:440–446, 1980.

51. Chen CH, Chen SC: Angiogenic activity of vitreous and retinal extract. Invest Ophthalmol Vis Sci 19:596–602, 1980.

52. Fenselau A, Mello RJ: Growth stimulation of cultured endothelial cells by tumor cell homogenates. Cancer Res 36:3269–3273, 1976.

53. Langer R, Folkman J: Polymers for the sustained release of proteins and other macromolecules. Nature 263:797–880, 1976.

54. Feinberg RN, Beebe DC: Hyaluronate in vasculogenesis. Science 220:1177–1179, 1983.

55. Chen CH, Patz A: Components of vitreous-soluble proteins: Effect of hyperoxia and age. Invest Ophthalmol 15:228–232, 1976.

56. Davis JL, Connor TB, Glaser BM: Purification of tissue plasminogen activator from vascular endothelial cells. Invest Ophthalmol Vis Sci 25[Suppl]:316, 1984.

57. Elstrow SF, Schor AM, Weiss JB: Bovine retinal angiogenesis factor is a small molecule (molecular mass <600). Invest Ophthalmol Vis Sci 26:74–79, 1985.

58. Hiscott PS, Grierson I, Trombetta CJ, Rahi AHS, Marshall J, McLeod D: Retinal and epiretinal glia—An immunohistochemical study. Br J Ophthalmol 68:698–707, 1984.

59. Eisenfeld AJ, Bunt-Milam AH, Sarthy PV: Muller cell expression of glial fibrillary acidic protein after genetic and experimental photoreceptor degeneration in the rat retina. Invest Ophthalmol Vis Sci 25:1321–1328, 1984.

60. Soong HK, Eller AW, Hirose T, Hanninen L, Kenyon KR: In situ actin distribution in excised retrolental membranes in retinopathy of prematurity. Arch Ophthalmol 103:1553–1556, 1985.

61. Finer NN, Schindler RF, Peters KL, Grant GD: Vitamin E and retrolental fibroplasia: Improved visual outcome with early vitamin E. Ophthalmology 90:428–435, 1983.

62. Phelps DL, Rosenbaum A, Isenberg SJ, Leake RD, Dorey FJ: Tocopherol efficacy and safety for preventing retinopathy of prematurity: A randomized, controlled, double-masked trial. Pediatrics 79:489–500, 1987.

63. Johnson L, Bowen FW, Abbasi S, Herrmann N, Weston M, Sacks L, Porat R, Stahl G, Peckham G, Delivoria-Papadopoulos M, Quinn G, Schaffer D: Relationship of prolonged pharmacologic serum levels of vitamin E to incidence of sepsis and necrotizing entercolitis in infants with birth weight 1,500 grams or less. Pediatrics 75:619–638, 1985.
64. Committee for the Classification of Retinopathy of Prematurity: An international classification of retinopathy of prematurity. Pediatrics 74:127–133, 1984.

Commentary and Questions: Session II

In the first module of this session, the focus was very much on ROP, the pathology of the disease, particularly in its late phases; the possibility that polypeptide growth factors, the same as or similar to those that play such a beneficent role in wound healing, play a devastating role in denouément of ROP. Finally, light, at once the adequate stimulus of the visual sense organ and probably the most ubiquitous form of energy in the universe, may have a down side in that it may, in the ambient concentrations in today's nursery, be toxic to the newly formed endothelium of retinal capillaries.

Dr. Foos, drawing on what is probably the finest collection of end-stage ROP pathologic specimens in the world, has reconstructed for us a coherent picture of their pathology, attempting (but not always completely succeeding) to overlay each stage of the new International Classification of ROP [1,2] with its corresponding pathology. In this process, much is to be learned from the light microscopic picture, but much needs to be added by the electron microscope and special histochemical stains.

Moving the stage of observation several orders of magnitude lower, Dr. Hjelmeland has spelled out in detail what is known about cellular growth factors and the role they play in normal wound repair. Contrasting with that role, these same factors have been identified as having a deleterious role in diabetic retinopathy. By extension, it appears that they may have a role as well in ROP, another vasoproliferative retinopathy. Obviously, few concrete data exist today on that point, but it will certainly prove a fertile field of basic scientific endeavor in times to come.

Finally, Dr. Glass reintroduced in this session the provocative role that light and its potentially toxic effects may play in the genesis of ROP. Because high levels of ambient light 24 hours per day are part of the picture in today's newborn intensive care unit, it becomes vital to reexamine the role of light under these circumstances.

Most of the questions in this session, as can well be imagined, were directed to Dr. Glass. Among the particular questions, the audience asked what are the light levels currently in use in today's nursery. Hard data on this subject are beginning to accumulate [3–9]. Mentioned also in this regard were two animal studies (unpublished by John T. Flynn and Dale L. Phelps) that failed to show any protective effect of dark-rearing on oxygen toxicity in

Birth Defects: Original Article Series, Volume 24, Number 1, pages 169–171

the kitten model of ROP. An interesting ethical issue was raised in that the experimenter (Dr. Glass) would have been in a difficult and tenuous position had the experiment had the opposite outcome, ie, had darkness proved to be toxic rather than light.

Questions directed toward Dr. Hjelmeland sought to bring out the tissue conditions necessary to bring about the release of growth factors. Dr. Hjelmeland, in reply, pointed out that the wound repair model with damaged tissue, lower oxygen tension, inciting effector cells, such as platelets, wound macrophages, and endothelial cells might be responsible for the release of growth factors. A second model, the fibrosis model, which applies to liver, lung, and bone marrow, calls upon such cells as lymphocytes, tissue macrophages, and fibrocytes to provide stimulation of endothelial cells to migrate and that this sort of model might be leading us to the effector cells.

The next module shifted the stage of observation to the retinal blood vessels. Dr. Flower reviewed his work on angioblasts, which, he hypothesizes, give rise to spindle cells *in situ with no migration* and those in turn to the endothelium of primitive capillaries. He stressed again the role of vasotonia as being protective in the presence of hyperoxia. Finally, he pointed out that high transluminal pressure in new formed capillaries may give rise to the retinal hemorrhages seen so commonly at the site of the shunt in ROP and emphasized the likelihood that factors other than oxygen exposure alone must be considered as significant in the pathogenesis of ROP.

Dr. Kretzer reviewed his anatomic work on spindle cells, which, he believes, *do migrate* on the basis of EM micrographs. With retinal photoreceptor maturation, an oxygen sink develops in the outer retinal layers, preventing choroidal oxygen from diffusing to the inner retina. Spindle cell stress of any kind (hyperoxia, hypoxia, cold, etc) results in increased gap junction formation, and accompanying this is an increase in the rough endoplasmic reticulum that synthesizes an angiogenic factor. This in turn brings about stacking of spindle cells and metaplasia to fibroblasts containing contractile protein filaments in the cytoplasm. These latter, in turn, invade the vitreous gel to form the membranes that are so devastating to the architecture and integrity of the eye. These hypotheses, as pointed out by Dr. Silverman in the discussion, give rise to many points and questions that are distinctly testable. This anatomic theory of the genesis of ROP on the ultrastructural level was then extended to explore its potential implications in two new, and as yet unproved treatments of ROP, vitamin E [10] and cryotherapy [11]. The illustrations of the chapter are magnificent, and there are many exciting times ahead as we work our way through this new idea.

Still another theory of angiogenesis, derived primarily from work on adult animal models, was presented by Dr. Bert Glaser. In the adult animal, new blood vessel formation is a multistep process. The first step is a breakdown of the extracellular matrix. The second is the migration of endothelial cells, and the third is the proliferation of these endothelial cells. Oxygen is an important inhibitor of endothelial cell proliferation but does not inhibit the first two steps of the process. Characteristic of the new blood vessel formation are gaps in adjacent endothelial cells. On a biochemical level, prostacyclin stimulates new blood vessel formation.

Missing, unfortunately, because of the press of time, was a far reaching discussion of the similarities and dissimilarities between these three theories of angiogenesis so ably presented by Drs. Flower, Kretzer, and Glaser. There are undoubted similarities between the three, but there are points of difference. The differences are significant, as the reader is undoubtedly aware from reading the chapters. Is adult new blood vessel formation the same as that in the infant? Where are angioblasts located? Do they migrate, or are they laid down in situ in the retina? What role does gap junction area play in beginning the cascade of events leading to new blood vessel formation? What role does prostacyclin formation play? All these and many other questions will undoubtedly occur to the reader, as they must have to our speakers. Unfortunately, an opportunity was missed to probe these areas at the conference.

REFERENCES

1. Committee on Classification of Retinopathy of Prematurity: An international classification of retinopathy of prematurity. Arch Ophthalmol 102:1130–1134, 1984.
2. Committee on Classification of Retinopathy of Prematurity: An international classification of retinopathy of prematurity. II. The classification of retinal detachment. Arch Ophthalmol 105:906–912, 1985.
3. Glass P, Avery GB, Subramanian KNS, Keys MP, Sostek AM, Friendly DS: Effect of bright light in the hospital nursery on the incidence of retinopathy of prematurity. N Eng J Med 313:401–404, 1985.
4. Gottfried AW, Wallace-Lande P, Sherman-Brown S, King J, Coen C: Physical and social environment of newborn infants in special care units. Science 214:673–675, 1981.
5. Hamer RD, Dobson V, Mayer MJ: Absolute thresholds in human infants exposed to continuous illumination. Invest Ophthalmol Vis Sci 25:381–388, 1984.
6. Korones S: Physical structure and functional organization of neonatal intensive care units. In Gottfried AW, Gaiter J (eds): "Infant Stress Under Intensive Care." Baltimore: University Park Press, 1985.
7. Lawson K, Daum C, Turkewitz G: Environmental characteristics of a neonatal intensive-care unit. Child Dev 48:1633–1639, 1977.
8. Lucey JF: Nursery illumination as a factor in neonatal hyperbilirubinemia. Pediatrics 44:155–157, 1969.
9. MacLeod P, Stern L: Natural variations in environmental illumination in a newborn nursery. Pediatrics 50:131–133, 1972.
10. Committee of the Institute of Medicine: "Vitamin E and Retinopathy of Prematurity. Washington, DC: National Academy of Medicine Press, 1986, pp 1–24.
11. Palmer EA, Phelps D: Multicenter trial of cryotherapy for retinopathy of prematurity (Editorial). Pediatrics 77:428–429, 1986.

V. CLINICAL DIAGNOSIS AND CONSERVATIVE MANAGEMENT OF RETINOPATHY OF PREMATURITY

An International Classification of Retinopathy of Prematurity: Development of the Classification of the Late Stages of Retinopathy of Prematurity

John T. Flynn, MD

Bascom Palmer Eye Institute, University of Miami Medical School, Miami, Florida 33101

With the publication in 1984 [1–3] of the new International Classification of Retinopathy of Prematurity (ICROP), a significant step foward was taken in our knowledge of ROP. Lacking, however, in that first effort at classification was any attempt to classify the late stages of the disease. This in no sense reflected a failure on the part of the original committee to recognize the need to extend the classification to its natural limits, end-stage disease or regression. Lacking, rather, was expertise in the make-up of that committee in the domain of severe end-stage retina-vitreous proliferative disease, the central problem to be solved in finishing the work of classification.

To meet this need, a new committee including some with retina-vitreous experience in the surgical treatment of the severe end stages of ROP was assembled. This was buttressed by the addition of some with pathologic expertise in the later proliferative phases of the disease. Enough of the membership of the International Committee was retained to maintain its distinctive flavor of international good will; a quasi-humorous approach in their discussion of what at times appeared to be insuperable obstacles, as a safety valve; and above all a dedication to a common end, the formulation of a new classification.

This study was supported in part by Public Health Service research grant EY03513 from the National Institutes of Health; the U.S. Department of Health and Human Services, Public Health Services Division of Maternal and Child Health, Bethesda, Maryland; The March of Dimes Birth Defects Foundation, White Plains, New York; The Macula Society; The Macula Foundation; The National Children's Eye Care Foundation; The Retina Society; The Vitreous Society; and The Gonin Society.

Birth Defects: Original Article Series, Volume 24, Number 1, pages 175–183
© **1988 March of Dimes Birth Defects Foundation**

THE CONCEPTION, PARTURITION, AND BIRTH OF THE CLASSIFICATION OF THE LATE STAGES OF ROP

A small working party comprising primarily American retina-vitreous surgeons, a pathologist, and other interested parties met in preliminary session in January, 1985, at Key Biscayne, Florida, for a working weekend. Discussion of the problems posed by extending the new classification were "full and frank" in diplomatic parlance. At the end of the weekend, however, consensus was achieved on several critical issues. 1) The focus of the classification of the end stages of ROP should be on the retinal detachment and its location, nature, and anatomy rather than on any other feature of end-stage disease. 2) The stages of ICROP must be expanded to five rather than four stages. 3) The signs of regression of ROP should be treated as a separate entity, existing beside but not becoming an intrinsic part of the classification.

From the working notes of that conference, a rough outline of the end-stage ROP classification emerged. The full committee, consisting of 21 members from seven countries (see Appendix), met in October of 1985 in San Francisco immediately after the American Academy of Ophthalmology annual meeting in that city. Once again, as with the smaller working party, the viewpoints of the membership were fully and frankly aired. Three issues, which were not resolved at the January meeting, were resolved at this meeting: first, the commitment to remain with the basic ICROP format of recording retinal involvement by zones and sectors; second, the need to organize the signs of regression into peripheral and central, vascular and retinal changes; and, third, to provide interested parties with a computer-compatible coding form that allowed full description of an end-stage eye. When that meeting adjourned, the committee took one final step, that of posing for a picture taken by Akio Majima, the group's indefatigable cameraman (Fig. 1).

Since broad agreement in principle on the contents of a new classification had been reached among the members, the task of writing the final document was simplified. This went through several drafts before emerging in publishable form; the latter occured in July, 1987 [4].

CLASSIFICATION OF THE LATE STAGES OF ROP

The system that emerged from the committee's deliberations made the morphology and location of the retinal detachment in the eye the centerpiece of the new classification. To accomplish this, stage IV of the old ICROP (retinal detachment) was renamed subtotal retinal detachment, and stage V, total retinal detachment, was added:

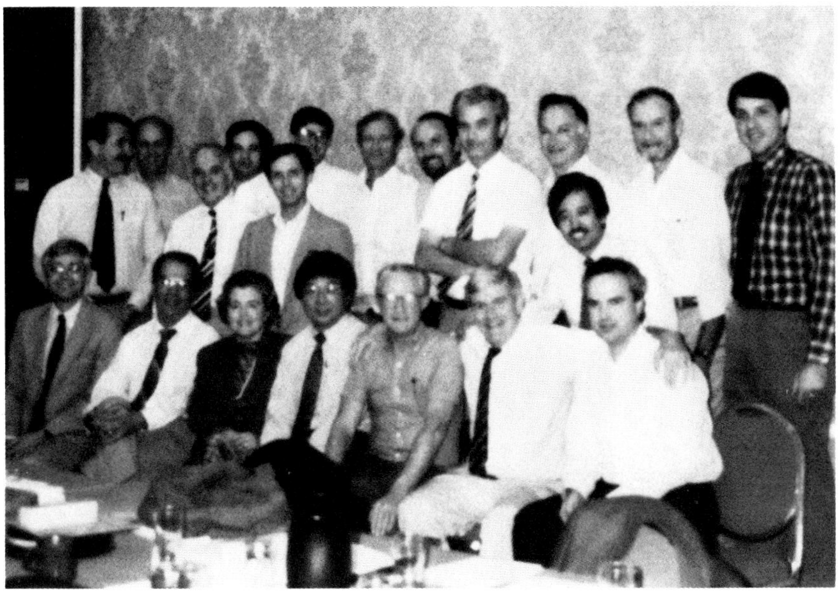

Fig. 1. Group photograph of the members of the International Committee at the end of the deliberations in San Francisco, October, 1985. Front row (left to right): T. Topping, R. Machemer, A. McPherson, T. Hirose, A. McCormick, J. Flynn, G. Quinn. Second row (left to right): M. Trese, A. Garner, T. Aaberg, F. Koerner, Y. Tanaka. Third row (left to right): S. Charles, B. Cohen, J. Clarkson, I. Ben-Sira, H. Paulmann, W. Tasman, R. Foos, J. Robertson. Not pictured: A. Majima, Cameraman.

Stage 4: Subtotal Retinal Detachment

This stage was further subdivided by whether involvement of the macula was recognized or not, for obvious reasons.

Subtotal retinal detachment without macular involvement (Fig. 2).

In essence, this is a peripheral, concave traction detachment, which, although it may exert traction on the posterior pole structures, such as vessels and macula, does not detach the latter. For this reason, the prognosis for vision is usually good. (See Color Section, page C2).

Subtotal retinal detachment with macular involvement (Fig. 3).

Here, the traction detachment extends to involve the macula in a typical fold. This severely limits the visual potential of the eye, although other areas of the retina may remain attached. (See Color Section, page C2).

Stage 5: Total Retinal Detachment (Fig. 4).

This most catastrophic outcome of ROP is characterized by a total traction detachment, which usually begins as a concave, open-funnel type. However because of complex, poorly understood traction forces developing in the vitreous gel of the eye, the retina oftens assumes a closed or partially closed configuration. The visual result is the same regardless of the retina's configuration, blindness or near blindness, with a total retinal detachment. (See Color Section, page C2).

REGRESSION (TABLE I)

Recognizing that the task would be left unfinished without describing the most common changes of ROP, the committee undertook to delineate the changes of regression. As mentioned above, regression and its accompanying changes were not considered an integral part of the ROP classification, directed as it was toward describing the detachment aspect of the disease. The committee chose to organize the description of these changes by separating peripheral from central and vascular from retinal changes. In so doing, it recognized that to separate them is to ignore the dynamic and interactive aspects of one of the most interesting phenomena connected with ROP and thereby to narrow the base of its description to a morphologic one. For simplicity, the committee opted for this latter solution, which, however, leaves room for patterns to emerge as data on many infants and children with regressed ROP are developed from the use of this system. The examiner can, using the simple ''check-off'' format, code his observations in a quick and complete manner.

THE ANTERIOR SEGMENT

Often neglected in any description of ROP are significant anterior segment changes, particularly in the end stages of severe ROP. To meet this need, the committee included in its description of the disease the condition of the cornea, the depth of the anterior chamber, and the conditions of the iris (Fig. 5—See Color Section, page C2), the lens, and the retrolenticular space (Fig. 6A,B—See Color Section, page C3). We also called attention to the intraocular pressure, an often overlooked cause of devastating loss. With this, the committee concluded its work by furnishing a computer-compatible form to aid in coding the disease (Fig. 7).

THE FUTURE

To what use should this now finished classification of ROP be put? The first stages of the classification found an immediate application in the current trial of cryotherapy in ROP [5]. With this new addition, a coherent picture has emerged of the end stage of the disease consistent with all that we know about it at present. In particular, the classification of the retinal detachment can serve as a basis for a rational approach to a study of the therapy of retinal

RETINOPATHY OF PREMATURITY (ROP) OPHTHALMIC EXAMINATION RECORD II

<u>BIOGRAPHICAL DATA</u>

Name________________________________ Hospital # __ __ __ __ __ __ __

Birthdate (MM/DD/YY) __ __/__ __/__ __   Sex (M=1, F=2) __

Birthweight (grams) __ __ __ __   Gestational Age (weeks) __ __

Multiple Births (Single-1, Twin=2, Triplet=3) __

<u>EXAMINATION:</u>

Date of Exam __ __/__ __/__ __   Examiner's Initials or # __ __ __

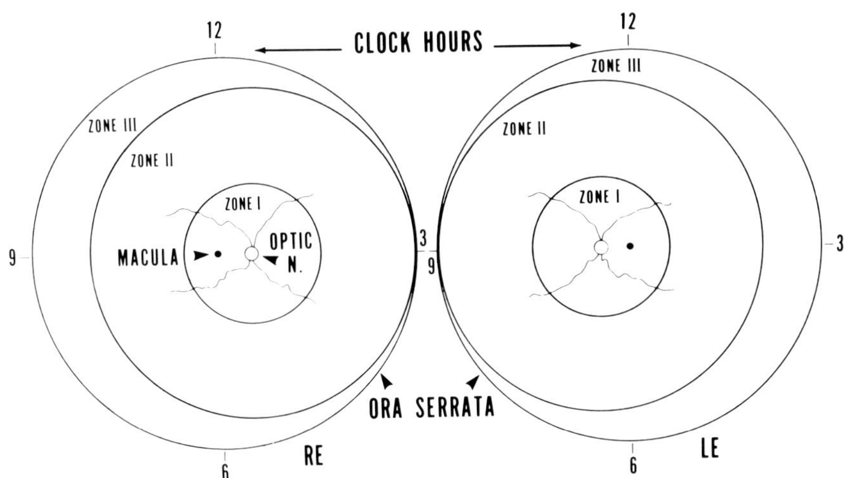

Fig. 7. Ophthalmologic examination form for retinopathy of prematurity.

detachment in this disease. There are many unanswered questions in this area, not the least of which is the fundamental one; namely, does this therapy help these infants see any better than they do without it? Suffice it to say that the completion of the classification comes at a most felicitous time in the development of our approach to end-stage ROP.

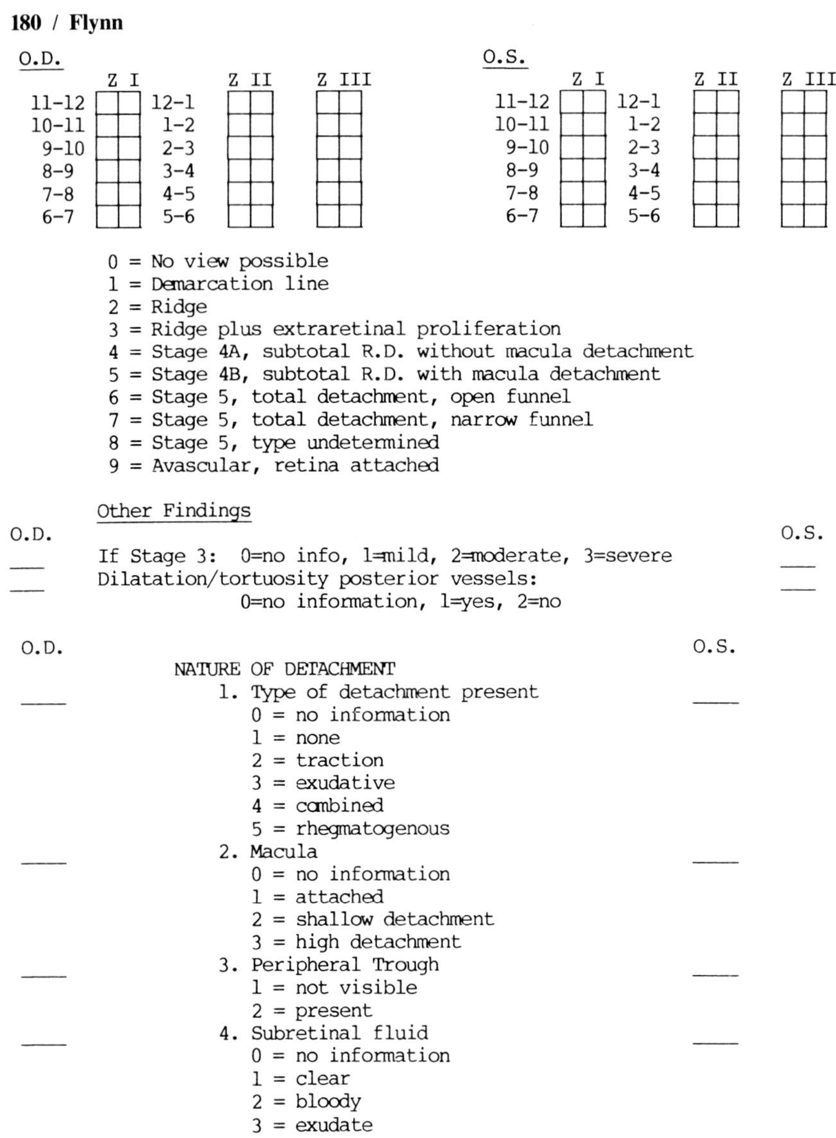

Fig. 7.   Ophthalmologic examination form for retinopathy of prematurity (Continued).

SUMMARY AND CONCLUSIONS

In another publication [6], an agenda for ROP was outlined for the future. High on that list was the completion of the task of classifying ROP. This has been accomplished, but it is obvious that no classification is any better than

```
                    ANTERIOR SEGMENT
                    (0 = no information, 1 = yes, 2 = no)

O.D.                1. Cornea                              O.S.
____                   Clear                               ____
                       Cloudy                              ____
                    2. Anterior chamber
____                   Normal depth                        ____
____                   Shallow                             ____
____                   Absent                              ____
                    3. Iris
____                   Normal                              ____
____                   Active vasculature                  ____
____                   Atrophy                             ____
____                   Synechiae                           ____
                    4. Pupil
____                   Normal                               ____
____                   Fixed                                ____
____                   Secluded                             ____
                    5. Lens
____                   Clear                                ____
____                   Cataract                             ____
                    6. Retrolental space
____                   Clear                                ____
____                   Vascularized membrane                ____
____                   Opaque membrane                      ____
                    7. Vitreous
____                   Clear                                ____
____                   Hemorrhage                           ____
```

Fig. 7.   Ophthalmologic examination form for retinopathy of prematurity (Continued).

the use to which it is put. This is the case with this work. Its implementation in a prospective, controlled trial of surgical therapy of end-stage ROP will more than justify the labors of all who participated in its development.

ACKNOWLEDGMENTS

We thank Allison Medical Illustrators, Inc. (Eric Grafman, MS, Barbara Cousins, and Leona M. Allison, MS), for the illustrations.

Table I. Regressed ROP.

(0 = No information, 1 = Present, 2 = Absent)

A. Peripheral Changes

<u>Vascular</u>

O.D.		O.S.
___	Failure to vascularize to ora	___
___	Abnormal branching	___
___	Vascular arcades	___
___	Telangiectatic vessels	___

<u>Retinal</u>

O.D.		O.S.
___	Pigmentary changes	___
___	V-R interface changes	___
___	Thin retina	___
___	Peripheral folds	___
___	Vitreous membranes	___

B. Posterior Changes

<u>Vascular</u>

O.D.		O.S.
___	Tortuosity	___
___	Straightening of vessels	___
___	Decrease in angle of insertion of major temporal arcade	___

<u>Retinal</u>

O.D.		O.S.
___	Pigmentary changes	___
___	Distortion/ectopia of macula	___
___	Fold of retina	___
___	V-R interface changes	___
___	Vitreous membranes	___
___	Dragging of retina over disc	___
___	Traction/rhegmatogenous retinal detachment	___

REFERENCES

1. The Committee for the Classification of Retinopathy of Prematurity: An international classification of retinopathy of prematurity. Arch Ophthalmol 102:1130–1134, 1984.
2. An International Classification of Retinopathy of Prematurity: Pediatrics 74:127–133, 1984.
3. Committee for the Classification of Retinopathy of Prematurity: An international classification of retinopathy of prematurity. Br J Ophthalmol 68:690–697, 1984.
4. The International Committee for the Classification of the Late Stages of Retinopathy of Prematurity: An international classification of retinopathy of prematurity: II. The classification of retinal detachment. Arch. Ophthalmol. 105:906–912, 1987.
5. Palmer EA, Phelps D: Multicenter trial for cryotherapy for retinopathy of prematurity (Editorial). Pediatrics 77:428–429, 1986.
6. Flynn JT: An international classification of retinopathy of prematurity. In Silverman WA, Flynn JT (eds): "Contemporary Issues in Fetal and Neonatal Medicine: Vol. 2: Retinopathy of Prematurity." Boston: Blackwell Scientific Publications, 1985, pp 1–17.

APPENDIX: COMMITTEE MEMBERS

Thomas Aaberg, M.D., United States
Isaac Ben-Sira, M.D., Israel
Steve Charles, M.D., United States
John Clarkson, M.D., United States
Ben Zane Cohen, M.D., United States
John Flynn, M.D., United States
Robert Foos, M.D., United States
Alec Garner, M.D., Ph.D., Great Britain
Tatsuo Hirose, M.D., United States
Fritz Koerner, M.D., Switzerland
Robert Machemer, M.D., United States
Akio Majima, M.D., Japan
Andrew McCormick, M.D., Canada
Alice McPherson, M.D., United States
Helge Paulmann, M.D., Federal Republic of Germany
Graham Quinn, M.D., United States
Joseph Robertson, M.D., United States
Yasuhiko Tanaka, M.D., Japan
William Tasman, M.D., United States
Trexler Topping, M.D., United States
Michael Trese, M.D., United States

Diagnosis and Early Follow-Up of Retinopathy of Prematurity

Robert E. Kalina, MD

Department of Ophthalmology, University of Washington, Seattle, Washington 98195

Modern techniques of neonatal intensive care have resulted in increased survival rates among low-birthweight infants at greatest risk of developing retinopathy of prematurity (ROP). A close working relationship should be established between ophthalmologists interested in ROP and the medical and nursing staffs of each neonatal unit housing premature infants. A comprehensive screening program should be established that will ensure identification of affected infants. Although results of treatment of ROP remain uncertain at this time, early and accurate diagnosis has great value in counseling parents about visual prognosis. Also, children with arrested ROP are at risk for later visual complications that may be preventable, and proper identification of such infants will permit proper referral and follow-up.

SELECTION OF INFANTS FOR ROP SCREENING

The incidence, and perhaps also the severity, of ROP is related inversely to birthweight [1]. A large collaborative study [2] found that birthweight was more reliable and correlated better with development or absence of development of ROP than did gestational age. Accordingly, a birthweight criterion for screening appears logical.

Any screening examination must balance effort and risks against benefits. In 1984, I surveyed ophthalmic experts interested in ROP and found that they used upper limit screening criteria ranging from 1,300 to 2,000 gm. My experience and that of others is that visually significant ROP is rare if birthweight exceeds 1,500 gm. Since risks of screening larger infants are small, it may be best to err on the larger rather than the smaller side.

It is of interest that none of the respondents to my survey used oxygen administration as a criterion to select infants for examination. This attitude reflects the modern belief that prematurity rather than oxygen administration is the most important factor in determining whether ROP will develop.

Birth Defects: Original Article Series, Volume 24, Number 1, pages 185–191
© **1988 March of Dimes Birth Defects Foundation**

However, certain infants above the birthweight screening criterion may have other risk factors for ROP, such as prolonged administration of supplemental oxygen [2] or general anesthesia with hyperoxygenization [3]. Such infants also should be selected for screening by the neonatal intensive care unit staff, but they rarely if ever will develop ROP. In light of present knowledge, many previously reported cases of what appeared to be ROP in term infants now must be suspected to have been a manifestation of autosomal dominant exudative vitreoretinopathy [4].

INITIAL EXAMINATION FOR ROP

The American Academy of Pediatrics [5] recommends an initial ophthalmoscopic screening examination for premature infants 6–8 weeks after birth. Palmer [6] studied this issue and found that an initial screening examination 7–9 weeks after birth was likely to identify most affected infants, while the disorder was still active but before it had gone on to severe proportions. The 1984 survey that I performed showed an acceptable range of 4–9 weeks for the initial screening examination. The collaborative CRYO-ROP study initiated calls for earlier first examination at 28–35 days after birth to study the natural history of ROP and to be certain that infants are identified immediately if they reach criteria for randomization to treatment [7].

It is important to recognize that the only eyes at risk for development of ROP are those in which the peripheral retina is incompletely vascularized. Whereas a timing criterion of an arbitrary number of weeks following birth is reasonable for infants remaining in the neonatal unit for extended periods of time, careful ophthalmoscopy will disclose younger infants who no longer are at risk for ROP and older infants who remain at risk. My own practice is to examine infants at the time of discharge or at 6 weeks of age, whichever occurs earlier.

A three-level regional network for perinatal care has been developed [8]. Premature infants managed acutely at a level-three medical center may be transferred to a level-two or a level-one community hospital after initial stabilization. Transfer may occur when the peripheral retina is incompletely vascularized and prior to the time when changes of ROP might be expected to be observed. The ophthalmologist at the level-three facility should establish a network of trained and interested ophthalmologists located near level-two and level-one facilities who are willing to take on the responsibility for ROP screening and follow-up.

Ophthalmoscopy while infants are receiving supplemental oxygen may show arterial constriction if the arterial oxygen concentration (PaO_2) is elevated [9]. These correlations are technically difficult, and modern techniques for monitoring PaO_2 have made such attempts obsolete. Ophthalmoscopy of critically ill newborn premature infants interferes with care, poses unnecessary hazards, and should not be performed.

EXAMINATION TECHNIQUE FOR ROP

The bright illumination and wide field provided by the binocular indirect ophthalmoscope makes it the instrument of choice for the examination of premature infants [10]. An eyelid speculum is essential. The eye often can be rotated into desired positions of gaze by use of the doll's head phenomenon. Scleral depression can be performed by use of a flat instrument such as a lens loop or paper clip placed directly in the conjunctival fornix. The scleral depressor used in conjunction with indirect ophthalmoscopy in adults is too bulky.

Although pupils generally dilate well in premature infants, the absolute pupillary size is small, and even maximal pharmacologic dilatation may provide only marginal visibility of the fundus. The combination of an anticholinergic and a sympathomimetic is required to achieve maximum dilatation. Although the risks of these agents are lessened when premature infants are not screened during the first few weeks of life, paralytic ileus [11] has been described following the use of anticholinergics, and significant blood pressure increases [12] may result from topical sympathomimetics. Accordingly, the lowest drug concentrations producing the desired results should be used. All respondents to my 1984 survey used a combination of an anticholinergic and a sympathomimetic. Many combinations were used, and complications reported were few.

We studied the effects of progressively dilute concentrations of mydriatics in premature infants and found that concentrations could be reduced to 0.4% cyclopentolate and 2.0% phenylephrine before effectiveness began to be lost (R. E. Kalina and E. F. Carpel, unpublished observations). No such preparation is commercially available, but this or a similar solution can be prepared easily. Two instillations at 5 minute intervals provide better pupillary dilatation than a single instillation. Although occlusion of the lacrimal puncta theoretically reduces systemic absorption, this procedure is technically cumbersome, and we have not found it effective. However, we do remove excess solution from the skin of the eyelids.

Ophthalmologists who undertake screening programs for ROP in neonatal units should become thoroughly familiar with the normal appearances of the premature infant's eye [10]. Opacities in the media include residual pupillary membrane strands, transient cataracts of prematurity, and hyaloid vascular remnants, with surrounding vitreous haze. The optic disk appears normal, but the macula is poorly formed. Retinal hemorrhages are frequent in all newborn infants examined soon after birth. Of greatest importance is the recognition that the normal incompletely vascularized peripheral retina is grey and opaque. The earliest signs of ROP appear at the junction of vascularized and nonvascularized retina.

REPEAT EXAMINATION FOR ROP

Infants in whom the peripheral retina has become completely vascularized no longer are at risk for ROP and need no further examination even if still requiring oxygen. Parents may be told that the child has escaped the risk of ROP but remains at risk for any other ocular disorders of childhood. Infants in whom the peripheral retina is incompletely vascularized or in whom active ROP is present need repeat examinations.

The timing of repeat examinations for infants with ROP is influenced heavily by attitude toward surgical intervention. Those who believe in the effectiveness of treatment for intermediate stages of ROP would recommend frequent examination for infants with early ROP. Those who believe that no treatment is effective or that late vitrectomy is the treatment of choice would advise less frequent examinations. The CRYO-ROP study [7] will require examination at intervals of 2 weeks or less until the process is shown to be resolving.

Whether cryotherapy or another form of treatment ultimately is shown to be effective for ROP, periodic reexamination of infants with active ROP should be performed until the process has resolved or stabilized. Information is collected that allows parental involvement and prognostication for vision and future complications. A reasonable and practical time to perform repeat examination is a range of 1 week for an infant with severe ROP to 6–8 weeks in an infant with limited neovascularization in the far periphery of the retina.

VISUAL PROGNOSIS IN ACUTE ROP

When a diagnosis of ROP is first made, parents and neonatal staff legitimately demand to know the severity of the problem and the prognosis for vision. Unfortunately, published studies that contain natural history data suffer from lack of uniformity of the examination techniques and grading systems used, and it is difficult to summate them to arrive at a prognosis for deterioration or recovery for a given infant. Widespread future use of the new international classification of ROP [13] should facilitate the development of more useful information.

Nevertheless, it is certain that the risk of visual impairment parallels the severity of acute ROP. Factors thought to carry a poor prognosis for spontaneous regression have included extensive peripheral neovascularization, posterior location of neovascularization, and vascular tortuosity and engorgement [14], but all these can regress spontaneously with few or no sequelae. My own experience, however, agrees with that of Tasman [15] in that eyes with peripheral retinal detachment nearly always develop permanent changes with visual signficance. However, peripheral retinal detachment often does resolve to leave an impaired but highly useful eye. The greater the extent of retinal detachment, the more grave the prognosis for vision, especially when the macula is involved.

Most parents can be informed that ROP is a potentially vision-threatening process but that the prognosis generally is favorable [2]. Published statistics may distort the incidence of blindness among infants affected by ROP since reported series often have been based on infants selected because they were at high risk for severe ROP [15,16].

With increased public awareness of the need for visual experience to stimulate development of vision, parents often ask whether ROP will interfere with visual maturation. Since the proliferative changes of ROP are in the retinal periphery, the developing visually functional retina in the posterior pole of the eye is not affected except in the most severe cases of ROP involving the macula. There is no clinical evidence that visual development is impaired in infants with spontaneously regressed peripheral ROP. However, such infants are at risk for amblyopia resulting from strabismus or asymmetric errors of refraction and require periodic ophthalmologic examination [17,18].

PREVENTION OF ROP

When the diagnosis of ROP is made, parents understandably ask whether it could have been prevented. They can and should be told that some very low-birthweight infants develop severe ROP in spite of the best medical care available. Incidence rates may vary somewhat because of geographic, ethnic, racial, or other unknown factors, but severe ROP continues to occur in every center caring for very small infants.

Although there is little doubt that oxygen administration in excess of need is related to ROP, most cases develop after provision of medical care entirely within the framework of good medical practice utilizing life-saving measures. Such infants typically require more intense care and longer durations of oxygen therapy than their unaffected peers [2]. Parents can be told without hesitation that prematurity is the most important factor in their child's illness.

Since ROP is related directly to prematurity and since the results of treatment of ROP are uncertain, what are the prospects for prevention? Considerable progress has been made in identification of high-risk mothers, such as those carrying twins. When identified early, these women can receive special prenatal attention and the infants can be delivered adjacent to a neonatal intensive care unit. However, prevention of prematurity is a social as well as a medical problem [19]. Incidence rates are highest among disadvantaged segments of the population, among whom nutrition and prenatal care may be inadequate. Cigarette smoking, on the increase among young women, has been associated with premature delivery, as has alcohol and drug abuse.

The very success of neonatal intensive care ensures a supply of patients. Cesarean sections are being performed to deliver distressed infants at ever earlier gestational ages [20]. Prior to modern neonatal intensive care, cesarean section often was not performed for such fetuses, since they could not be expected to survive.

Physicians, scientists, and other members of the health care team should continue laboratory and clinical studies that will contribute to the survival of premature infants and preservation of their vision. They should also be aware of their broader societal role in preventing premature birth.

SUMMARY

Low-birthweight premature infants should be screened for ROP by indirect ophthalmoscopy. Repeat examination should be performed until retinal vascularization is complete, regression and stabilization have occurred, or surgical intervention is recommended. Parents should be informed of the diagnosis early and counseled periodically regarding prognosis. Infants with arrested cicatricial changes of ROP should have periodic ophthalmologic examinations for late complications. The emergence of low birthweight as the single most important factor causing ROP calls for societal efforts to reduce the incidence of premature birth.

REFERENCES

1. Kalina RE, Karr DJ: Retrolental fibroplasia: Experience over two decades in one institution. Ophthalmology 89:91–95, 1982.
2. Kinsey VE, Arnold HJ, Kalina RE et al: PaO$_2$ levels and retrolental fibroplasia: A report of the cooperative study. Pediatrics 60:655–668, 1977.
3. Betts EK, Downes JJ, Schaffer DB et al: Retrolental fibroplasia and oxygen administration during general anesthesia. Anesthesiology 47:518–520, 1977.
4. van Nouhuys CE: "Dominant Exudative Vitreoretinopathy and Other Vascular Developmental Disorders of the Peripheral Retina." The Hague: W. Junk NV Publishers, 1982.
5. American Academy of Pediatrics: "Guidelines for Perinatal Care." Evanston, IL: American Academy of Pediatrics, 1983.
6. Palmer EA: Optimal timing of examination for acute retrolental fibroplasia. Ophthalmology 88:662–668, 1981.
7. "Manual of Procedures: Multicenter Trial for Cryotherapy for Retinopathy of Prematurity." Bethesda, MD: National Eye Institute, 1985.

8. McCormick MC, Shapiro S, Starfield BH: The regionalization of perinatal services. Summary of the evaluation of a national demonstration program. JAMA 253:799–804, 1985.

9. Patz A: New role of the ophthalmologist in prevention of retrolental fibroplasia. Arch Ophthalmol 78:565–568, 1967.

10. Kalina RE: Examination of the premature infant. Ophthalmology 86:1690–1694, 1979.

11. Bauer CR, Trottier MCT, Stern L: Systemic cyclopentolate (cyclogyl) toxicity in the newborn infant. J Pediatr 82:501–505, 1973.

12. Borromeo-McGrail V, Bordiuk JM, Keitel H: Systemic hypertension following ocular administration of 10% phenylephrine in the neonate. J Pediatr 51:1032–1036, 1973.

13. The Committee for the Classification of Retinopathy of Prematurity: An international classification of retinopathy of prematurity. Arch Ophthalmol 102:1130–1134, 1984.

14. Flynn JT: An international classification of retinopathy of prematurity: Clinical experience. Ophthalmology 92:987–994, 1985.

15. Tasman W: The natural history of active retinopathy of prematurity. Ophthalmology 91:1499–1503, 1984.

16. Flynn JT, Cassady J, Essner D et al: Fluorescein angiography in retrolental fibroplasia: Experience from 1969 to 1977. Ophthalmology 86:1700–1723, 1979.

17. Kushner BJ: Strabismus and amblyopia associated with regressed retinopathy of prematurity. Arch Ophthalmol 100:256–261, 1982.

18. Schaffer DB, Quinn GE, Johnson L: Sequelae of arrested mild retinopathy of prematurity. Arch Ophthalmol 102:373–376, 1984.

19. Rinke CM: Infant mortality and the low birth weight infant (editorial). JAMA 253:826, 1985.

20. Danforth DN: Cesarean section. JAMA 253:811–818, 1985.

Long-Term Follow-Up of Regressed Retinopathy of Prematurity

Burton J. Kushner, MD

Department of Ophthalmology, University of Wisconsin School of Medicine, Madison, Wisconsin 53706

The milder stages of retinopathy of prematurity (ROP) typically do not lead to serious cicatricial disease yet may result in a number of ocular problems requiring attention. A number of factors influence the appropriate follow-up protocol for infants with ROP. These include gestational age at birth, stage of ROP at the time of discharge from the nursery, rapidity of the evolution of the lesion ROP, and the possible development of ocular complications of regressed ROP. In addition, various factors influence the appropriate follow-up of the premature infants found in the nursery not to have ROP.

FOLLOW-UP OF THE PREMATURE INFANTS NOT HAVING ROP

It has been suggested that the ideal time to examine the premature infant for ROP is at 7–9 weeks of age [1]. Frequently, infants are being discharged from, or transferred from, the infant intensive care unit (ICU) prior to that recommended age. If an infant is discharged from the infant ICU prior to 7 weeks of age, and if the ocular examination does not show ROP prior to discharge, a follow-up examination should be carried out between 7 and 9 weeks of age unless the retinal periphery is completely, or almost completely, vascularized. If it is, the infant is not at risk for developing ROP. Similarly, if an examination in the nursery does not show the presence of ROP at 7–9 weeks of age and if the retina is completely, or almost completely, vascularized, a follow-up examination is not necessary. If the retina is incompletely vascularized, outpatient follow-up should be arranged and continued until vascularization is complete. Generally, a follow-up examination in 4–6 weeks is adequate. The more posterior the anterior edge of the developing vasculature lies, the more at risk the child is for developing ROP. Very incomplete vascularization at the time of discharge may suggest earlier follow-up. Also, the longer the time that has elasped since an infant

Birth Defects: Original Article Series, Volume 24, Number 1, pages 193–199

has been exposed to situations that increase the risk of ROP (respiratory problems, exchange transfusions, etc), the less the risk of developing ROP. An infant who has been exposed to such factors shortly prior to a normal predischarge examination, may possibly need to be seen sooner in follow-up.

FOLLOW-UP OF INFANTS WITH MILD ROP

The initial postdischarge follow-up examination for a child with mild ROP should be influenced by the location of the disease and the speed with which it is evolving. The more posterior, the greater the risk that it will progress to severe ROP. Also, disease that is located more posteriorly may tend to deteriorate more rapidly. When ROP regresses, it tends to do so slowly; when it deteriorates, it tends to do so rapidly. Therefore, if an infant has been seen several times prior to discharge, and the disease is relatively anterior (zone 3), and it has evolved slowly over several examinations, an outpatient follow-up examination can be recommended in 5–6 weeks. If an infant had not been seen several times prior to discharge, yet if the disease is mild and relatively anterior (zone 3), follow-up may be somewhat earlier, such as at 4–5 weeks. If, however, the disease is fairly posterior (zone 1 or early zone 2), yet still mild, and the examiner does not have a good feel for the rapidity with which a particular infant's disease is evolving, follow-up in 2–3 weeks would be appropriate. Once it is determined that the disease is not deteriorating, the frequency of the examinations can be spread out until total regression of the active lesion occurs.

THE CHILD WITH SEVERE ROP

Frequently, an infant is medically ready for discharge from the infant ICU around the time when the diagnosis of severe ROP is made. The principles indicated above influence the appropriate follow-up time. The more posterior the disease, and the more rapidly it is evolving, the earlier the infant should be examined after discharge. The more anterior the disease, and the slower it is evolving, the more time that can elapse before follow-up. A child with "plus" disease, and the more advanced stage of ROP, may need to be seen in several days to one week. This may necessitate the infant staying in the hospital longer.

FOLLOW-UP AFTER TOTAL REGRESSION OF ROP

It has been found that infants who develop even the most mild forms of ROP, and in whom the lesion totally regresses, have a significant incidence of high refractive errors, amblyopia, and strabismus [2]. Once the lesion of

ROP regresses, infants should be followed as one would follow a child who is at high risk for developing a disorder of binocular vision. Although it may be expedient to have an infant dilated prior to seeing the ophthalmologist while the active lesion of ROP is being followed, once it has regressed the child should be seen prior to dilatation, with careful attention paid to fixation behavior and ocular motility. This frequently involves seeing the child at intervals of 3–6 months after resolution of the lesion of ROP, during the first year of life, with a gradual increase in the time between visits approaching yearly. It is recommended that the child be followed as a strabismus or amblyopia suspect, until he or she is literate and is confirmed as having normal visual acuity.

FOLLOW-UP OF CHILDREN DEVELOPING MILD CICATRICIAL DISEASE

Numerous ocular complications occur in infants who develop even mild forms of cicatricial disease. In such children, follow-up should include careful assessment of ocular motility and refractive error, with the timing for follow-up visits being influenced by the specific findings.

High refractive errors, typically myopia, are frequent in infants who develop even mild cicatricial changes after ROP. Often, very high myopic refractive errors can accompany a nearly normal-appearing retina. Because ROP is often asymmetric, the subsequent high refractive errors are often asymmetric, leading to anisometropic amblyopia.

Not only is there a high incidence of strabismus in infants with regressed ROP, the types of strabismic conditions occurring tend to be complicated. Even after mild ROP regresses, leaving a nearly normal-appearing retina, there is a higher than normal incidence of strabismus with ``A'' or ``V'' patterns, nystagmus, or the nystagmus compensation syndrome [3]. Nevertheless, these motility disorders, as well as the frequently associated amblyopia, tend to respond well to standard amblyopia and strabismus management.

With the presence of cicatricial disease, management of strabismus can become more complicated. A null-point nystagmus is frequently present, resulting in a head turn (Fig. 1). Because the disease is often asymmetric, the nonfixing eye frequently has much poorer vision than the fixing eye, resulting in the necessity to perform surgery on the patient's ``good eye.'' In one large series of patients with abnormal head postures resulting from nystagmus, almost one-fourth of the patients had nystagmus associated with ROP [4]. Surgery of the Kestenbaum type can be helpful for these patients.

If the cicatrization results in a dragging of the macula temporally, and if the patient has good enough visual acuity to fixate in the macular area, he or

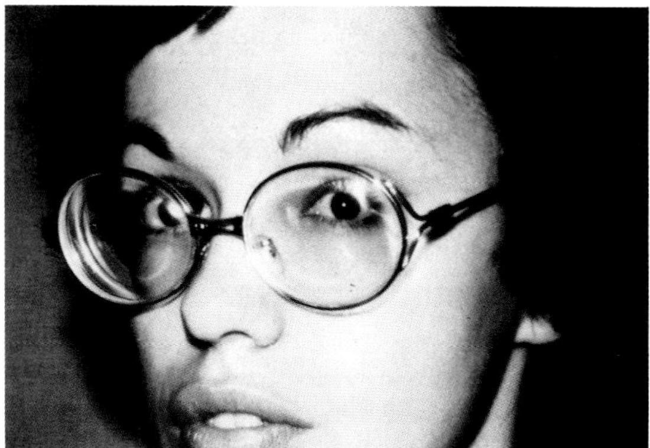

Fig. 1. Patient with mild cicatricial retrolental fibroplasia in her right eye fixates with a marked face turn to the right to put the eye in the null point of her nystagmus. Her left eye has minimal visual function. Her preferred head posture has her looking through the periphery of her highly myopic lens, which furthers decreases her visual acuity. (Reproduced with permission from Blackwell Scientific Publications, Inc., from "Retinopathy of Prematurity," edited by W.A. Silverman and J.T. Flynn.)

she may have the appearance of having an exotropia when in fact this technically is not so (positive angle kappa, Fig. 2). This can produce some very difficult-to-treat cosmetic problems. In some instances, the use of prisms may improve cosmesis; however, this may be at the expense of visual acuity and may result in there being no adequate solution of the problem [5].

In many instances, the amblyopia associated with regressed ROP is due to anisometropia or strabismus and responds to standard amblyopia management. It is therefore critical that careful attention be paid to visual acuity or fixation behavior in infants with ROP.

Even mild-to-moderate degrees of cicatrization from ROP can result in a predisposition for developing acute angle closure glaucoma secondary to the narrow angle pupil block mechanism [6]. Because this has been recognized only recently, many patients from the retrolental fibroplasia (RLF) epidemic of the 1940s and 1950s are unaware that they are at significant risk for having this complication and are not receiving regular ophthalmologic care. As many of the older RLF patients from that epidemic are now in their 30s and 40s, it has been estimated that the occurrence of acute angle closure glaucoma in these patients will become more frequent. This is particularly serious because acute angle closure glaucoma is treatable and preventable with iridectomy, either surgical or laser. The problem is compounded by the fact that many of these patients who are predisposed to this complication have a fellow eye that is blind.

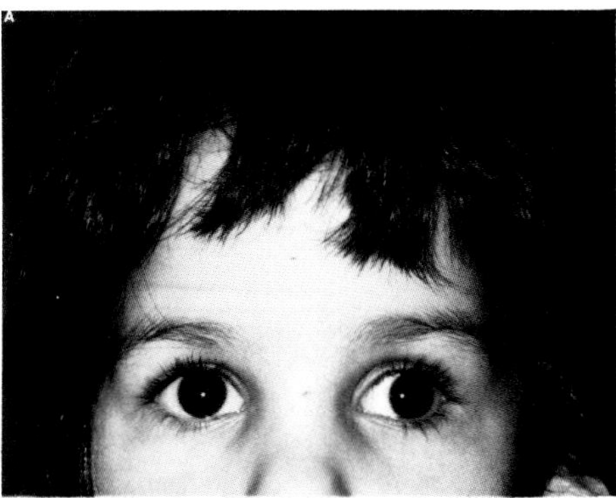
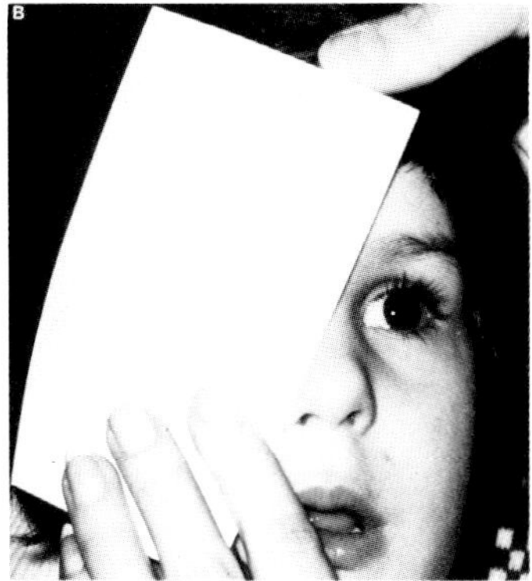
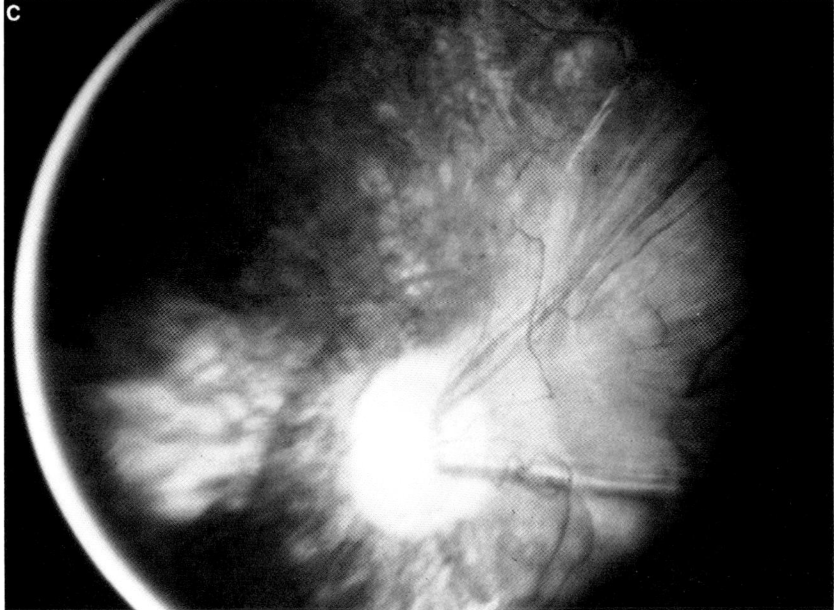

Fig. 2. A: A child with what appears to be a left exotropia. B: Actually, she is fixing with her left eye, which looks exotropic because of a positive angle kappa. Her right eye has minimal visual function. C: Fundus of left eye showing significant dragging of vessels temporally, which resulted in temporal displacement of the fovea. (Reproduced with permission from Blackwell Scientific Publications, Inc., from ''Retinopathy of Prematurity,'' edited by W.A. Silverman and J.T. Flynn.)

There appears to be an unexplained predisposition for the development of ciliary block glaucoma (malignant glaucoma) in eyes with mild degrees of cicatrization from ROP [7]. This association is important for ophthalmologists caring for these patients; appropriate recognition of ciliary block glaucoma is the key to its management.

Cataract formation has long been recognized as a complication of severe cicatricial RLF. It also has an increased incidence in eyes that have regressed ROP in which only mild cicatrization occurs. Because many of these patients have compromised visual acuity from other factors such as retinal abnormalities, amblyopia, or nystagmus, the development of a cataract may seriously compromise visual acuity.

Infants that have mild cicatricial changes from ROP have an increased incidence of peripheral retinal breaks, even if the posterior pole is normal [7]. All such patients should be advised of their being at risk for late retinal detachment. Many patients with these retinal abnormalities, possibly in their better or only seeing eye, are unaware that they are at risk for developing serious retinal problems and are not receiving routine ophthalmologic care. Patients should be instructed about the signs and symptoms of impending retinal detachment.

Some patients with only minimal signs of cicatricial disease appear to have markedly decreased visual acuity. Although nystagmus frequently accompanies the decreased visual acuity, many of these patients have marked abnormalities of their electroretinogram, suggesting a diffuse abnormality of rod and cone function. The exact mechanism of this finding is unclear.

EDUCATIONAL REQUIREMENTS

A number of factors go into determining the educational needs of a child with visual impairment. Two children with identical visual acuity may have very different needs depending on the presence of other neurologic abnormalities or handicapping conditions, intelligence, and environment. Presently, the laws mandate that school districts provide for the educational requirements of children with special needs.

In general, children with visual acuity between 20/30 and 20/80 can function in a normal class room setting, provided that they are neurologically normal, are of average intelligence, and have no other serious handicapping conditions. They may benefit from input from a vision consultant within the school who can work with the classroom teacher defining the child's special needs. This may include seating the child both near the front of the class and also where the lighting is optimum. Certain physical education activities may prove difficult, particularly those that involve seeing a fast-moving ball, especially if a visual field defect is present. Generally, large-print books are not necessary, and magnification or merely holding the text material closely can aid in near work.

Often children with visual acuity less than 20/80, and even down to no light perception, can function in a local school with aid of the "resource room" concept. This involves having several children with serious vision impairment spend part of the school day in a resource room supervised by a teacher specially trained in working with vision-impaired students. Often, they will go to regular classes in the school for many subjects but get additional one-on-one aid from the resource room teacher. Frequent dialogue between the resource room teacher and the regular classroom teacher is important. The use of specialized low-vision aids in the form of telescopes or magnification for reading may be helpful. The resource room concept works better in more densely populated areas. Even so, children frequently need to be bussed to the one school within their area that has a resource room program.

The decision to send a child to a resident school for the vision impaired is often based on many factors. A child coming from a rural area, where the availability of a resource room program may not exist, may be more likely to benefit from attending a resident school for the vision impaired than a child with a resource room program in his community. The child of below normal intelligence, or with other handicapping conditions, may be more in need of attending a resident school.

REFERENCES

1. Palmer EA: Optimal timing of examination for acute retrolental fibroplasia. Ophthalmology 88:662–668, 1981.
2. Kushner BJ: Strabismus and amblyopia associated with regressed retinopathy of prematurity. Arch Ophthalmol 100:256–261, 1982.
3. Kushner BJ: Ocular causes of abnormal head postures. Ophthalmology 86:2115–2125, 1979.
4. Foster RS, Metz HS, Jampolsky A: Strabismus and pseudostrabismus with retrolental fibroplasia. Am J Ophthalmol 79:985–989, 1975.
5. Smith J, Shivitz I: Angle-closure glaucoma in adults with cicatricial retinopathy of prematurity. Arch Ophthalmol 102:371–372, 1984.
6. Kushner BJ: Ciliary block glaucoma in retinopathy of prematurity. Arch Ophthalmol 100:1078–1079, 1982.
7. Tasman W: Late complications of retrolental fibroplasia. Ophthalmology 86:1724–1740, 1979.

COLOR SECTION

Classification of Late Stages of ROP—Flynn

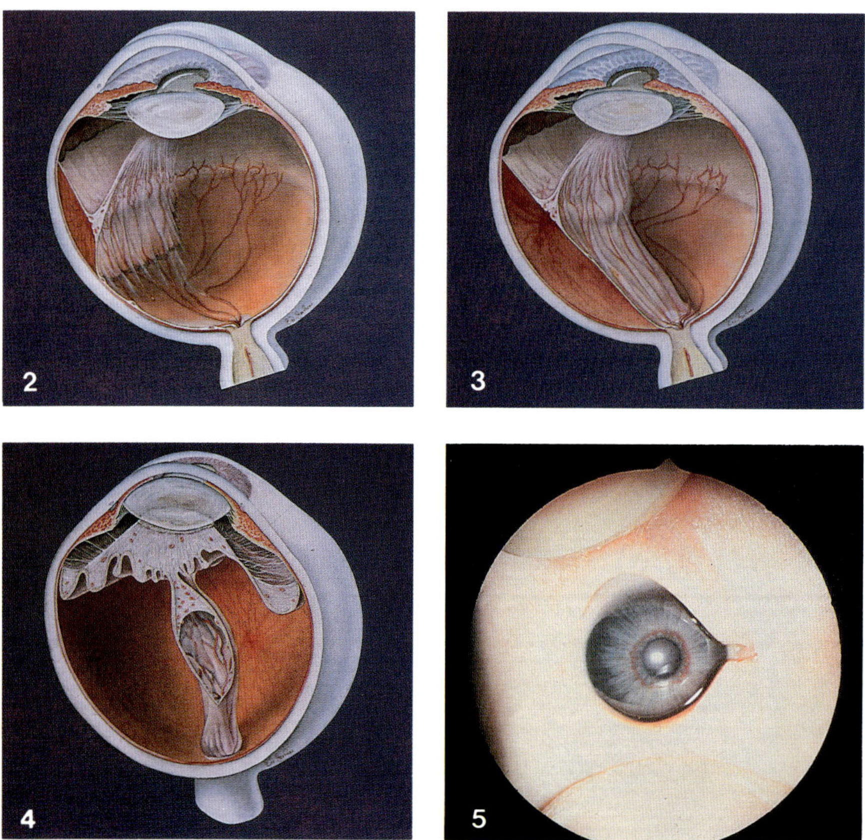

Fig. 2. Stage IV A. Subtotal retinal detachment, peripheral in type, exerting traction on the macula and vessels in the posterior pole without detaching them (See page 177).

Fig. 3. Stage IV B. Subtotal retinal detachment with extension of a fold into the macula. Traction is pulling the retina over the optic disc. (Page 177).

Fig. 4. Stage V. Total retinal detachment, funnellike in shape, extending from the optic disc to the retrolenticular space (Page 177).

Fig. 5. Marked engorgement of the iris vasculature, a grim prognostic sign of severe disease in the posterior pole (See page 178).

Classification of Late Stages of ROP

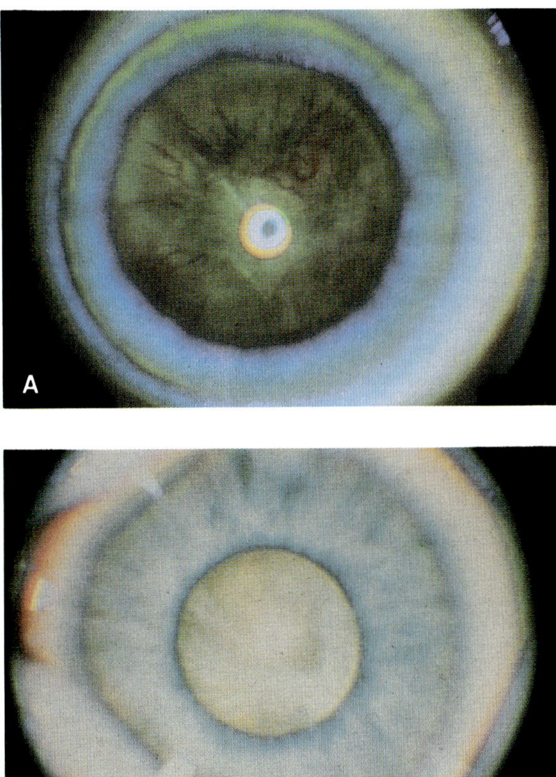

Fig. 6. **A:** Avascular membrane covering surface of totally detached retina in retrolenticular space. **B:** Totally detached retina, located behind lens, covered with translucent membrane containing retinal blood vessels (See page 178).

Pathogenesis of Late Stages of ROP—Machemer

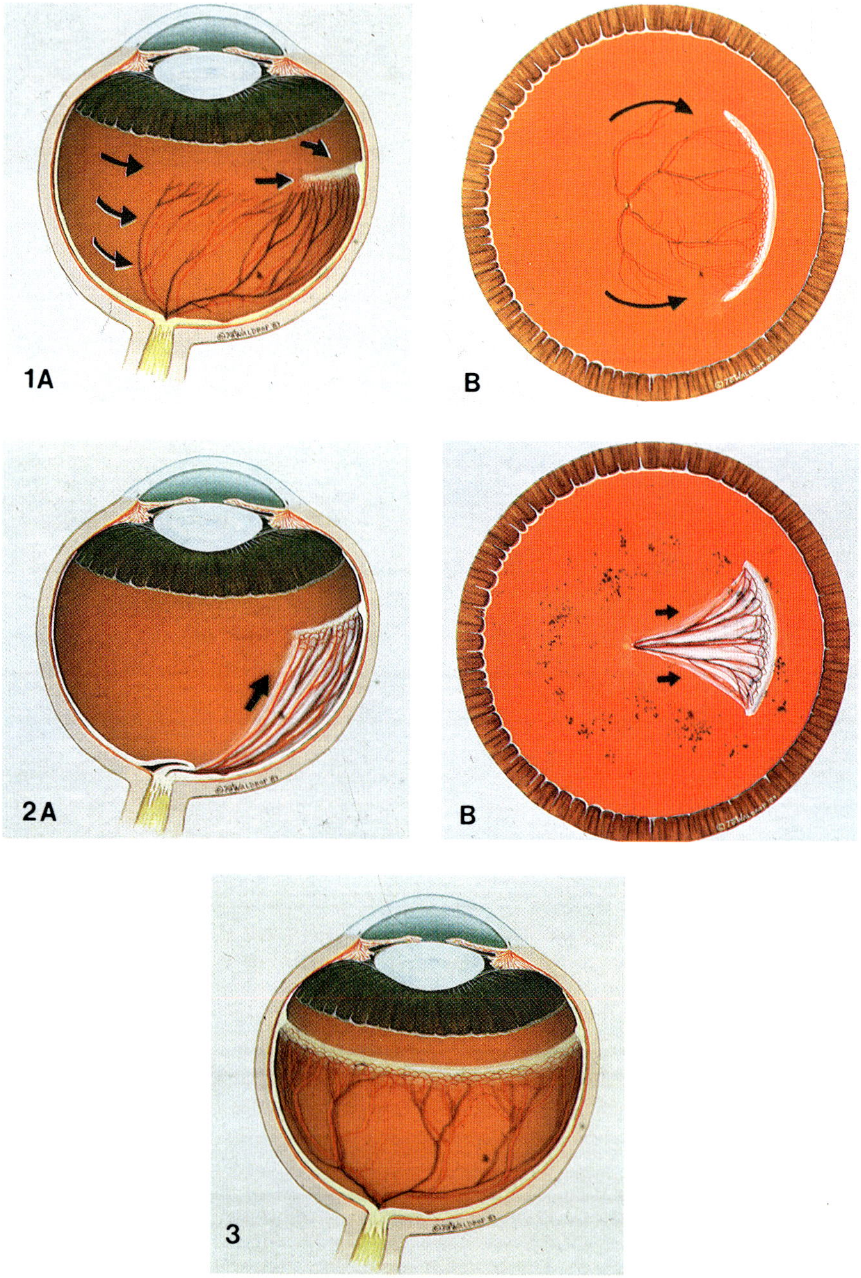

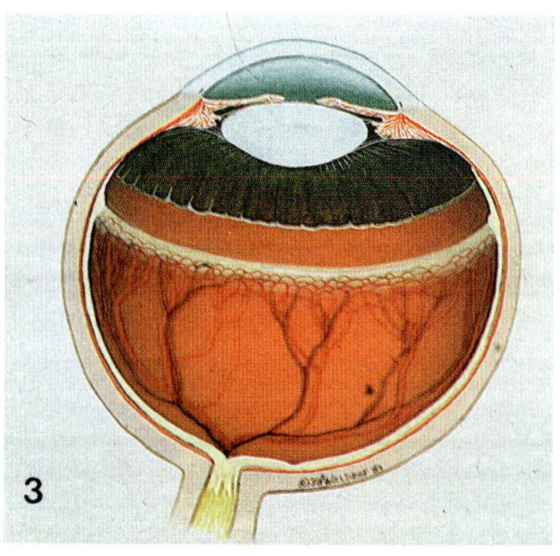

Pathogenesis of Late Stages of ROP

Fig. 1.   Schematic cross section **(A)** and fundus view **(B)** of an eye with a localized shunt area. With contraction of the shunt, avascular retina on the nasal side stretches, and vessels are dragged toward the temporal side (See page 276).

Fig. 2.   Schematic cross section **(A)** and fundus view **(B)** of an eye in which the temporal shunt area has pulled all vascularized retina toward the temporal side. Redundant vascularized retina is thrown into folds, and the avascular retina has been extremely stretched. Vessels from the nasal side of the disk have been ulled temporally, causing a retinal fold. The irregular pigmentation of the fundus is a sign of pigment epithelium irritation during the retinal stretching and migration (See pages 276–277).

Fig. 3.   Anteriorly located circular shunt in an ROP eye before contraction has occurred. Note that all the retina posterior to the shunt remains vascularized (See page 277).

Pathogenesis of Late Stages of ROP

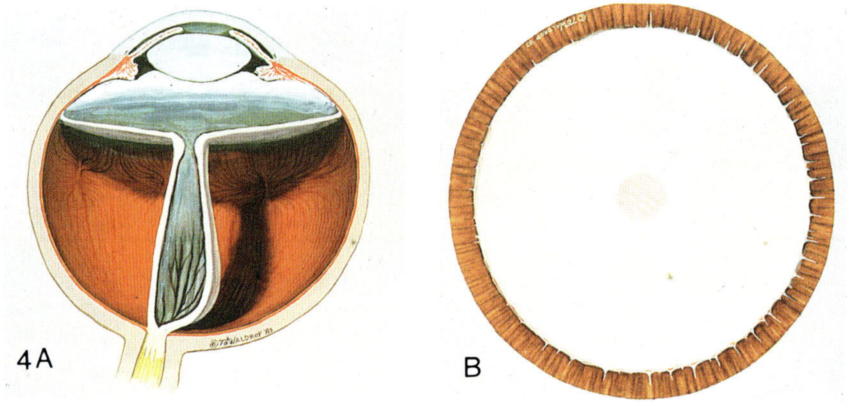

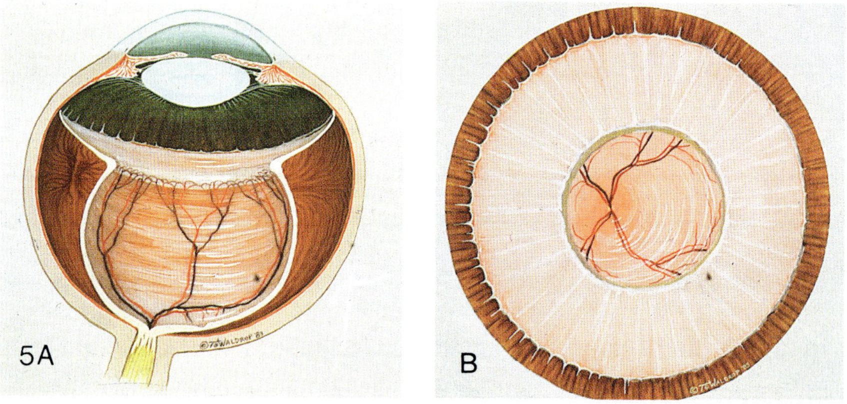

Fig. 4.   Cross section (**A**) and fundus view (**B**) of an eye after complete contraction of the anterior circular shunt. Note the total detachment of the retina and the formation of a narrow funnel, with vascularized retina. Sometimes, a subtle red reflex is seen if the posterior retina is not too far away from the underlying choroid (See page 277).

Fig. 5.   Cross section (**A**) and fundus view (**B**) of an eye with incomplete contraction of the anterior circular shunt. There is total retinal detachment, but a red reflex persists because of the flat detachment posteriorly (See page 277).

Pathogenesis of Late Stages of ROP

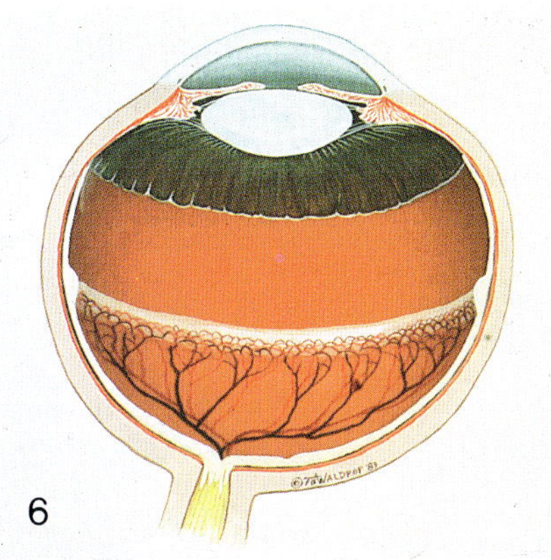

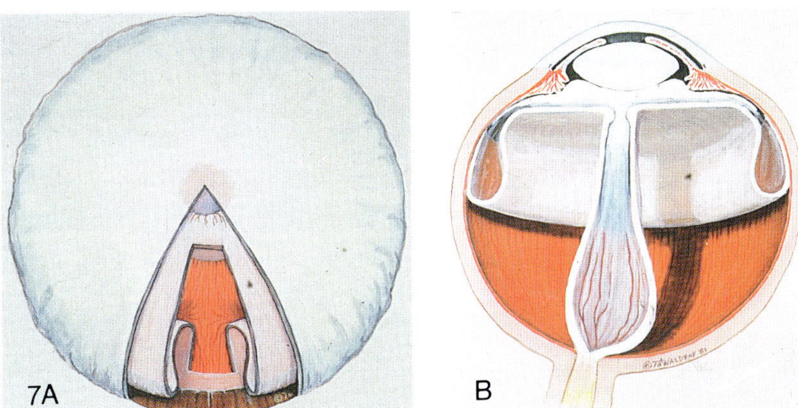

Fig. 6. Equatorial circular shunt in an ROP eye before contraction has occurred (See page 278).

Fig. 7.   Cross section **(A)** and cut-away frontal view **(B)** of fundus in an eye after complete contraction of the equatorial circular shunt. Anterior avascular retina is very stretchable. A peripheral trough (arrow) of redundant avascular peripheral retina has formed. Some of this retina is attached, giving a red peripheral reflex. The central funnel of detached vascularized retina is quite narrow; therefore, only a subtle red reflex can be seen through the retrolental scar tissue (See page 278).

Pathogenesis of Late Stages of ROP

8

9A B

10 A B

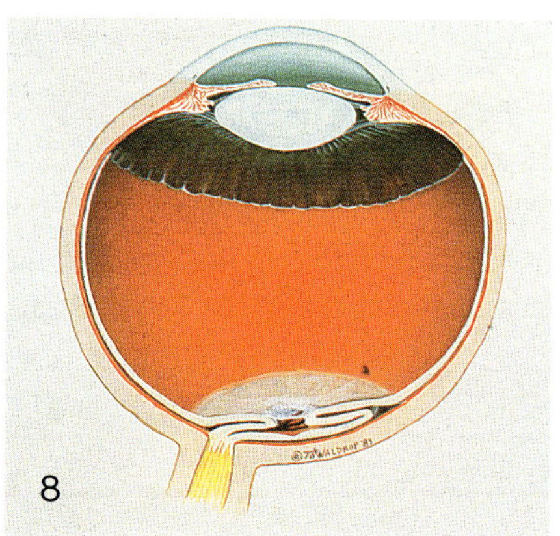

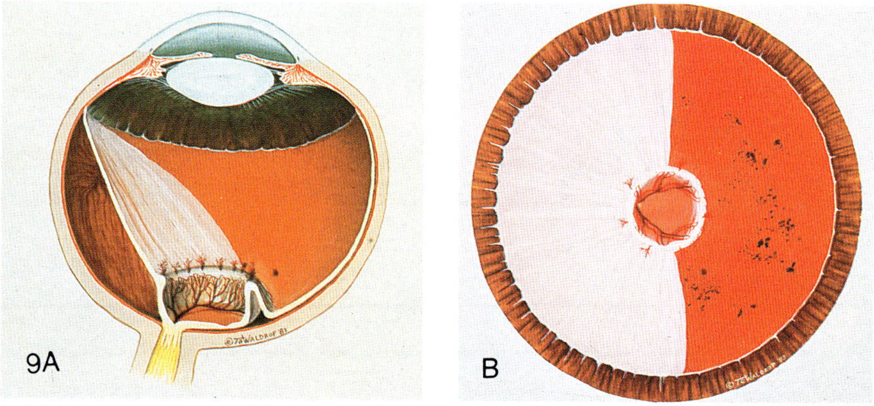

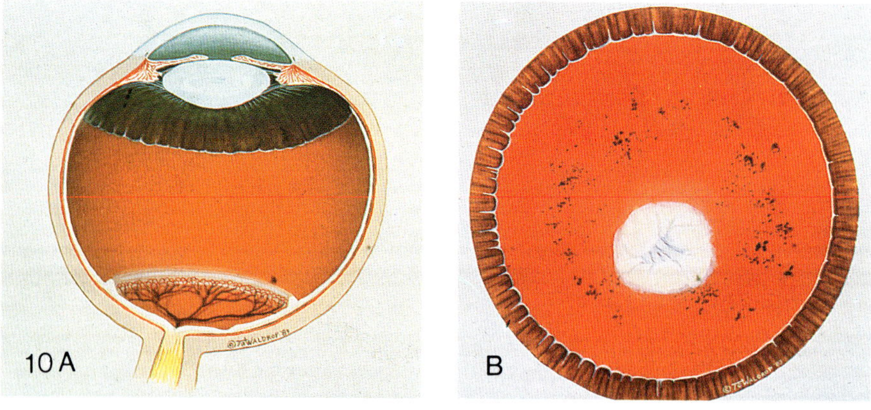

Pathogenesis of Late Stages of ROP

Fig. 8. Posteriorly located circular shunt in an ROP before contraction has occurred (See page 279).

Fig. 9.   Cross section **(A)** and fundus view **(B)** in an eye after partial contraction of posterior shunt. Cuplike traction detachment surrounds the posterior pole (See page 279).

Fig. 10.   Cross section **(A)** and fundus view **(B)** with complete contraction of posterior shunt. Collapsed retina forms a fold over a small area of vascularized retina; the remainder of the retina is avascular (See page 279).

Surgical Pathoanatomy in Stage 5 ROP—de Juan, Machemer, Flynn, and Green

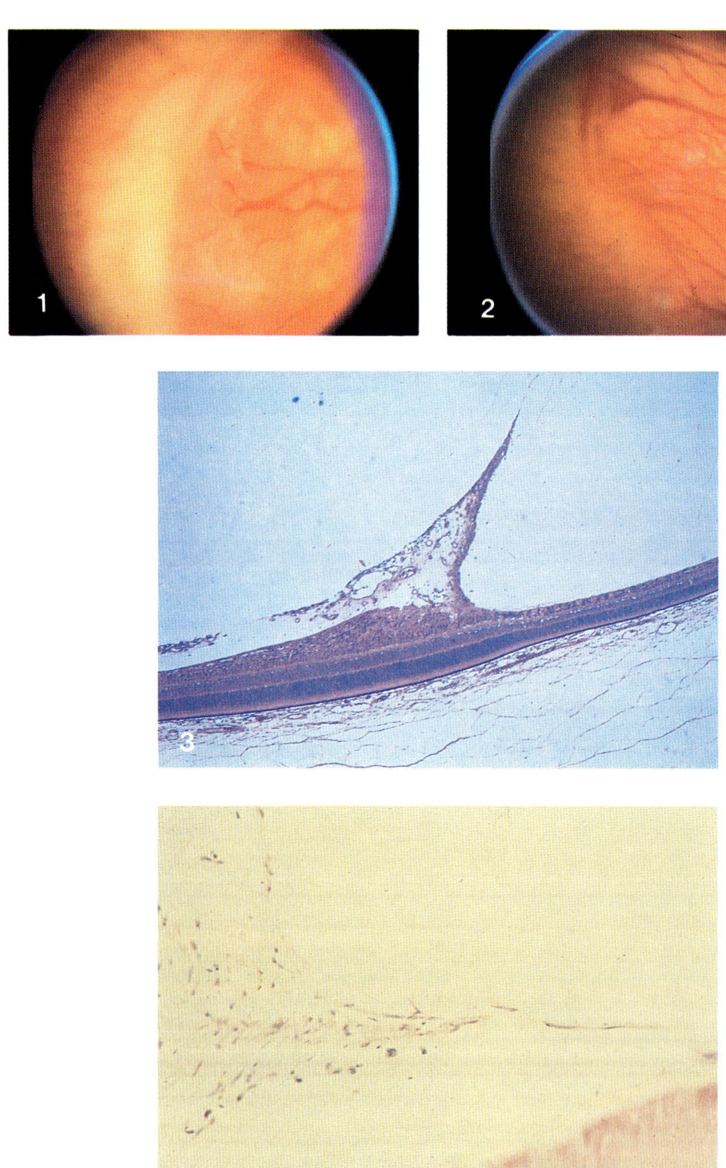

Surgical Pathoanatomy in Stage 5 ROP

Fig. 1. Fundus photograph of patient with stage 3 ROP. Active disease; note lush brush border (See page 282).

Fig. 2. Stage 3 ROP. Proliferations appear relatively avascular and have extended posteriorly over the retinal surface (See page 282).

Fig. 3. Photomicrograph of a section of an eye with stage 3 ROP. Proliferation extends anteriorly and toward the lens. Also, the proliferation can be seen extending posteriorly over the retinal surface. Angioblasts extend directly into the vitreous rather than along the hyaloid surface. Periodic acid Shiff. ×40. (See page 282).

Fig. 4. Photomicrograph demonstrating cells growing toward the lens capsule from the retina. Hematoxylin and eosin. ×100. (See page 282).

Surgical Pathoanatomy in Stage 5 ROP

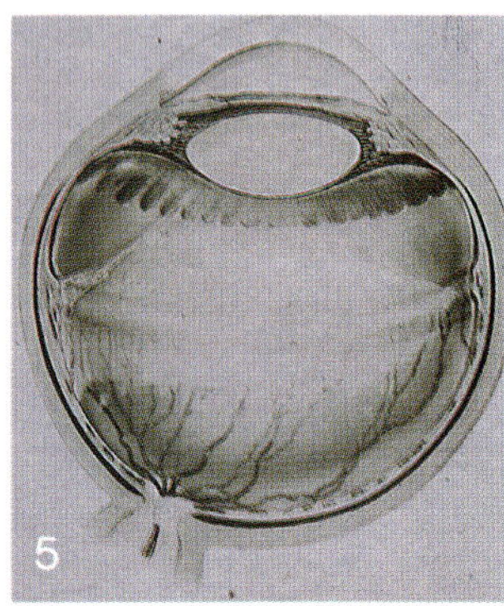

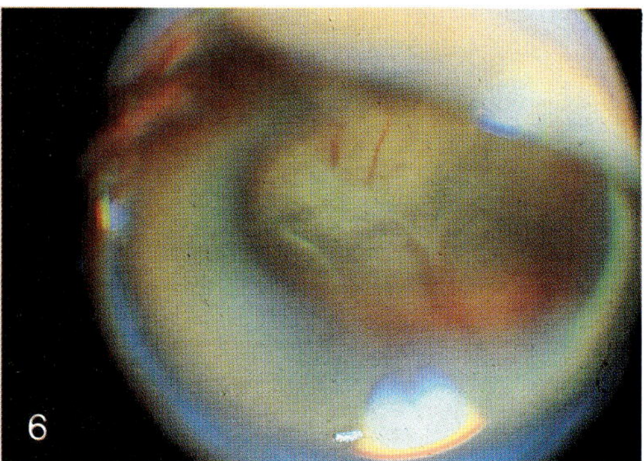

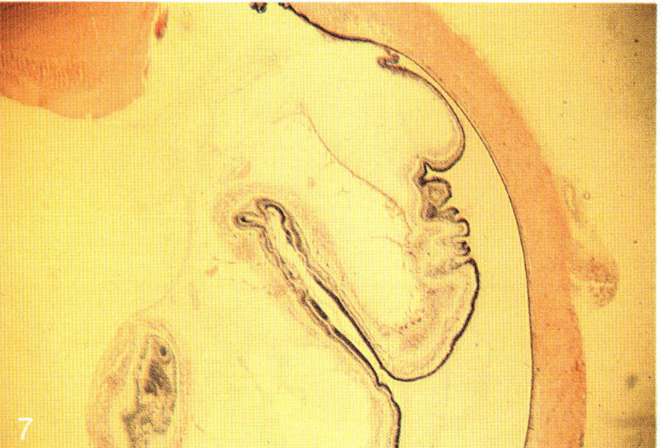

Fig. 5. Drawing showing a three-dimensional conception of the vitreous ''veil'' extending from the elevated ridge in stage 3 ROP. The drawing also demonstrates proliferation growing posteriorly over the retinal surface (See page 282).

Fig. 6. Fundus photograph showing an avascular vitreous veil extending toward the lens in patient with a tractional retinal elevation (See page 282).

Fig. 7. Photomicrograph of eye with stage 5 ROP. Note large retinal folds with proliferations growing from broad, plaque-like areas over the retinal surface both at the edge of the fold and also deeper in the troughs of the folds. Hematoxylin and eosin. ×10. (See page 282).

Surgical Pathoanatomy in Stage 5 ROP

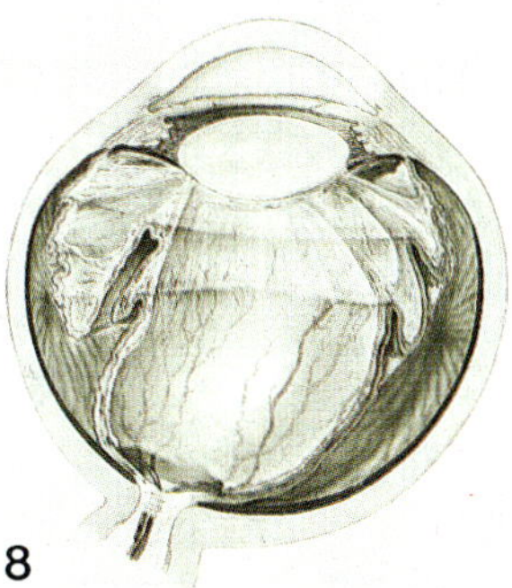

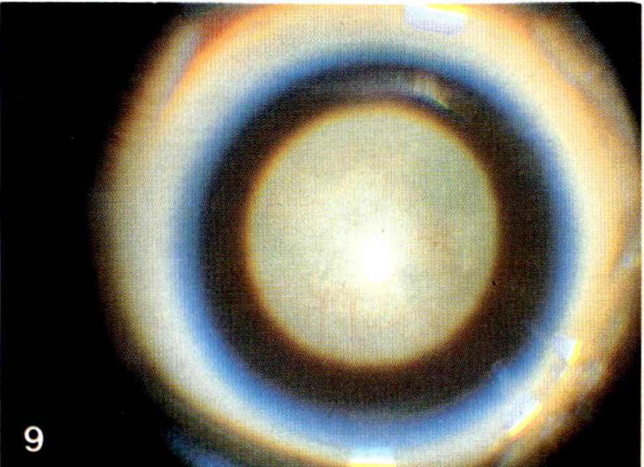

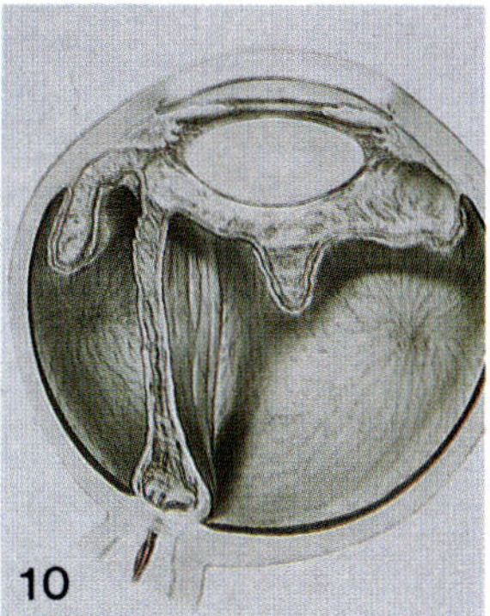

Fig. 8. Drawing demonstrating three-dimensional view of retina pulled into multiple folds from proliferations contracting anteriorly and circumferentially causing both narrowing of the funnel as well as multiple folds in the retina (See page 282).

Fig. 9. Clinical photograph showing typical appearance of a white vascularized retrolental mass in patient with severe stage 5 ROP (See page 282).

Fig. 10. Drawing demonstrating three-dimensional view of severe stage 5 ROP with closed funnel detachment (See page 282).

Surgical Pathoanatomy in Stage 5 ROP

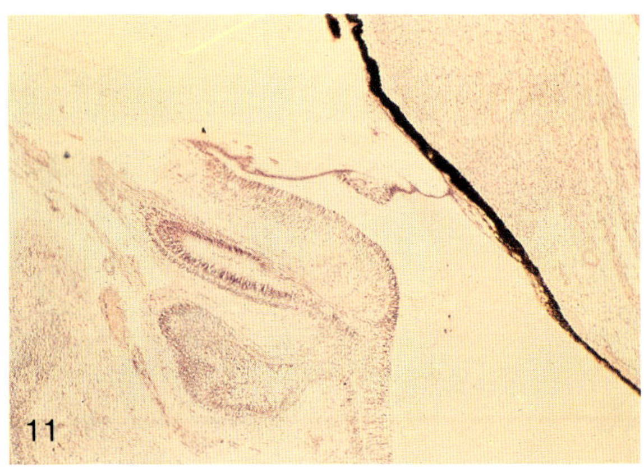

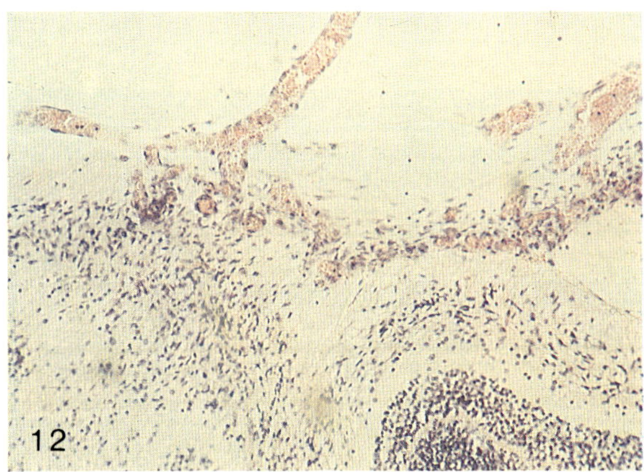

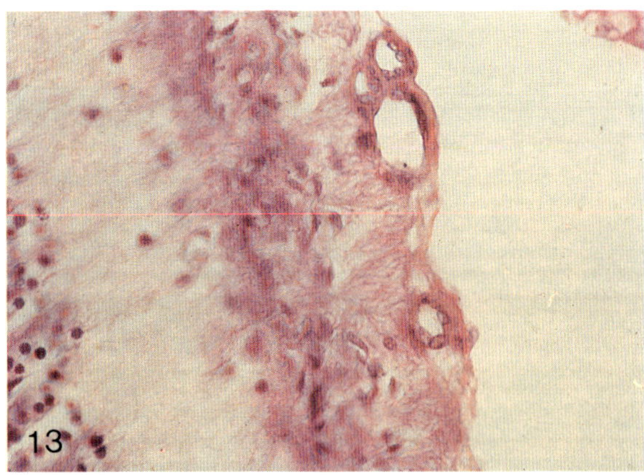

Surgical Pathoanatomy in Stage 5 ROP

Fig. 11. Photomicrograph showing pars plana detachment, as well as multiple peripheral folds in the retina, with dragging of the retina and preretinal tissue anteriorly and toward the lens. Hematoxylin and eosin. ×40. (See page 283).

Fig. 12. Photomicrograph showing retinal vessels exiting the retinal tissue in a broad, plaque-like manner. There is moderate intraretinal gliosis. No clear anatomic plane can be distinguished between preretinal and retinal tissue. Hematoxylin and eosin. ×100. (See page 284).

Fig. 13. Photomicrograph of developing vessels within the retinal tissue. Again, no clear anatomic plane is present separating preretinal membrane from retinal tissue. Hematoxylin and eosin. ×400. (See page 284).

Surgical Pathoanatomy in Stage 5 ROP

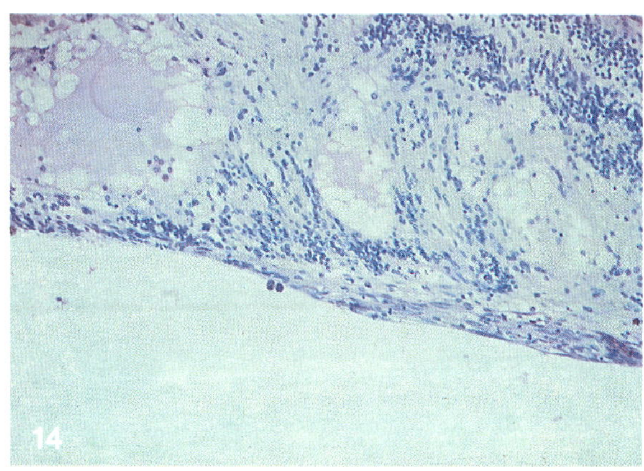

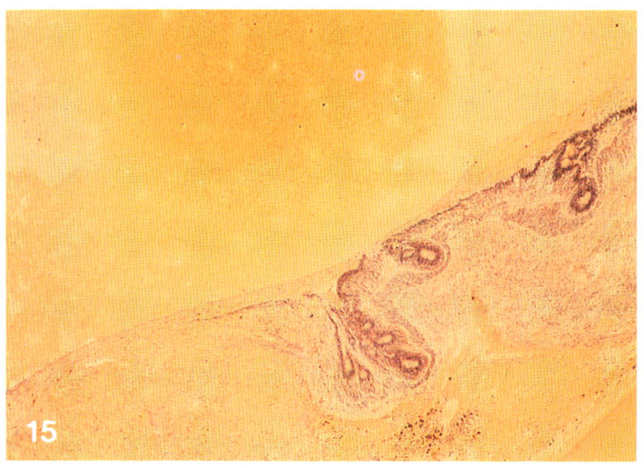

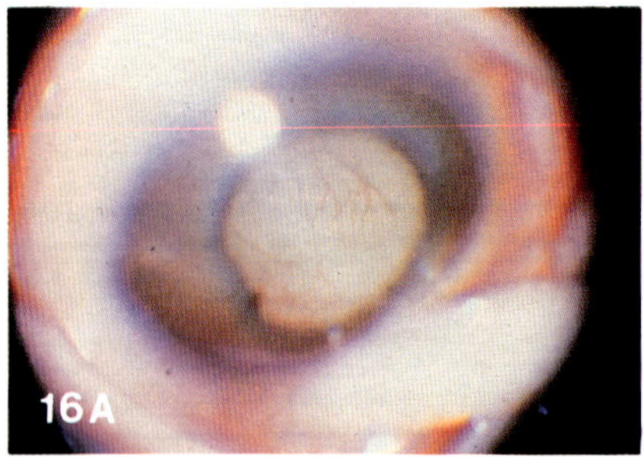

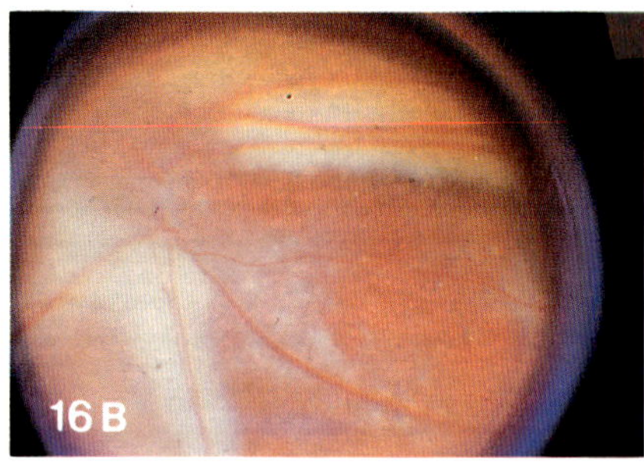

Surgical Pathoanatomy in Stage 5 ROP

Fig. 14. Photomicrograph of developing vessels within the retinal tissue. Again, no clear anatomic plane is present separating preretinal membrane from retinal tissue. Hematoxylin and eosin. ×400. (See page 284).

Fig. 15. Photomicrograph showing severe subretinal scarring, posterior retinal folds, subretinal membrane formation, and severe intraretinal gliosis with subretinal hemorrhage in advanced stage 5 ROP. Hematoxylin and eosin. ×40. (See page 284).

Fig. 16. **A:** Clinical photograph demonstrating vascularized retrolental fibrous tissue in patient with closed-funnel stage 5 ROP. **B:** Postoperative appearance of fundus, showing reattached retina and accumulation of subretinal lipid, possibly old blood associated with the tractional retinal elevation (See page 284).

VI. THE OXYGEN HYPOTHESIS, ANTI-OXYGEN THERAPY IN THE NURSERY

The Oxygen Hypothesis: Fruitful Predictor or Narrow Dogma?

William A. Silverman, MD

*Columbia University College of Physicians and Surgeons, New York,
New York 10032*

It has been said that "nothing is so dangerous as an idea—when it's the
only one you've got." The hazard is exemplified perfectly in the experience
with a three-decade-old idea holding that supplemental-oxygen treatment is
the sole necessary and sufficient cause of the retinopathy that affects
premature infants (ROP). In the mid-1950s this supplemental-oxygen hypothesis led to changes in medical management practices and to a sharp
reduction in the occurrence of ROP [1], but, we can see with the clear vision
of hindsight, what was once hailed as a "medical victory" has turned out to
be merely the opening skirmish in a long battle to dispel ignorance about the
eye-damaging disorder.

Argument about the "cause" of ROP virtually ceased after a 1953–1954
multicenter, randomized, clinical trial disclosed convincing evidence [2] that
a policy of prolonged exposure to high concentrations of oxygen (FIO_2
>50% for 28 days) in the management of small infants (<1.5 kg birth-
weight) tripled the risk of the retinal damage. What followed was a
phenomenon that might be called the "failure of success." Over a 20-year
period, the "restrict-supplemental-oxygen" thesis was transformed into a
rigid dogma reinforced by the written and oral proscriptions of respected
authorities [3]. An incriminatory attitude protected the dogma against
criticism—every instance of retrolental fibroplasia (RLF) blindness was
taken as proof of mismanagement in the use of supplemental oxygen. During
this "dark age," there was little if any heretic dissent, and original
investigation proceeded at a snail's pace. Slowly, questions about the
limitations of the supplemental-oxygen explanation multiplied, and there is
now hope that we are on the verge of an age of enlightenment (Fig. 1) [4].
At present, there is general agreement that supplemental oxygen is merely
one (and now, arguably, the least important) of a number of determinants
affecting the risk of retinal damage in premature infants.

Birth Defects: Original Article Series, Volume 24, Number 1, pages 203–207
© **1988 March of Dimes Birth Defects Foundation**

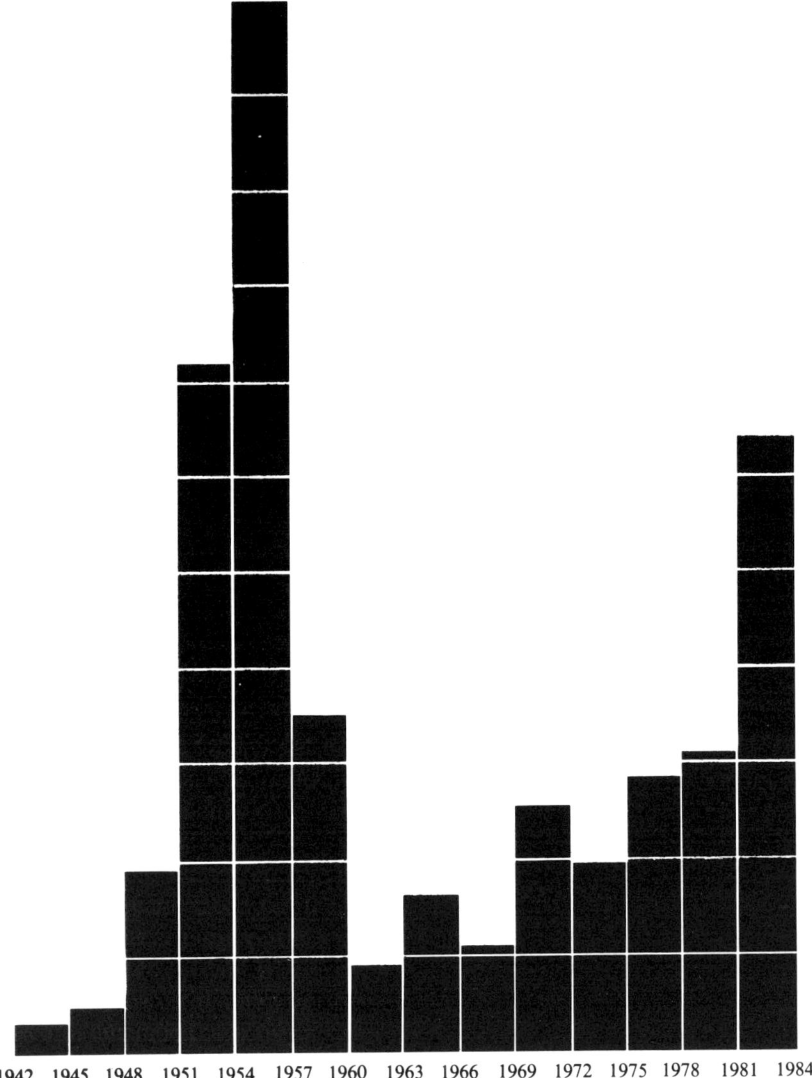

Fig. 1. Number of ROP articles in 3-year intervals, 1942–1984. (Reproduced from Silverman et al [13], with permission of the publisher.)

THE KINSEY STUDY

We need to recall, painfully, that many important practical questions were raised by the circumstantial evidence obtained when the data collected in the large study of 1953–1954 were dredged. The questions, however, were never subjected to a rigorous, prospective "trial by fire." For example, it was observed [2] that eye damage seemed to occur more frequently with increasing duration (during the first 1–2 weeks of treatment) but not with increasing concentration of the therapeutic gas. The interesting findings were reported as "conclusions" of (and were widely interpreted as proved by) the controlled trial. Readers were not warned about the weakness of this evidence obtained by retrospective search for associations carried out in clinical experience with oxygen treatment prescribed by physicians within two broadly limited trial conditions. (In the "routine oxygen" arm of the trial, oxygen—FIO_2 >50% p.r.n.—both duration and concentration between 21% and 50% were prescribed according to clinical judgment). Interpretation of the precise connection between dosage of oxygen and retinal risk was undermined by confounding influences: The sickest infants (in both arms of the trial) received oxygen treatment for the longest periods and in the highest concentrations. Ethical constraints blocked all thought of using a direct approach—a new focused clinical trial—to test the limits of the important duration-of-exposure question *suggested* by the association found after the fact in the just-completed management policy exercise. For more than 30 years, the issue has remained unsettled.

ROP RISK TODAY

It is now quite clear that the risk of retinal damage among premature infants breathing only 21% oxygen in room air is not zero. Huge malpractice awards to the contrary notwithstanding, there is no battle-tested evidence to support the claim that the room air baseline risk is increased after moderate hyperoxia induced by exposure to supplemental oxygen (especially when hyperoxia is intermittent) in the first few days after premature birth. It is time to admit that the shape of the oxygen dose: ROP risk curve is not known, and to acknowledge that the many observational studies over the past 30 years have pointed to, but have failed to resolve, the duration-of-exposure question. Survey after survey of clinical experience [5–7] has been unable to establish the limits of the supplemental-oxygen effect, because it is impossible to untangle the relationship between oxygen treatment, infant's state of health, and ROP risk. Without such critical information, physicians have had to rely on crude guesses when faced with the need to balance the trade-off risks of eye damage, brain damage, and death in the management of premature infants.

The convincing positive results of studies of supplemental oxygen exposure have tended to obscure the fact that few other associations have been subjected to rigorous examination. Over 50 separate "causes" of ROP were proposed over the years since it was first described in 1942 [8,9]. Very few of these proposals were formally evaluated, and we can see in retrospect that virtually all the negative-result trials of suspected determinants had little power of disclosure (they were much too small to rule out important effects). The most encouraging aspect of the current resurgence of interest in ROP is the fact that multiple influences (vitamin E treatment, hypercapnea, light exposure, etc) are once more under active consideration.

CONCLUSIONS

ROP is a disease that stubbornly refuses to go away, but the flip side of the unhappy experience has been the valuable lessons learned about the kinds of traps and practical difficulties that stand in the way of solutions to problems faced daily by doctors. The experience with the disorder makes a powerful case for the general proposition that all knowledge claims in medicine must be subjected to unrelenting criticism. There is no other way of detecting our mistakes and profiting from them. For example, there is little question that uncritical acceptance in the 1940s of the declarations that asymptomatic premature infants breathe ''. . . in a more normal manner in an oxygen enriched atmosphere'' [10] and that many premature infants may be in a state of ''subcyanotic anoxia'' [11] led to overuse of supplemental oxygen, with tragic consequences, throughout the world for a period of 12 years. Similarly, for many years, there was underuse of the valuable gas and dire consequences because of failure to test the limits of the restrictive policy adopted to end the 1942–1954 ROP epidemic.

Information about complex events that make up medical experience is never complete. Modern medicine does not have the property of finality—a fixed body of undoubted knowledge and a limited set of unquestioned concepts. It is, rather, an evolving, open-ended search; moreover, the uncertainties are taken as a given condition of the enterprise. As a result (and in the interest of safeguarding patients), there must be tentative acceptance of only those claims and hypotheses that have survived the toughest critical tests we can devise [12]. A strong challenge to current oxygen treatment practices in the care of newborn premature infants is long overdue.

REFERENCES

1. Yankauer A et al: The rise and fall of retrolental fibroplasia in New York State: A preliminary report. NY State J Med 56:1474–1477, 1956.
2. Kinsey VE: Retrolental fibroplasia. Cooperative study of retrolental fibroplasia and the use of oxygen. AMA Arch Ophthlalmol 56:481–543, 1956.
3. Guy LP et al: The possibility of total elimination of retrolental fibroplasia by oxygen restriction. Pediatrics 17:247–249, 1956.

4. Silverman WA, Flynn JT: Overview: A "developmental" retinopathy reconsidered. In Silverman WA, Flynn JT (eds): "Contemporary Issues in Fetal and Neonatal Medicine: Volume 2, Retinopathy of Prematurity." Boston: Blackwell Scientific Publications, 1985, pp xi–xxiii.

5. Kinsey VE, et al: PaO_2 levels and retrolental fibroplasia: A report of the cooperative study. Pediatrics 60:655–668, 1977.

6. Payne JW, Patz A: Current status of retrolental fibroplasia. The retinopathy of prematurity. Ann Clin Res 11:205–221, 1979.

7. Lucey JF, Dangman B: A re-examination of the role of oxygen in retrolental fibroplasia. Pediatrics 73:82–96, 1984.

8. Zacharias L: Retrolental fibroplasia: A survey. Am J Ophthalmol 35:1426–1454, 1952.

9. Silverman WA: "Retrolental Fibroplasia. A Modern Parable." New York: Grune & Stratton, 1980.

10. Wilson JL, et al: Respiration of premature infants. Response to variations of oxygen and to increased carbon dioxide in inspired air. Am J Dis Child 63:1080–1085, 1942.

11. Smith CA, Kaplan E; Adjustment of blood oxygen levels in neonatal life. Am J Dis Child 64:843–859, 1942.

12. Silverman WA: "Human Experimentation: A Guided Step Into the Unknown." Oxford: Oxford University Press, 1985.

13. Silverman WA et al (eds): "Retinopathy of Prematurity: Current Controversies." Boston: Blackwell Scientific Publications, 1985.

Vitamin E and Retinopathy of Prematurity: The Clinical Investigator's Perspective on Antioxidant Therapy: Side Effects and Balancing Risks and Benefits

Dale L. Phelps, MD

Department of Pediatrics, University of Rochester School of Medicine, Rochester, New York 14642

METHODS FOR THE CLINICAL INVESTIGATOR

It has been said that all physicians are clinical investigators, that each patient and his therapy are an experiment. However, we must not confuse the art of practicing medicine, which is the wise application of scientific facts and accumulated experience, with the science of medicine, which is the systematic application of the scientific method to clinical questions [1,2]. When using the scientific method, the investigator forms a hypothesis, tries it in the toughest and most unbiased test that he can apply, and records systematic, rigidly defined, prospective data for statistical analysis. The hypothesis may be developed from many different sources—from as ''little'' as inductive reasoning alone to as much as years of bench work followed by cell culture tests and finally physiologic animal model studies, which then bring the question to the threshold of the clinical arena.

The randomized clinical trial (RCT) is the most powerful tool we have available for this testing process. Although it has been widely hailed as such, the technical and practical difficulties of applying the complex technique of the RCT have interfered with its general use. Additionally, its incomplete use or misuse has led to many disappointments and misunderstandings of its power. Only scattered true RCTs were published through the 1950s, 1960s, and 1970s. However, as with so much of our complex modern technology, their use has increased with the accumulation of investigators familiar with their limitations and strengths. The 1980s have seen not only the much wider and wiser application of the RCT technique but finally the publication of several excellent instructional articles [3–5] and a regular periodical [6] on its use. Dr. Silverman's recent text is another shining light to guide those who desire to learn [2].

Birth Defects: Original Article Series, Volume 24, Number 1, pages 209–218

The most difficult first task for most of us to face is accepting that *we do not know* if our hypothesis is true. Once we overcome the hurdle of acknowledging that our pet idea may not prove to be efficacious, or if it is efficacious that it might not be safe, we are at least on our way to becoming good clinical investigators [7].

WHY THE CLINICAL INVESTIGATION OF VITAMIN E?

How did we come to the testing of vitamin E for the possible prevention of retinopathy of prematurity (ROP)? Based on the 1956 RCT of prolonged vs curtailed oxygen administration, oxygen was clearly identified as having some role in this disorder, since the infants randomly assigned to receive the routine prolonged administration of oxygen had more cases of serious vision loss than those receiving the experimental curtailed administration of oxygen [8]. Since oxygen seems to exert its toxic effects elsewhere in the body, and in tissue culture, through free oxygen radicals and activated oxygen species, it seemed reasonable inductively that an antioxidant would provide some protective effect.

Vitamin E, one of the fat-soluble vitamins, seemed like an excellent candidate in that premature infants are born with low plasma and tissue levels compared to adult norms, although these rise promptly when feedings are begun [9]. Vitamin E's natural function appears to be to protect unsaturated fats against peroxidative damage initiated by activated oxygen species. Early clinical trials of vitamin E were conducted in 1949 [10], prior to oxygen being suspected as a potential contributing factor, and in 1974 [11]. Both these trials suggested that there may be a clinical benefit, but neither was statistically significant at the usually accepted levels of confidence.

ANIMAL STUDIES OF VITAMIN E AND OXYGEN-INDUCED RETINOPATHY

The kitten has an incompletely vascularized retina at birth and develops an acute proliferative retinopathy when exposed for 3–7 days to 70–100% oxygen during the first 7 days after birth. This retinopathy can be seen 2–4 weeks later, but, unlike the human disorder, the oxygen-induced retinopathy in the kitten always regresses; that is, it always heals without apparent sequelae. Therefore, this model is best referred to as oxygen-induced retinopathy, and *not* as a model of ROP. It is useful for the testing of novel ideas, but results from this model must never be uncritically accepted for direct application to the human.

Using the oxygen-induced retinopathy model, vitamin E was tested as parenteral tocopherol acetate [12] given to the kittens from the day of birth through 3 weeks of age. The animals received 80% inspired oxygen for 48–80 hours beginning on day 3, and the retinas were removed at 3 weeks of age. The abnormal growth of the vessels was scored by examining the india ink-injected vessels of these flat-mounted retinas. A quantitative retinal scoring system was developed to score each retina, and it was found that vitamin E-treated kittens had less severe retinopathy than their littermates who had received the same oxygen exposure but only placebo injections [12].

EFFICACY OF VITAMIN E IN ROP

There seemed to be sufficient clinical, inductive, and experimental background to begin randomized controlled trials. Six of these have been described in the literature [13–18]. The following chapter deals with an assessment of the data for efficacy of tocopherol (vitamin E) in the prevention of ROP in human premature infants; therefore, efficacy will not be discussed here. The evaluation of any potential therapy for general use, however, requires that its risks be assessed, and each of the reported RCTs of tocopherol in premature infants can be examined for these potential risks, remembering, of course, that we are limited by what the investigators have thought to look for.

SIDE EFFECTS OF TOCOPHEROL ADMINISTRATION

Drug Formulations and Animal Toxicology Studies

Vitamin E is normally present in our diets as free tocopherol, a long-chain fatty alcohol; however, when provided pharmaceutically, an ester is preferred because of its longer shelf-life. The most common ester synthesized is tocopherol acetate, but others are made as well. Table I lists several of the formulations of tocopherol that recently have been available.

When administered orally, the free tocopherol, or its ester, is partially absorbed into the body with dietary fats. The ester is hydrolyzed off of the tocopherol before it reaches the plasma. With the oral administration of tocopherol acetate, only the free tocopherol appears in the plasma and body tissues [19]. To date, it has not been possible to give a dose of *oral* tocopherol (or tocopherol acetate) in animals that was high enough to be fatal, although changes in hepatic findings have been noted in rabbits fed an atherogenic diet and high doses of oral tocopherol acetate [20]. Two of the RCTs of tocopherol in premature infants used oral tocopherol in the free form, and these two did not report any toxicity [13,14].

When tocopherol or tocopherol acetate is administered parenterally, there is obligatory complete absorption compared to the incomplete absorption

TABLE I. Tocopherol Formulations

Oral
  Free tocopherol in oil ("natural vitamin E")
  Tocopherol acetate (or other ester) in emulsifiers, "water-soluble"
  Free tocopherol adsorbed onto a powder
  Tocopherol acetate present in small quantities in many solid and liquid vitamin
    preparations
Parenteral
  Tocopherol acetate as emulsified in multivitamin IV preparations
  Tocopherol, free in alcohol and emulphor (investigational new drug status) tested for both
    IV and IM administration
  Tocopherol acetate as a single IV preparation in polysorbates (recalled by FDA—April,
    1984)
  Tocopherol acetate in sesame oil (recently removed from market)

observed from the gastrointestinal tract. Also, with parenteral tocopherol acetate, the acetate is now found in the plasma and tissues [19,21]. As a single dose, parenteral free tocopherol has an LD^{50} of 440 mg/kg in mice when formulated in ethanol and propylene glycol [22]. In animals given prolonged, large, daily doses of parenteral tocopherol, primarily hepatic changes have been observed [12,23], although, at doses of 200 mg/kg/day of the free tocopherol, death associated with lethargy, coma, and seizures occurred [23].

The mean plasma level of tocopherol in kittens treated with 50 mg/day subcutaneously (SQ) (about 500 mg/kg/day) of tocopherol acetate was 7 mg/dl. The side effects noted in these animals were hepatosplenomegaly and loss of subcutaneous tissue, with fixation of the kitten's normally loose and mobile skin to the underlying tissues [12]. It would appear that the formulation of the tocopherol used is important, at least for the side effects data, and that includes the various emulsifiers used to make it possible to inject it.

Human Studies

There have been anecdotal reports of lethargy in humans taking oral vitamin E and the enhancement of the effect of coumadin in an adult human [24], which was reproduced in dogs [25]. However, until parenteral tocopherol began to be used in large doses in premature infants, no systematically documented, serious side effects had been noted. With the reported randomized trials, however, large doses of parenteral tocopherol, and even oral tocopherol or tocopherol acetate, have been found to be associated with a number of problems, including local reactions to injection, late-onset sepsis [26], necrotizing enterocolitis [26,27], increased retinal hemorrhages when ROP does occur [28], and intraventricular hemorrhage [29].

The most confusing is the effect on intraventricular/periventricular hemorrhage (IV/PVH). Two studies have suggested that IV/PVH is reduced by the early prophylactic administration of tocopherol: One study used IM free tocopherol as a supplement to oral free tocopherol powder in MCT oil [30], and the other IM tocopherol acetate [31]. In contrast to this, another study using the same free tocopherol parenteral preparation as used by Speer et al [30] but using it with a slow intravenous infusion, found that severe IV/PVH occurred at a significantly higher rate in tocopherol-treated infants of under 1 kg birthweight than in placebo-treated controls [29]. None of these studies had been designed to test the effect of tocopherol on IV/PVH, but they found the effect in a retrospective review. Each observed statistically significant differences, and it seems extremely important that this question be subjected to further testing as soon as possible.

Johnson and coworkers [26] found that the use of IV and oral free tocopherol in doses that were adjusted to a 3.5–4.0 mg/dl target level, and achieved actual mean plasma levels of 4.8 mg/dl, resulted in significantly more late-onset sepsis and necrotizing enterocolitis in the treated infants of under 1.5 kg birthweight than in the controls. Phelps and coworkers [32] did not encounter this problem treating infants with the same formulation, but at lower mean plasma levels of only 2.8 mg/dl, power 93%. Therefore, it is possible that this finding is dose-related and possibly preventable by monitoring plasma levels.

The deaths of several infants in association with the use of an IV preparation of tocopherol acetate in polysorbate merit further mention here. The manner in which the drug was marketed and used is an important lesson for all clinicians in the approach to a newly available drug. Two major flaws probably led to the misadventure: 1) the new formulation was never tested in animals (either at all or in the recommended doses), and 2) the formulation was marketed as a nutritional supplement, but no testing had been done to determine the amount needed to restore tissue or plasma levels of tocopherol to normal in a fasting infant or a newborn animal. As a result, large doses (25–100 mg/day) were given IV on a daily basis. The infants who died developed hepatic and renal failure in association with plasma tocopherol levels over 12 mg/dl [33,34], and it has yet to be sorted out whether the responsible toxic agent is the tocopherol acetate, the tocopherol, a component of the emulsifiers used to dissolve the drug, or some other agent [35].

BALANCING THE RISKS AND THE BENEFITS

To make the decision whether to use a new treatment that has been shown to be effective requires a recognition, evaluation, and acceptance of the risks

TABLE II. Estimating Numbers of Infants in One Year

Birthweight (kg)	No. born	No. surviving (% of births)	No. cicatricial (% of survivors)	No. blind (% of survivors)
<1	19,000	7,200 (38)	2160 (30)† 700 (5–10)†	361 (5)
1–1.5	23,000	19,000 (83)	420 (2.2)	95 (0.5)

†The published literature [37–39] is at variance with the experience reported in this volume, so both are used.

of that treatment. A particularly useful approach in this case when the treatment must be applied prophylactically to infants before it is known if they will get the disease is to estimate the absolute number of patients at risk and therefore the number who will have to be treated compared to the number who will suffer the disease and therefore could benefit. Table II shows the estimate, for a single year, of the number of verylow-birthweight infants born in the United States and their estimated survival and the incidence of ROP. The projection is based on 42,000 deliveries of infants weighing less than 1,500 gm in 1985 and calculated, as previously described, by pooling the findings in several single centers and projecting these averages on national natality statistics [36].

Looking at this table, it is apparent that infants of under 1 kg birthweight are projected to contribute the majority of infants with cicatricial ROP. The two estimates shown of 2,160 and 700 infants are at variance because of the literature reports that an average of 30% of under 1 kg survivors will have cicatricial disease [37–39] vs more recent experience, presented in this volume, that only 5–10% of survivors under 1 kg will have cicatricial disease. However, it remains apparent that the smallest infants should be our target of greatest concern. Unfortunately, almost all the reported toxicity has also occurred in these smallest infants. Perhaps, however, the ratio of 7,200 survivors to 2,160 (or 700) with cicatricial disease, that is, 3.3:1 (or 10:1), would justify taking a moderate treatment risk for each of 3.3 (or 10) infants, knowing that, on average, one might benefit. This would be true only if there were evidence of efficacy for infants of under 1 kg birthweight. In addition, if we believe that monitoring of plasma levels can eliminate most of the toxicity, it would be even more reassuring and reasonable to use the treatment.

However, the situation is somewhat different for those infants born weighing over 1 kg. Because most of these larger of the small premature infants survive, and only a few have serious ROP, there would have to be 45 infants treated prophylactically for each one that was going to develop cicatricial ROP, (19,000:420). Certainly, the evidence for safety would have

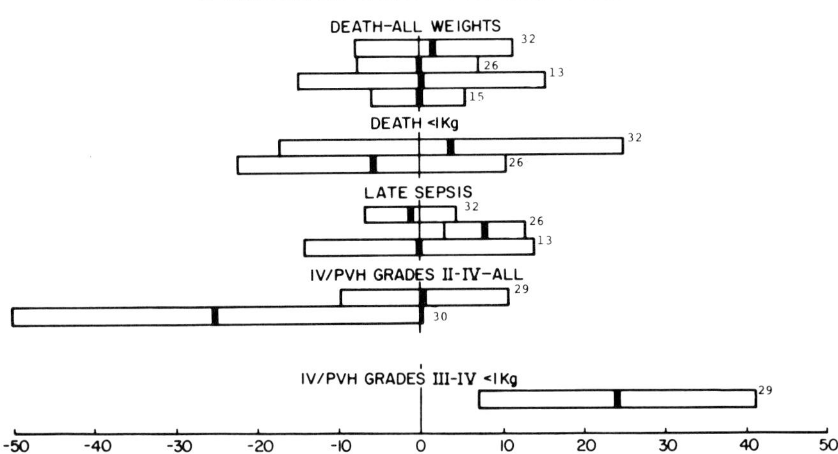

Fig. 1. Bars represent the 95% confidence interval surrounding the difference between the incidence of the indicated side effect in the tocopherol group and the placebo group in randomized controlled trials of tocopherol in premature infants [40]. The small numbers on the bars correspond to the reference for that particular study.

to be extremely strong to justify the use of the drug in these larger infants, and our confidence in being able to minimize the side effects should be greater as well.

Although we will never be certain what the true incidence of side effects or benefits are, we can reduce our uncertainty by looking at the estimates of side effects that we observe across several RCTs. Unfortunately, the side effects data have not usually been reported in sufficient detail to permit careful comparisons, particularly as broken down by birthweight. Figure 1 shows an attempt to place the reported side effects data in perspective utilizing a bar graph with 95% confidence intervals around the differences observed. To do this, the incidence of the side effect observed in the placebo group is subtracted from the incidence of the side effect observed in the tocopherol group in the same RCT and is drawn as a single heavy vertical line. The 95% confidence interval around that estimated difference is calculated [40] and is drawn in the figure as a horizontal bar. If the difference between the tocopherol and control groups is significantly different from zero at the 5% level, the span of the 95% confidence interval bar does not cross the zero line. The larger the sample size, the narrower the width of the confidence interval bar.

In four studies reporting death statistics, there is no difference between the two groups [13,15,26,32]. In the two studies that reported death in infants of under 1 kg birthweight, death occurred a little more frequently in one study and a little less frequently in the other, neither being significantly different from no difference [26,32]. This tends to make one reasonably comfortable that mortality, at least, is not affected by tocopherol treatment as it has been used in the RCTs being discussed.

Late-onset sepsis also presents a reasonably compact set of confidence intervals. Two studies, one using IV free tocopherol [32] and one using oral free tocopherol [13], showed no effect on late-onset sepsis. However, as discussed above, the third [26], using free tocopherol parenterally at higher plasma levels, did show a significant increase in sepsis among the tocopherol-treated infants.

The IV/PVH data are far more mixed, and the figure demonstrates these results graphically. Both significantly increased and significantly decreased morbidity have been observed. In a placebo-controlled RCT, IV free tocopherol in infants born weighing under 1 kg resulted in an increase of severe IV/PVH [29]. On the other hand, decreased IV/PVH and death were observed in infants born weighing under 1 kg with oral plus IM free tocopherol compared to oral alone [30]. Only additional, tightly controlled RCTs will be able to settle this issue.

CONCLUSIONS

The question of whether IM tocopherol truly reduces IV/PVH and mortality in infants of under 1 kg birthweight or IV tocopherol increases it must be studied urgently. The pharmacokinetics of tocopherol outside the plasma compartment are just beginning to be studied, and this knowledge will be critical to our being able to use tocopherol safely in the premature infant, should it prove beneficial. Tentatively, if there is evidence for efficacy in the infants of under 1 kg birthweight, tocopherol use might be justified with careful plasma monitoring, since it is anticipated that onc of three to ten infants of this birthweight will have cicatricial ROP. In infants at birthweights of 1–1.5 kg, even if there is evidence of efficacy, tocopherol would have to be used extremely cautiously, since the ratio of 45 infants treated with prophylactic tocopherol for every one affected with cicatricial ROP requires us to be most careful with these infants who have little to gain.

Note: Since this manuscript was accepted, a RCT with favorable outcome for the prevention of IV/PVH has been published. Intramuscular tocopherol acetate started on day 1 significantly reduced the incidence of IV/PVH. [Sinha S, Davies J, Toner N, Bogle S, Chiswick M: Vitamin E supplementation reduces frequency of periventricular haemorrhage in very premature babies. Lancet 1:466–471, 1987].

REFERENCES

1. Menachof L: Corticosteroids in croup: Reply from ground level. Pediatrics 49:154, 1972.
2. Silverman WA: "Human Experimentation: A Guided Step Into the Unknown." Oxford: Oxford Medical Publications, 1985.
3. Pocock SJ: "Clinical Trials." New York: John Wiley and Sons, 1983.
4. Chalmers TC: Randomization of the first patient. Med Clin North Am 59:1035–1038, 1975.
5. Meinert C: Toward more definitive clinical trials. Controlled Clin Trials 1:249–261, 1980.
6. "Controlled Clinical Trials: Design, Methods, and Analysis. From 1980."
7. Ederer F: Randomized controlled clinical trials. National Eye Institute for Ophthalmologists. Why do we need controls? Why do we need to randomize? Am J Ophthalmol 79:758–762, 1975.
8. Kinsey VE, Jacobus JT, Hemphill FM: Retrolental fibroplasia: Cooperative study of retrolental fibroplasia and the use of oxygen. Arch Ophthalmol 56:481–543, 1956.
9. Bucher JR, Roberts RJ: Alpha tocopherol (vitamin E) content of lung, liver, and blood in the newborn rat and human infant: Influence of hyperoxia. J Pediatr 98:806–811, 1981.
10. Owens WC, Owens EU: Retrolental fibroplasia in premature infants: II. Studies on the prophylaxis of the disease: The use of alpha tocopheryl acetate. Am J Ophthalmol 32:1631–1637, 1949.
11. Johnson L, Schaffer D, Boggs TR Jr: The premature infant, vitamin E deficiency and retrolental fibroplasia. Am J Clin Nutr 27:1158–1173, 1974.
12. Phelps DL, Rosenbaum AL: The role of tocopherol in oxygen-induced retinopathy: Kitten model. Pediatrics 59[suppl]:998–1005, 1977.
13. Hittner, HM, Godio LB, Rudolph AJ et al: Retrolental fibroplasia: Efficacy of vitamin E in a double-blind clinical study of preterm infants. N Engl J Med 305:1365–1371, 1981.
14. Milner RA, Watts JL, Paes B et al: RLF in 1500 gram neonates: Part of a randomized clinical trial of the effectiveness of vitamin E. "Retinopathy of Prematurity Conference Syllabus," Washington DC, December 4–6, 1981, Vol 2, pp 703–716.
15. Finer NN, Schindler RF, Peters KL, Grant GD: Vitamin E and retrolental fibroplasia: Improved visual outcome with early vitamin E. Ophthalmology 90:428–435, 1983.
16. Puklin JE, Simon RM, Ehrenkranz RA: Influence on retrolental fibroplasia of intramuscular vitamin E administration during respiratory distress syndrome. Ophthalmology 89:96–103, 1982.
17. Schaffer DB, Johnson L, Quinn GE, Weston M, Bowen FW: Vitamin E and retinopathy of prematurity: Follow-up at one year. Ophthalmology 92:1005–1011, 1985.
18. Phelps DL, Rosenbaum AL, Isenberg SJ, Leake RD, Dorey F: Effect of IV tocopherol (Vit E) on retinopathy of prematurity (ROP). Pediatr Res 19:357A, 1985.
19. Knight ME, Roberts RJ: Disposition of pharmacologic doses of vitamin E in newborn rabbits. Pediatr Res 18:154A, 1984.
20. Awad AB, Gilbreath RL: Hypervitaminosis E in atherosclerotic rabbits. Nutr Rep 11:409–417, 1975.
21. Bauernfeind, JC, Newmark H, Brin M: Vitamins A and E nutrition via intramuscular or oral route. Am J Clin Nutr 27:234–253, 1974.
22. Hoffmann-La Roche: "Vitamin E Information Brochure for Clinical Investigators." Nutley, NJ, 1976.

23. Phelps DL: Local and systemic reactions to the parenteral administration of vitamin E. Dev Pharmacol Ther 2:156–171, 1981.
24. Corrigan JJ Jr, Marcus FI: Coagulopathy associated with vitamin E ingestion. J Am Med Assoc 230:1300–1301, 1974.
25. Corrigan JJ Jr: Coagulation problems relating to vitamin E. Am J Pediatr Hematol Oncol 1:169–173, 1979.
26. Johnson L, Bowen FW Jr, Abbasi S, Herrmann N, Weston M, Sacks L, Porat R, Stahl G, Peckham G, Delivoria-Papadopoulos M, Quinn G, Schaffer D: Relationship of prolonged pharmacologic serum levels of vitamin E to incidence of sepsis and necrotizing enterocolitis in infants with birth weights 1,500 grams or less. Pediatrics 75:619–638, 1985.
27. Finer NN, Peters KL, Hayek Z, Merkel CL: Vitamin E and necrotizing enterocolitis. Pediatrics 73:387–393, 1984.
28. Rosenbaum AL, Phelps DL, Isenberg SJ, Leake RD, Dorey F: Retinal hemorrhage in retinopathy of prematurity associated with tocopherol treatment. Ophthalmology 92:1012–1014, 1985.
29. Phelps DL: Vitamin E and CNS hemorrhage (editorial). Pediatrics 74:1113–1114, 1984.
30. Speer ME, Blifeld C, Rudolph AJ, Chadda P, Holbein ME, Hittner HM: Intraventricular hemorrhage and vitamin E in the very low-birth-weight infant: Evidence for efficacy of early intramuscular vitamin E administration. Pediatrics 74:1107–1112, 1984.
31. Chiswick ML, Johnson M, Woodhall C, Gowland M, Davies J, Toner N, Sims DG: Protective effect of vitamin E (DL-alpha-tocopherol) against intraventricular haemorrhage in premature babies. Br Med J 287:81–84, 1983.
32. Phelps DL, Rosenbaum A, Isenberg S, Leake RD, Dorey F: Safety of intravascular tocopherol in a randomized double blind trial in premature infants. Pediatr Res 18:158A, 1984.
33. Roberts RJ, Knight ME, Mortensen ML, Martone W, Phelps DL, Sinha SN, Frank DJ, Vidyasagar D: Vitamin E content of tissues obtained from human infants given pharmacologic doses of tocopherol or tocopheryl acetate intravenously. Pediatr Res 19:178A, 1985.
34. Bodenstein CJ: Intravenous vitamin E and deaths in the intensive care unit (letter). Pediatrics 73:733, 1984.
35. Phelps DL: E-ferol: What happened and what now? Pediatrics 74:1114–1116, 1984.
36. Phelps DL: Retinopathy of prematurity: An estimate of vision loss in the United States— 1979. Pediatrics 67:924–926, 1981.
37. Gunn TR, Easdown J, Outerbridge EW et al: Risk factors in retrolental fibroplasia. Pediatrics 65:1096–1100, 1980.
38. Bauer CR: The occurrence of retrolental fibroplasia in infants of birth weight 1000 g and less. Clin Res 26:824A, 1978.
39. Shahinian L Jr, Malachowski N: Retrolental fibroplasia: A new analysis of risk factors based on recent cases. Arch Ophthalmol 96:70–74, 1978.
40. Detsky AS, Sackett DL: When was a "negative" clinical trial big enough? How many patients you needed depends on what you found. Arch Intern Med 145:709–712, 1985.

Vitamin E and Retinopathy of Prematurity: The Ophthalmologist's Perspective

David B. Schaffer, MD, Lois Johnson, MD, Graham E. Quinn, MD, Soraya Abbasi, MD, Chari Otis, MS, and Frank W. Bowen, MD

Departments of Ophthalmology (D.B.S., G.E.Q.), Pediatrics (L.J.), Pediatrics and Obstetrics (S.A., F.W.B.), and Biostatistics (C.O.), University of Pennsylvania School of Medicine, Philadelphia, Pennsylvania 19104

The possible benefit of vitamin E (alpha tocopherol) in the prevention of the blinding sequelae of retinopathy of prematurity (ROP) was first reported in 1949 (Table I) by Owens and Owens [1]. With the identification of oxygen as the supposedly "prime" etiologic factor [2] and the failure of the medical community to corroborate the Owens' initial observations with further clinical trials, interest in vitamin E waned [3].

Over the next 20 years, improvements in both the delivery and monitoring of oxygen and the many advances in neonatal intensive care permitted the survival of increasingly smaller infants who were at the greatest risk for developing ROP. Despite these advances, premature infants continued to develop blinding ROP, and we began a reexamination of the efficacy of vitamin E in both the prevention and treatment of ROP in the early 1970s. Our initial controlled, masked pilot study reported on only a small number of infants [4]. Nonetheless, the 1972–1974 study suggested a vitamin E benefit on the incidence of ROP in infants less than 1,500 gm (Table II). In addition, using a derived severity index and considering all infants, it appeared that the severity of ROP was also affected favorably by vitamin E (Table III). Our initial conclusions were subsequently supported by the kitten studies of Phelps and Rosenbaum [5].

Since these reports, several centers have undertaken clinical trials with vitamin E, and the preliminary abstracts from some of them [6–10] seemed encouraging. In late 1981, Hittner et al [11], using oral vitamin E in a randomized, double-blind trial, reported a significant reduction in the severity, but not the incidence, of ROP in 50 treated compared to 51 control infants with birthweights below 1,500 gm. Puklin et al [12], using intramuscular (IM) vitamin E within the first 24 hours of life to study its effect on the respiratory distress syndrome (RDS), found no reduction in the incidence of

Birth Defects: Original Article Series, Volume 24, Number 1, pages 219–235

TABLE I. Effect of Vitamin E on the Incidence of Retrolental Fibroplasia (RLF) in Premature Infants [1]

Group	(Infants all < 1,360 gm birthweight)		
	(N = 101)	No. RLF	Percent RLF
No vitamin E	78	17	21.8
Vitamin E Rx	23	1	4.4
			P = 0.06

TABLE II. Influence of Parenteral Vitamin E on the Incidence of Retrolental Fibroplasia (RLF) [4]

	Infants < 2,001 gm birthweight			Infants < 1,501 gm birthweight		
	(N = 81)	No. RLF	Percent RLF	(N = 33)	No. RLF	Percent RLF
No E	40	15	37.5	17	12	70.5
E Rx	41	9	22.0	16	6	37.5
			P ≤ 0.1*			P ≤ 0.06*

*Fisher's exact probability test (2 × 2 contingency table).

TABLE III. Influence of Parenteral Vitamin E on the Derived Severity/Incidence Index[†] of RLF by Birthweight [4]

	Infants < 2,001 gm				Infants < 1,501 gm			
	Vitamin E		Placebo		Vitamin E		Placebo	
	OD	OS	OD	OS	OD	OS	OD	OS
No. eyes Grade 1 RLF	6	5	8	9	3	3	7	8
No. eyes Grade 2 RLF	3	3	7	6	3	3	5	4
Abnormal points/ No. of infants	23/41		43/40		18/16		33/17	
RLF index	0.56		1.08		1.12		1.94	
			P < 0.05*				P = 0.08*	

[†]Severity/incidence index, each infant's RLF score = the sum of the highest stage of RLF in each eye. Individual scores for each weight group are totalled and divided by the number of infants in that group.
*Student's t test comparing levels of severity with pooled variance estimate.

ROP in 37 vitamin E-treated (mean weight 1,484 ± 73 gm) compared to 37 placebo-treated infants (mean weight 1,540 ± 85 gm) receiving standard care consisting of oral vitamin E drops of 30–55 IU/day. Finer et al [13], in a series of 99 surviving infants weighing less than 1,500 gm, reported that early IM administration of vitamin E did not affect the incidence of ROP but, using multiple linear regression analysis, did significantly reduce the severity of subsequent eye damage. Milner et al [14] could not detect any statistically significant benefit of oral vitamin E in 225 surviving infants (114 controls, 111 vitamin E-treated) also weighing less than 1,500 gm at birth. However, in this study, ophthalmoscopy could not be performed at a frequency that would allow for the assessment of the incidence of low-grade ROP. Because of the infrequency of severe acute ROP and the even lower incidence of its cicatricial retrolental fibroplasia (RLF) residua, the relatively small sample sizes in these clinical studies did not allow for statistically convincing evidence that vitamin E was beneficial.

Possible additional corroboration of the influence of vitamin E on the development of ROP was presented by Kretzer et al [15] in 1982. In infants of over 27 weeks of gestational age, they showed ultrastructural evidence that the increase in gap junction formation between spindle cells seen in these babies born with immature retinas is decreased by elevated plasma vitamin E levels achieved early in neonatal life. Kretzer et al postulated that the increased gap junction area and other spindle cell abnormalities caused a cessation of the normal orderly vascularization of the peripheral retina and resulted in the vascular changes of ROP [16,17].

The spindle cell hypothesis has not been independently verified, and it is questioned by several investigators [18,19]. In addition, the subsequently reported [20,21] toxic side effects of an increased incidence of sepsis and late-onset necrotizing entercolitis (NEC) associated with high serum vitamin E levels used prophylactically placed the role of the vitamin in controversy [3,22]. The status of vitamin E was further complicated by other contradictory reports of additional effects of the vitamin, both beneficial and harmful [23–32], on the newborn infant.

MATERIALS AND METHODS
Study Design

Our study at the University of Pennsylvania School of Medicine nursery complex (Pennsylvania Hospital, The Children's Hospital of Philadelphia, and University of Pennsylvania Hospital) enrolled 914 infants from January, 1979, to May, 1981. Those eligible had to be younger than 6 days old and have a birthweight less than 2,001 gm. Initially, we also included those over 2,000 gm if their gestation age was less than 37 weeks and oxygen was used for 24 hours or more. After the first 18 months of enrollment, the unqualified upper limit for birthweight was reduced to 1,750 gm because of the very low incidence of ROP found in infants born above this weight. The final enrollment consisted of 369 infants >1,500 gm, 216 with birthweights of 1,251–1,500 gm, 183 weighing 1,001–1,250 gm and 146 infants weighing <1,001 gm at birth. Complete details of both the randomization and extensive masking procedures have been reported previously [29].

TABLE IV. Mean (± SD) Serum Vitamin E Levels (mg/dl) in Placebo-Treated Infants < 1,251 gm Birthweight

	1,001–1,250 gm (N = 77)	< 1,001 gm (N = 41)
Entry	0.54 ± 0.21	0.56 ± 0.23
Day 1	0.71 ± 0.38	0.58 ± 0.29
Days 1–7	0.80 ± 0.41	0.72 ± 0.23
Days 1–14	0.83 ± 0.31	0.81 ± 0.22
Days 1–28	0.86 ± 0.28	0.86 ± 0.23
Days 1–56	0.93 ± 0.30	0.95 ± 0.27

As soon as possible after admission to the nursery, consent was obtained and an initial blood sample was drawn for analysis of the serum vitamin E levels prior to any supplemental vitamin or the placebo. The target serum vitamin E level of 5 mg/dl was then established rapidly using the dl-alpha tocopherol free alcohol preparation (50 mg/dl) supplied by Hoffmann LaRoche and given either orally, IM, or by a slow IV infusion over 6–8 hours. Serum levels were monitored daily at first, then twice weekly while the infants were still in the nursery. All total tocopherol concentrations were determined by the ultramicrocolorimetric method of Hashim and Schuttringer [33] on 50 lambda of serum.

After infants were discharged from the hospital, vitamin E levels were measured and adjusted at the time of each eye examination at Children's Hospital to maintain the serum vitamin E at 5 mg/dl until the retinas were judged mature or any ROP had resolved. Vitamin E or the placebo was stopped unless there were any residual funduscopic findings, in which case treatment was continued to maintain the serum vitamin E level at 3 mg/dl until the 1-year examination. As is indicated in Table IV, the placebo group, especially the smaller infants, were initially in the vitamin E-deficient range, but the serum vitamin E gradually increased to near-sufficient levels on standard dietary formulas by about 2 weeks of age.

Ophthalmologic Examination

Each infant enrolled in the study underwent the initial eye examination as soon as the neonatologist judged that the infant's condition permitted it safe, even if it was on the first day of life. Pupillary dilatation was accomplished with 1.0% tropicamide and 2.5% phenylephrine HCl, one drop of each instilled into each eye at 15-minute intervals for three doses. Funduscopy was performed 15 minutes after the last drops using a binocular indirect ophthalmoscope with a 30 diopter lens. Lid speculums and scleral depression were used as required, but this was not found routinely necessary. These

TABLE V. Similarities of Classification Systems

GEQ/DBS ROP classification (1982)	ICROP classification (1984)
G 1 ROP = abnormal intraretinal vascular changes	Not classified as ROP
G 2 ROP = line or ridge	{ S 1 ROP = demarcation line { S 2 ROP = ridge
G 3 ROP = ridge + ERNV[†]	S 3 ROP = ridge + ERNV
G 4 ROP = partial RD[‡]	S 4 ROP = any RD
G 5 ROP = total RD	

[†]ERNV, extraretinal neovascularization.
[‡]RD, retinal detachment.

examinations were repeated every 1–2 weeks until retinal vascular maturity was observed or until regression of any active ROP was well established. During this period of ROP resolution, the eye evaluations were continued as frequently as was indicated by the child's ocular status. Infants with normal, mature eyes and those with resolved ROP were seen at 3, 6, and 12 months from the estimated date of term delivery and according to need thereafter. Any infant who progressed to our grade 3+ ROP was treated with vitamin E at the target level of 5 mg/dl regardless of study medication assignment. If the retinopathy progressed to posterior detachment (grade 4 ROP), consultation was obtained with an experienced vitreoretinal surgeon. Cryotherapy was recommended and successfully performed on one eye of only one patient.

All eye examinations were performed by either D.B.S. or G.E.Q. using our previously published classification of acute ROP [34–36], which was specifically developed in 1979 for this study and which is almost identical (Table V) to the International Classification of Retinopathy of Prematurity (ICROP) published in 1984 [37,38]. Furthermore, in addition to the stage of ROP, we also prospectively recorded the presence or absence of plus disease, the A-P location by retinal drawings, and the circumferential extent of the retinal disease by quadrant (Fig. 1). Although most infants were seen by only one of the authors (D.B.S. or G.E.Q.), periodic cross-checks for possible drift were performed on approximately 25% of the cases. Repeated analyses showed that diagnostic agreement was maintained between the two observers at over 95% for grade 1 ROP and over 99% for grade 2 or higher. In addition, an outside retinal specialist examined about 10% of randomly chosen infants to corroborate the findings.

Our protocol also planned for a 1–2-year follow-up eye examination that would yield a stable cicatricial RLF grading by the Reese classification [39].

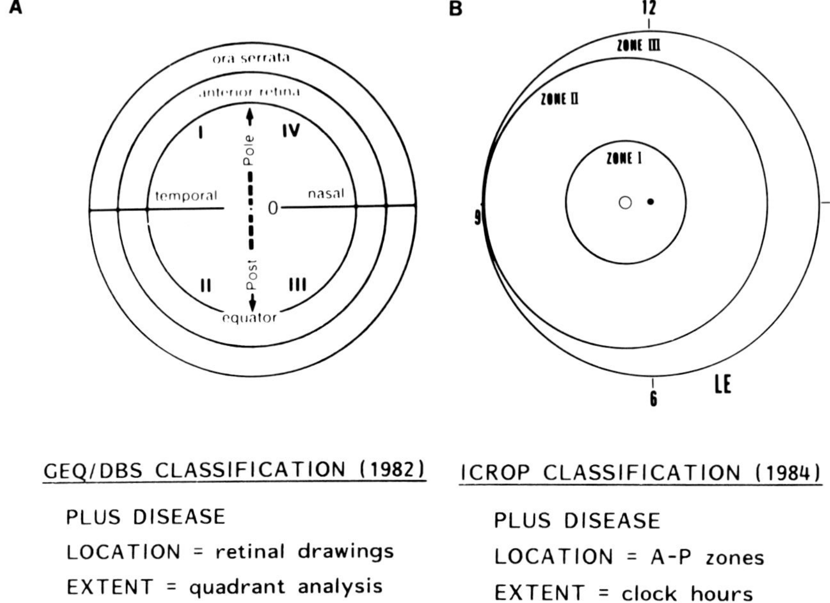

Fig. 1. A: Example of retinal diagram used for recording the results in the Philadelphia study. B: Retinal diagram recommended by the ICROP. Both are almost identically capable of indicating the presence or absence of + disease, the anterior-posterior location, and the circumferential extent of ROP.

Furthermore, since sequelae of arrested mild ROP [40,41] might also be affected, we assessed visual acuity and analyzed the range of refractive errors, anisometropia, strabismus, and amblyopia at that point. The methods particular to the 1–2-year follow-up examination as well as some of the results have been previously reported [40,42].

RESULTS

Morbidity and Mortality

Our results reveal excellent randomization for demographic variables (Table VI) and for many correlates of illness (Table VII). We paid close attention to the amount of blood received as well as to a number of oxygen and metabolic variables as indices of illness and found no statistical differences between the vitamin E and placebo groups (Table VII). We did find a significantly increased incidence of vitamin E-related bacterial sepsis

TABLE VI. Comparison of All (N = 914) Placebo-and Vitamin E-Treated Infants at Enrollment Into the Study*

| | Infants > 1,500 gm | | Infants < 1,501 gm | |
	Placebo (N = 185)	Vitamin E (N = 184)	Placebo (N = 275)	Vitamin E (N = 270)
Sex				
Male	108	98	149	146
Female	77	86	126	124
Race				
White	107	101	126	126
Black	79	71	139	127
Other	9	12	10	17
Birthweight in gm				
(mean ± SD)	1,870 ± 306	1,900 ± 336	1,156 ± 232	1,162 ± 230
Gestational age in weeks				
(mean ± SD)	33.8 ± 1.6	33.6 ± 1.5	30.2 ± 2.8	30.1 ± 2.3
Intrauterine growth				
retardation	9	5	38	35
Apgar score				
1 min < 5	31	37	108	121
5 min < 7	28	31	91	99
In-born	108	109	174	173

*There are no significant differences between treatment groups for any of the variables lists (P > 0.1).

TABLE VII. Comparison of Placebo and Vitamin E Treatment Groups in Infants Born Weighing < 1,501 gm (N = 424) With Respect to 10 Correlates of Illness*

Variable	Placebo ($\bar{X}$ ± SE; N = 216)	Vitamin E ($\bar{X}$ ± SE; N = 208)
Blood (ml/kg BW)	165 ± 16	179 ± 13
Days FiO$_2$ > 22%	22.1 ± 2.0	24.1 ± 2.1
Days on ventilator	12.6 ± 1.7	11.8 ± 1.6
Hours PaO$_2$ 40–54 Torr	19.5 ± 2.0	17.4 ± 1.7
Hours PaO$_2$ > 110 Torr	11.5 ± 1.0	11.1 ± 0.9
Hours pCO$_2$ > 55 Torr	10.4 ± 1.6	9.8 ± 1.4
Hours pCO$_2$ < 30 Torr	9.7 ± 1.1	7.1 ± 0.7
Hours − BE > 5 mg/liter	41.1 ± 4.3	28.0 ± 2.6
pH < 7.25	17.7 ± 2.1	14.3 ± 1.7
Days in hospital	70.2 ± 2.3	76.4 ± 2.9

*P = NS between treatment groups for all variables listed.

and late-onset NEC confined to infants <1,501 gm and have reported this dose-related toxicity [21,29]. Other investigators [23–26,30,31] have reported varying effects of vitamin E on both mortality and intraventricular

TABLE VIII. Infant Mortality Through Age 1 Month by Birthweight Group

Birthweight group (gm)	Placebo No.	(%)	Vitamin E No.	(%)
1,501–2,000	6	(3.2)	8	(4.3)
1,251–1,500	4	(3.6)	10	(9.4)
1,001–1,250	12	(13.4)	15	(16.3)
< 1,001	30	(40.5)	22	(30.6)
				P > 0.1

TABLE IX. Proven Intraventricular Hemorrhage by Birthweight Groups

Birthweight group (gm)	Placebo No.	(%)	Vitamin E No.	(%)
1,501–2,000	5	(2.7)	8	(4.4)
1,251–1,500	5	(4.6)	5	(4.8)
1,001–1,250	15	(17.1)	19	(20.7)
< 1,001	24	(32.4)	19	(26.8)
				P > 0.1

TABLE X. Incidence and Severity of ROP: Placebo- (P) vs Vitamin E-Treated (E) Infants (All infants N = 755)

	P	E
No ROP	261	271
Mild ROP	99	74
Moderate ROP	16	22
Severe ROP	9	3
	P = 0.05	

hemorrhage (IVH). Because of the obvious importance of these considerations, we examined the mortality (Table VIII) and IVH status (Table IX) in our study by birthweight groups. As shown, we found no statistical difference between the two study groups.

Ophthalmic Results

Of the 914 infants enrolled in the study, complete acute-stage eye data were obtained in 755 babies, of whom 424 weighed <1501 gm at birth. Our data showed a significant benefit (P = 0.05) of prophylactic high-dose vitamin E therapy when considering all infants and increasing severity of ROP (Table X) categorized as none, mild, moderate, and severe. When the data on the 755 infants were analyzed by specific birthweight groups, a favorable effect of vitamin E on the incidence of ROP was apparent (P = 0.01) in the larger infants, all of whom had low-grade disease (Table XI).

TABLE XI. Incidence and Severity of ROP by Birthweight: Placebo- (P) vs Vitamin E-Treated (E) Infants

	Infants > 1,500 gm (N = 331)			Infants > 1,501 gm (N = 424)	
	P	E		P	E
No ROP	154	158	No ROP	107	113
Mild ROP	15	4	Mild ROP	84	70
			Moderate ROP	16	22
			Severe ROP	9	3
	P = 0.01			P = 0.15	

TABLE XII. Incidence and Severity of the ROP by P/E Groups: A Comparison of All Study Infants vs Only Early Enrollment

	Infants enrolled on days 0–5				Infants enrolled on days 0–1			
	All infants (N = 755)		Infants < 1,501 gm (N = 424)		All infants (N = 510)		Infants < 1,501 gm (N = 288)	
	P	E	P	E	P	E	P	E
Incidence of ROP								
No ROP	261	271	107	113	181	187	71	85
Any ROP	124	99	109	95	83	59	76	56
	P = 0.10		P = 0.32		P = 0.06		P = 0.04	
Incidence and severity of ROP								
No ROP	261	271	107	113	181	187	71	85
Mild ROP	99	74	84	70	67	43	60	40
Moderate ROP	16	22	16	22	9	13	9	13
Severe ROP	9	3	9	3	7	3	7	3
	P = 0.05		P = 0.15		P = 0.07		P = 0.05	

However, the smaller babies, who had the more severe eye disease, did not seem to be significantly helped by vitamin E.

We did not limit enrollment to the first 48 hours because the largest of our three nurseries serves an entirely out-born population, and such a restriction would have seriously decreased the sample size available for study. Since age at which treatment begins was expected to be a major variable, the study was designed to allow a subset analysis of early vitamin E treatment by prospectively documenting both the time of enrollment and initiation of study medication. We analyzed the data for all eligible infants and for all infants enrolled by calendar age 1 day (Table XII). Table XII (top) presents the incidence of ROP as a yes/no variable; the bottom reports the severity variable. Considering the entire early enrolled population, borderline significance (P = 0.06) in favor of vitamin E is found for incidence. Most importantly, early vitamin E prophylaxis significantly decreased both the incidence (P = 0.04) and severity (P = 0.05) of ROP in the infants born weighing <1,501 gm.

Although vitamin E has been hypothesized to influence the events that initiate the disease [15–17], no one has clearly shown a vitamin E effect on the incidence of ROP in the smaller infants until this study. It is thought that this effect was finally noticed because of the enrollment of a large number of very-small-birthweight infants combined with the plan of treating them with supplemental vitamin E as early after enrollment as possible. Moreover, the studies showing a vitamin E benefit have demonstrated an effect on the severity of ROP [11,13], perhaps indicating that vitamin E plays a role in modifying the progression of the fibrovascular proliferation. Indeed, in this study also, severe ROP resulted from moderate ROP more frequently in the placebo infants (P <0.025), although the incidence of moderate ROP or worse (Table X) was the same in both groups (25 placebo and 25 vitamin E) when considering all the infants and ignoring the time of the initial vitamin E treatment. The progression to more severe ROP occurred in 36% (9/25) of the placebo infants and in only 12% (3/25) of the vitamin E-treated babies.

Still to be considered is whether vitamin E could also alter the events involved with scarring, as was previously suggested by Johnson et al [43]. We now have 1–2-year follow-up eye data on all the birthweight groups. Residual cicatricial disease occurred only in the infants with birthweights <1,501 gm, and no statistical difference was found between the incidence of cicatricial RLF in the placebo- and the vitamin E-treated groups. Of the 331 infants in this weight category for whom complete information is available, 13 of 164 (7.9%) placebo-treated and 13 of 167 (7.8%) vitamin E-treated had visible scars.

Since grade 1 cicatricial RLF is associated mainly with refractive errors and peripheral retinal abnormalities [39,41], we separated it from the more severe grades of cicatricial RLF that show anatomic changes in the posterior retina. As was previously reported [42], we noted only a trend (P = 0.07) toward a vitamin E benefit. However, comparing the severity of the cicatricial disease (by both eyes or by worse eye grade) among only those infants who had visible ocular residua (Table XIII), the benefit of vitamin E was found to be significant (P < 0.025). In the vitamin E-treated group, nine infants had grade 1 cicatricial RLF, three had grade 2 RLF, and only one had worse than grade 3 RLF. In the placebo infants, four had only grade 1, four had grade 2, and five had grade 3 cicatricial RLF or worse.

Finally, in addition to the effect we found vitamin E to have on ROP, we also discovered another ocular anomaly (Fig. 2) of lesser importance associated with sustained pharmacologic vitamin E serum levels. Transient neonatal lens vacuoles occurred more frequently (Table XIV) in the vitamin

TABLE XIII. Comparison of the E/P Severity of Cicatricial RLF Among Infants Who Had Visible Residua (Grade of cicatricial RLF outcome by eye)[†]

P		E	
OD	OS	OD	OS
0	1	1	0
1	1	1	1
1	1	1	1
1	1	1	1
1	2	1	1
2	1	1	1
2	2	1	1
2	2	1	1
2	3	1	1
3	1	1	2
1	5	2	2
5	1	2	2
5	5	3	5
		P < 0.025*	

[†]Table includes infants with 1-year follow-up data and three additional infants with severe disease (two placebo, one vitamin E-treated) who died with definite cicatricial disease before age 1 year.
*Sign test.

E-treated group (11.1%) than in the placebo-treated infants (3.5%), and this was statistically significant (P <0.005). However, in all cases, the vacuoles disappeared sometime during the first year of life without any dire consequences.

DISCUSSION: COMPARISON OF SIX STUDIES

From 1977 through 1983, prophylactic vitamin E and its effect on ROP has been studied in six randomized and prospective clinical trials [11–14,29,32]. The Mantel-Haenszel statistical technique [44] can be used to pool results, maximizing the available data when the trials are appropriately comparable. There are also the obvious advantages of increasing the sample size, placing in better perspective a particular outlyer trial, and minimizing sampling errors related to unknown and/or uncontrollable risk factors, including the poorly understood, multifactorial etiology of ROP and its even less well understood cicatricial results.

These six trials are sufficiently similar. They were all randomized, prospective, double-masked studies with simultaneous controls. Though it was not always clear in the original papers, subsequent reports [32,45] (also,

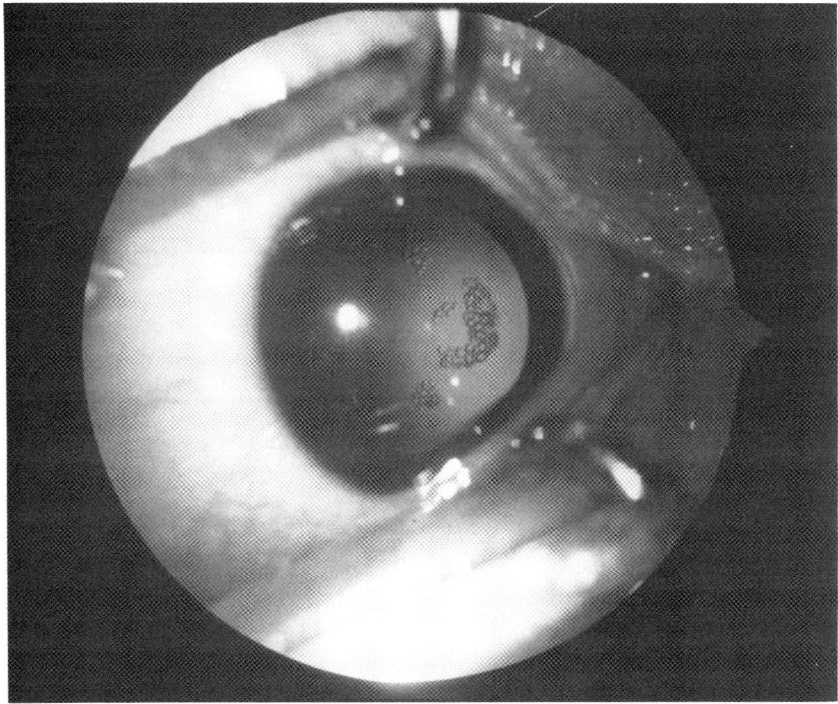

Fig. 2. Transient neonatal lens vacuoles. Photograph of vacuoles found at 4 weeks of age that subsequently disappeared.

TABLE XIV. Incidence of Transient Lens Vacuoles in Placebo- and Vitamin E-Treated Infants

	Placebo	Vitamin E-treated
Absent	368	329
Present	17	14
		$P < 0.005$

R.A. Ehrenkranz, personal communication) have made it possible to identify those infants born weighing below 1,501 gm in each study, thereby allowing for pooled analysis of those infants at greatest risk for severe ROP.

Although the target vitamin E level was attained within the first week of life in all the studies, there were differences in the criteria for enrollment, in the routes of administration of the vitamin and its placebo, and in the timing

TABLE XV. Comparison of the Six Prospective Trials of Prophylactic Vitamin E (All infants < 1,501 gm birthweight)

Study	Placebo		Vitamin E	
	Total No.	Severe ROP	Total No.	Severe ROP
Hittner et al [11]	51	5	50	0
Milner et al [14]	114	5	111	3
Erhenkranz and Puklin [45] (also, personal communication)	20	1	22	0
Finer et al [13]	51	4	48	2
Phelps [32]	99	1	97	1
Johnson et al [32]	216	9	208	3
Totals	551	25	536	9
Percent severe ROP	4.5		1.8	
	P < 0.01 (Mantel-Haenszel)			

of the initial dose. For example, the Finer et al study [13] required enrollment within the first 12 hours of life, the Hittner et al [11] and Puklin et al [12] studies by age 24 hours; the others [14,29,32] set later limits.

All the studies aimed for and achieved vitamin E levels at least in the 1–2 mg% range, and most, ours included, had higher serum E goals. The control populations exhibited different levels of vitamin E nutrition; however, they all had significantly lower serum vitamin E levels than the vitamin E-treated infants.

Although different, the ROP classifications were clearly stated, and after personal communication with several of the investigators (Finer, Ehrenkranz, Milner), we believe that similarly severe ROP (3 + ROP or worse) is identifiable, although mild ROP is not. The eye exams were performed frequently enough to be sure that severe ROP was not missed. However, the different examination schedules preclude comparison of the incidence of mild ROP between the studies. Furthermore, we cannot compare the acute ROP greater than stage 3 + or any final cicatricial RLF grades because of the various therapeutic interventions used for severe disease. As previously mentioned, we started all placebo infants on high-dose vitamin E at that point, and one child also received cryotherapy. Others [11,13] intervened with cryotherapy and/or scleral buckling procedures.

Reviewing the results from the infants with birthweights less than 1,501 gm (Table XV) shows that, in fact, in none of the studies did the vitamin E-treated infants have more severe ROP. Furthermore, by applying the Mantel-Haenszel technique, it does appear that comparison of severe disease in the treated vs control neonates in the six trials indicates a significant benefit for vitamin E (P < 0.01).

CONCLUSIONS

The results of our studies at the University of Pennsylvania, along with the analysis of the available data from the other trials, seem to suggest a beneficial effect on ROP obtained by maintaining serum vitamin E levels in the physiologic range of 1.0–2.5 mg/dl from the first or second day after birth. Our neonatologists therefore recommend this as a treatment goal. Serially monitoring serum vitamin E levels is an integral part of this recommendation because of the relatively mild ocular and definitely more serious systemic side effects that appear to be related to prolonged, high-dose vitamin E prophylaxis in infants weighing <1,501 gm at birth.

ACKNOWLEDGMENTS

The authors acknowledge the invaluable contribution of the late Thomas R. Boggs Jr., M.D., the study's original principal investigator. Also, the kind help extended by the Data and Safety Monitoring Committee: Drs. Henry Baird and Thomas Sisson, cochairman; Argye Hillis, Ph.D., Consultant Statistician; Gary Aden, Esq.; Ernest Harding, D.D.; Joanne Moriconi, R.N., M.S.; Helen Preston, M.B.A.; William Tasman, M.D., and Israel Goldberg, Ph.D, N.E.I. We thank enormously Drs. Linda Sachs, Rachel Porat, Elizabeth Fong, Maria Delivoria-Papadopoulos, George Peckham, and Stephen Sinclair for their participation, clinical expertise, and valuable consultations. We appreciate the fine statistical guidance from Marion Weston, M.S.; Nira Herrmann Ph.D.; and Donald Goldstein, M.S. We deeply thank all the neonatal fellows, residents, nurses, and pharmacists who were integral to the study's success, with particular praise for both Drs. D. Dransfield and V. Sakata. Our very special gratitude goes to Dorothy Neff, our administrative assistant. No study of this size can be accomplished without the dedication of innumerable other assistants, and we are especially thankful for the help given by Fred Cook, Kathy Cronin, Beverly Harrison, David Newman, Vince Sardi, Kevin Waninger, Mary Jo Mathis, Chris Dalin, Rosemary Dworanczyk, Mary Grous, Rita Divers, MariAnne Campbell, Mary Lou Walsh, and Anita Raj. Our thanks also to our secretarial staff, Margaret Walsh, Tricia Lawler, and Anne Skinner. Hoffmann-LaRoche generously provided the support of research staff (particularly Drs. M. Brin, J. Bauerfeind, and H. Bhagavan), the parenteral and oral preparations of vitamin E and their placebos, and additional funds for statistical analysis.

Finally, we are grateful to Pennsylvania Hospital for making available its mainframe computer facilities.

REFERENCES

1. Owens WC, Owens EU: Retrolental fibroplasia in premature infants. II. Studies on the prophylaxis of the disease: The use of alpha tocopheryl acetate. Am J Ophthalmol 32:1631–1637, 1949.
2. Kinsey VE: Retrolental fibroplasia: Cooperative study of retrolental fibroplasia and the use of oxygen. Arch Ophthalmol 56:481–543, 1956.
3. Phelps DL: Vitamin E and retrolental fibroplasia in 1982. Pediatrics 70:420–425, 1982.
4. Johnson L, Schaffer D, Boggs TR Jr: The premature infant, vitamin E deficiency and retrolental fibroplasia. Am J Clin Nutr 27:1158–1173, 1974.
5. Phelps DL, Rosenbaum AL: The role of tocopherol in oxygen-induced retinopathy: Kitten model. Pediatrics 59[Suppl]:998–1005, 1977.
6. Johnson LH, Schaffer DB, Rubenstein D, Crawford CS, Boggs TR: The role of vitamin E in retrolental fibroplasia. Pediatr Res 10:425A, 1976.
7. Johnson LH, Schaffer DB, Goldstein DE, Boggs TR: Influence of vitamin E treatment (Rx) and adult blood transfusions on mean severity of retrolental fibroplasia (MS-RLF) in premature infants. Pediatr Res 11:535A, 1977.
8. Milner RA, Bell E, Blanchette V, Ling E, Watts JL, Zipursky A: Vitamin E supplement in under 1500 gram neonates. Pediatr Res 13:501A, 1979.
9. Johnson L, Schaffer D, Boggs T, Quinn G, Mathis M: Vitamin E Rx of retrolental fibroplasia (RLF) grade III or worse. Pediatr Res 14:601A, 1980.
10. Ehrenkranz RA, Puklin JE, Warshaw JB: Effectiveness of vitamin E (E) administration during respiratory distress syndrome (RDS) in preventing retrolental fibroplasia (RLF). Pediatr Res 15:659A, 1981.
11. Hittner HM, Godio LB, Rudolph AJ et al: Retrolental fibroplasia: Efficacy of vitamin E in a double-blind clinical study of preterm infants. N Engl J Med 305:1365–1371, 1981.
12. Puklin JE, Simon RM, Ehrenkranz RA: Influence on retrolental fibroplasia of intramuscular vitamin E administration during respiratory distress syndrome. Ophthalmology 89:96–103, 1982.
13. Finer NN, Schindler RF, Grant G et al: Effect of intramuscular vitamin E on the frequency and severity of retrolental fibroplasia: A controlled trial. Lancet 1:1087–1091, 1982.
14. Milner RA, Watts JL, Paes B et al: RLF in 1500 gram neonates: Part of a randomized clinical trial of the effectiveness of vitamin E. In: "Retinopathy of Prematurity Conference Syllabus," Washington, DC, December, 1981, Vol 2, pp 703–716.
15. Kretzer FL, Hittner HM, Johnson AT, Mehta RS, Godio LB: Vitamin E and retrolental fibroplasia: Ultrastructural support of clinical efficacy. Ann NY Acad Sci 393:145–166, 1982.
16. Hittner HM, Godio LB, Speer ME et al: Retrolental fibroplasia: Further clinical evidence and ultrastructural support for efficacy of vitamin E in the preterm infant. Pediatrics 71:423–432, 1983.
17. Kretzer FL, Hittner HM: Initiating events in the development of retinopathy of prematurity. In Silverman WA, Flynn JT (eds): "Contemporary Issues in Fetal and Neonatal Medicine: Vol 2. Retinopathy of Prematurity." Boston: Blackwell Scientific Publications, 1985, pp 121–152.
18. Cole GA, Skinner JM, Henderson DW, Mukherjee TM: Vitamin E effect questioned. Pediatrics 73:734, 1984.

19. Cole GA, Skinner JM, Henderson DW, Mukherjee TM: Vitamin E and retinopathy of prematurity revisited. Pediatrics 75:1166–1167, 1985.

20. Sobol S, Gueriguian J, Troendle G, Nevius E: Letter to the editor. N Engl J Med 306:867, 1982.

21. Johnson L, Bowen FW, Herrmann N et al: The relationship of prolonged elevation of serum vitamin E levels to neonatal bacterial sepsis and necrotizing enterocolitis. Pediatr Res 17:319A, 1983.

22. Committee on Fetus and Newborn: Vitamin E and the prevention of retinopathy of prematurity. Pediatrics 76:315–316, 1985.

23. Bodenstein CJ: Intravenous vitamin E and deaths in the intensive care unit (letter). Pediatrics 73:733, 1984.

24. Chiswick ML, Johnson M, Woodhall C et al: Protective effect of vitamin E (dl-alpha-tocopherol) against intraventricular haemorrhage in the newborn. Ciba Foundation Symp 101:186–200, 1983.

25. Speer ME, Blifield C, Rudolph AJ, Chadda P, Holbein B, Hittner HM: Intraventricular hemorrhage and vitamin E in the very low-birth-weight infant: Evidence for efficacy of early intramuscular vitamin E administration. Pediatrics 74:1107–1112, 1984.

26. Phelps DL: Vitamin E and CNS hemorrhage. (Editorial). Pediatrics 74:1113–1114, 1984.

27. Phelps DL: E-ferol: What happened and what now? Pediatrics 74:1114–1116, 1984.

28. Finer NN, Peters KL, Hayek Z, Merkel CL: Vitamin E and necrotizing enterocolitis. Pediatrics 73:387–393, 1984.

29. Johnson L, Bowen FW, Abbasi S et al: Relationship of prolonged pharmacologic serum levels of vitamin E to incidence of sepsis and necrotizing enterocolitis in infants with birth weight 1500 grams or less. Pediatrics 75:619–638, 1985.

30. Rosenbaum AL, Phelps DL, Isenberg SJ, Leake RD, Dorey F: Retinal hemorrhage in retinopathy of prematurity associated with tocopherol treatment. Ophthalmology 92:1012–1014, 1985.

31. Lorch V, Murphy D, Hoersten LR, Harris E, Fitzgerald J, Sinha SN: Unusual syndrome among premature infants: Association with a new intravenous vitamin E product. Pediatrics 75:598–602, 1985.

32. Phelps DL: Vitamin E and retinopathy of prematurity. In Silverman WA, Flynn JT (eds): "Contemporary Issues in Fetal and Neonatal Medicine: Vol 2. Retinopathy of Prematurity." Boston: Blackwell Scientific Publications, 1985, pp 181–205.

33. Hashim SA, Schuttringer GR: Rapid determination of tocopherol in macro- and micro-quantities of plasma: Results obtained in various nutrition and metabolic studies. Am J Clin Nutr 19:137–145, 1966.

34. Schaffer DB, Johnson L, Quinn GE, Boggs TR Jr: A classification of retrolental fibroplasia to evaluate vitamin E therapy. Ophthalmology 86:1749–1760, 1979.

35. Quinn GE, Schaffer DB, Johnson LH: Classification of retinopathy of prematurity as a predictive tool: A re-evaluation. "Retinopathy of Prematurity Conference Syllabus," Washington, DC, December, 1981, Vol 1, pp 303–317.

36. Quinn GE, Schaffer DB, Johnson L: A revised classification of retinopathy of prematurity. Am J Ophthalmol 94:744–749, 1982.

37. Committee for the Classification of Retinopathy of Prematurity: An international classification of retinopathy of prematurity. Pediatrics 74:127–133, 1984.

38. Committee for Classification of Retinopathy of Prematurity: An international classification of retinopathy of prematurity. Arch Ophthalmol 102:1130–1134, 1984.

39. Reese AB, King MJ, Owens WC: A classification of retrolental fibroplasia. Am J Ophthalmol 36:1333–1335, 1953.

40. Schaffer DB, Quinn GE, Johnson L: Sequelae of arrested mild retinopathy of prematurity. Arch Ophthalmol 102:373–376, 1984.
41. Kushner BJ: Strabismus and amblyopia associated with regressed retinopathy of prematurity. Arch Ophthalmol 100:256–261, 1982.
42. Schaffer DB, Johnson L, Quinn GE, Weston M, Bowen FW Jr: Vitamin E and retinopathy of prematurity: Follow-up at one year. Ophthalmology 92:1005–1011, 1985.
43. Johnson L, Schaffer D, Quinn G et al: Vitamin E supplementation and the retinopathy of prematurity. Ann NY Acad Sci 393:473–495, 1982.
44. Fleiss JL: "Statistical Methods for Rates and Proportions, 2nd Ed." New York: John Wiley and Sons, 1981.
45. Ehrenkranz RA, Puklin JE: Reply to "Letter to the Editor." Ophthalmology 89:988–989, 1982.

Autoxidative Damage to the Retina: Potential Role in Retinopathy of Prematurity

Martin L. Katz, PhD, and W. Gerald Robison, Jr., PhD

Department of Ophthalmology, University of Missouri School of Medicine, Columbia, Missouri 65212 (M.L.K.); Section of Ocular Pathology, National Eye Institute, National Institutes of Health, Bethesda, Maryland 21224 (W.G.R.)

A number of medical advances have led to an increasing ability to maintain the survival of preterm infants. However, premature birth requires that a number of developmental stages occur in an environment quite unlike that of the womb in which early development normally takes place. This alteration in environment can adversely affect certain developmental processes, among which is the vascularization of the neural retina. Abnormal retinal vascularization following premature birth, termed retinopathy of prematurity (ROP), frequently results in severe visual defects.

A variety of experimental evidence suggests that ROP develops as a consequence of the higher oxygen tension to which infants are exposed in the typical hospital nursery relative to that in utero. Protection against the development of ROP by vitamin E has been suggested in a number of clinical trials [1–3], giving rise to the hypothesis that oxygen promotes ROP by inducing autoxidative tissue damage. Apparently, normal protective mechanisms against autoxidative damage are not fully developed in the premature infant [4–6], so that damage can occur to an extent great enough to affect normal developmental processes adversely. In this chapter, the molecular mechanisms of autoxidative damage to cells and tissues are reviewed. Normal protective mechanisms against autoxidative tissue damage are discussed. Finally, the hypothesis that autoxidation of cellular components plays a direct role in the development of ROP is presented.

MOLECULAR MECHANISMS OF AUTOXIDATIVE DAMAGE TO CELLS AND TISSUES

Oxygen is necessary for the maintenance of most forms of life; it is the energy derived from the reactions between oxygen and certain organic molecules that drives most metabolic processes. However, reactions of oxygen in biologic systems, outside of those controlled by enzymes, often

Birth Defects: Original Article Series, Volume 24, Number 1, pages 237–248

$$O_2 \xrightarrow{\;e^-\;} O_2^{\cdot-} \xrightarrow{\;e^-+2H^+\;} H_2O_2 \xrightarrow{\;e^-+H^+\;} \begin{array}{c} OH^{\cdot} \\ H_2O \end{array} \xrightarrow{\;e^-+H^+\;} H_2O$$

Fig. 1. Production of reactive oxygen-based free radicals by sequential one-electron reductions of oxygen. Transfer of a single electron to molecular oxygen produces superoxide anion ($O_2^-\cdot$). Reduction of superoxide produces hydrogen peroxide (H_2O_2). Hydroxyl radical (OH•) and water are produced by one-electron reduction of H_2O_2. Finally, hydroxyl radical reduction produces a second molecule of water.

$$H_2O_2 + Fe^{2+} \longrightarrow OH^{\cdot} + OH^- + Fe^{3+}$$

$$RH + Fe^{3+} \longrightarrow R^{\cdot} + Fe^{2+} + H^+$$

Fig. 2. Iron-catalyzed decomposition of H_2O_2. Ferrous iron (Fe^{2+}) can donate an electron to H_2O_2, producing the hydroxyl radical and hydroxide ion. The resultant ferric form of iron (Fe^{3+}) can then be reduced back to Fe^{2+} by a variety of organic reductants. Other transition metal ions are also capable of catalyzing H_2O_2 decomposition to produce hydroxyl radicals.

prove deleterious. The reduction of oxygen to water during normal mito-chondrial metabolism occurs via a series of one-electron transfers (Fig. 1) in which two highly reactive radical species, superoxide anion ($O_2^-\cdot$) and the hydroxyl radical (OH•), are formed. Hydrogen peroxide in turn can be broken down in the presence of reducing agents and trace amounts of metal ions to produce hydroxyl radicals (Fig. 2). Normally, the sequential steps involved in mitochondrial electron transport are tightly coupled so that partially reduced forms of oxygen are not released. However, a certain amount of leakage of these intermediates apparently does occur [7], resulting in the potential for damage to cellular macromolecules through reactions with the free radical species of partially reduced oxygen. These partially reduced forms of oxygen can also be generated by a variety of enzymatic processes in addition to mitochondrial electron transport [8], suggesting that the potential for free radical-mediated oxidative damage to cells is quite substantial.

Polyunsaturated fatty acids (PUFAs), particularly those of membrane phospholipids, appear to be primary targets for damage by oxygen-based radicals. This is because reaction of a single free radical species with a PUFA moiety can trigger a chain reaction in which many PUFA moieties partake (Fig. 3), resulting in a process called autoxidation. Although the variety and complexity of reactions involved in PUFA autoxidation are immense, a relatively small number of end-products of this process have been identified in biologic systems. Among these are conjugated dienes (Fig. 4), short-chain

PUFA Autoxidation

Initiation:

$$RH + OH\cdot \longrightarrow R\cdot + H_2O$$

$$RH + O_2^- + H^+ \longrightarrow R\cdot + H_2O_2$$

$$RH + X\cdot \longrightarrow R\cdot + X\cdot$$

Propogation:

$$R\cdot + O_2 \longrightarrow ROO\cdot$$

$$ROO\cdot + RH \longrightarrow ROOH + R\cdot$$

Chain Branching:

$$ROOH + M^{n+} \longrightarrow RO\cdot + OH^- + M^{(n-1)+}$$

Chain Termination:

$$R\cdot + ROO\cdot \longrightarrow ROOR$$

$$R\cdot + RO\cdot \longrightarrow ROR$$

$$R\cdot + R\cdot \longrightarrow RR$$

$$X\cdot + AH \longrightarrow XH + A\cdot$$

Fig. 3. Chemistry of PUFA autoxidation. Autoxidation is initiated by the abstraction of hydrogen from a PUFA molecule by a free radical (eg, OH•). The resultant PUFA radical (R•) reacts with oxygen to form a peroxy radical (ROO•), which in turn can abstract hydrogen from another PUFA molecule. This cycle can continue until one of a number of chain-terminating events occurs. The PUFA hydroperoxides (ROOH) generated during PUFA autoxidation can be decomposed via transition metal ion catalysis to produce organic oxyradicals (RO•).

alkanes (ethane and pentane), and malonaldehyde. The latter compound, a three-carbon dialdehyde, can cause further molecular damage to cells by reacting with amino groups on a variety of molecules and thereby cross-linking them (Fig. 5).

Direct damage by oxygen-based radicals to other cellular components, in addition to PUFAs, undoubtedly takes place, although it is often more difficult to demonstrate. For example, Cathcart and colleagues [9] have linked oxidative damage of thymine bases in DNA to reactions with oxygen-based radicals. Essentially all cellular components are potential

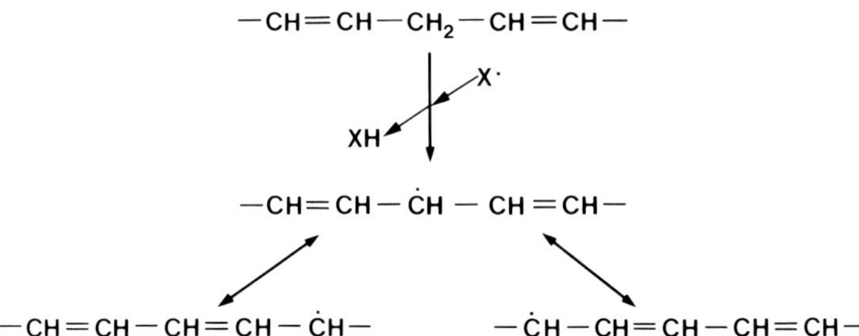

Fig. 4. Mechanism of conjugated diene formation during PUFA autoxidation. Double bonds in mammalian PUFA molecules are always separated by single methylene groups. Hydrogen abstraction from such a methylene group produces a delocalized free radical. Reduction of this radical at either end of the delocalized system produces a conjugated diene.

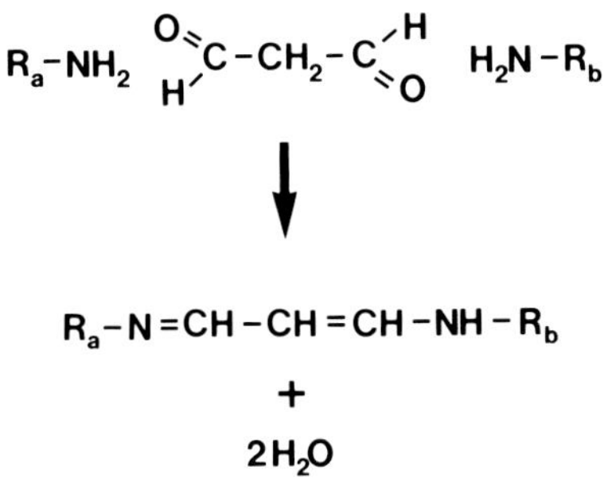

Fig. 5. Mechanism of malonaldehyde cross-linking of molecules with primary amino groups.

targets for damage by oxygen-based radicals, since the latter, particularly the hydroxyl radical, are highly reactive and nondiscriminatory.

PROTECTIVE MECHANISMS AGAINST AUTOXIDATIVE TISSUE DAMAGE

A variety of mechanisms have evolved to protect biologic systems from the potentially damaging effects of oxygen-based free radicals. Among these are the superoxide dismutase, catalase, and peroxidase enzymes as well as free radical scavengers such as vitamin E.

Superoxide Dismutases

The importance of the superoxide dismutases in protecting against oxygen toxicity is suggested by the fact that virtually every organism that undergoes aerobic metabolism synthesizes one or more forms of this enzyme, whereas obligate anaerobes in general do not [8]. A number of facultative organisms have been found to synthesize superoxide dismutase in response to exposure to oxygen, and blocking such synthesis rendered these organisms susceptible to oxygen toxicity [10]. Further evidence of the importance of superoxide dismutases in the biologic defense against oxygen toxicity is provided by studies in mammals and birds. In general, eukaryotes synthesize two distinct forms of superoxide dismutase. One is a copper- and zinc-containing enzyme localized in the cell cytosol and intermembrane spaces of mitochondria; the other form contains manganese and is localized in the mitochondrial matrix [11]. DeRosa and colleagues [12] found that feeding animals diets deficient in manganese resulted in a significant lowering of tissue levels of the manganese-containing superoxide dismutase and a concomitant elevation in the activity of the copper- and zinc-containing enzyme. Compensatory changes in the activities of these two enzymes suggest that their syntheses are probably regulated via a common mechanism that is dependent on intracellular $O_2^-\cdot$ concentrations, and thus illustrates the biologic importance of regulating cellular $O_2^-\cdot$. Further evidence that superoxide dismutase serves to protect against oxygen toxicity is provided by the demonstration that exposure of rats to high concentrations of oxygen leads to an increase in tissue superoxide dismutase activity and a concomitant increased tolerance of high oxygen concentrations [13].

Catalase

Catalase could potentially protect organisms from oxygen-based free radical damage by catalyzing the decomposition of H_2O_2. The enzyme can accomplish this via two possible mechanisms. In the first, one molecule of H_2O_2 is oxidized while a second H_2O_2 molecule is reduced (Fig. 6). Catalase also has peroxidatic activity since it can catalyze the reduction of H_2O_2 using a variety of electron donors. Apparently, the peroxidatic activity of catalase predominates in vivo in most cases [14]; this enzyme has a low affinity (high K_m) for H_2O_2 and is therefore ineffective at decomposing H_2O_2 via the catalatic mechanism at the low H_2O_2 concentrations found in most tissues. Catalase has a quite limited specificity for electron donors when acting as a peroxidase [7], and, since most of these potential donors are rarely present in significant amounts in tissues, the importance of the peroxidative activity of catalase in protecting against H_2O_2 toxicity is questionable. Further doubt about the significance of catalase in preventing H_2O_2 toxicity arises from the fact that most of the catalase in eukaryotic cells is localized in small organelles known as peroxisomes [14]. While peroxisomes contain some H_2O_2-generating oxidase enzymes, many such enzymes as well as other H_2O_2-generating systems are found in parts of the cell other than the

Biologic Antioxidant Mechanisms

Superoxide dismutases

$$O_2^{\cdot-} + O_2^{\cdot-} + 2H^+ \longrightarrow H_2O_2 + O_2$$

Catalases

$$H_2O_2 + H_2O_2 \longrightarrow 2H_2O + O_2$$

Peroxidases

$$H_2O_2 + RH_2 \longrightarrow 2H_2O + R$$

Radical scavengers

$$X^\cdot + SH \longrightarrow XH + S^\cdot$$

Fig. 6. Biologic mechanisms by which reactive oxygen species and free radicals are detoxified. Superoxide dismutase converts superoxide anions to H_2O_2 and molecular O_2. Catalase can catalyze the conversion of H_2O_2 to water and molecular O_2 by using one molecule of H_2O_2 as an electron donor to reduce another molecule of H_2O_2. Catalase is also capable of acting as a peroxidase. Peroxidases catalyze the reduction of H_2O_2 to H_2O using a variety of organic electron donors. Free radical scavengers (SH) can reduce free radicals via one-electron transfers. In the process, the scavenger becomes a free radical that is relatively stable and that does not propagate free radical chain reactions.

peroxisomes. Because of its localization and kinetics, catalase would not be expected to be highly effective at eliminating most cellular H_2O_2, and a variety of evidence suggests that in many cases it is not essential to the lives of cells or protection against oxygen toxicity. For example, humans suffering from an inborn error of metabolism that results in abnormally low catalase activities generally show minor, if any, harmful effects [15].

Peroxidases

Whereas catalase is apparently ineffective in maintaining intracellular levels of H_2O_2 at low levels, a variety of peroxidase enzymes exist that apparently play more important roles in decomposing H_2O_2 at low concentrations. Some of the most thoroughly studied of these enzymes are the glutathione peroxidases, which catalyze the reduction of H_2O_2 and organic hydroperoxides using glutathione as the electron donor (Fig. 7). Glutathione peroxidases examined to date contain selenium [16,17], which is essential to the catalytic activity of the enzyme. Tissue levels of glutathione peroxidase decrease dramatically in animals maintained on selenium-free diets [18,19].

Degradation of Peroxides by Glutathione Peroxidase

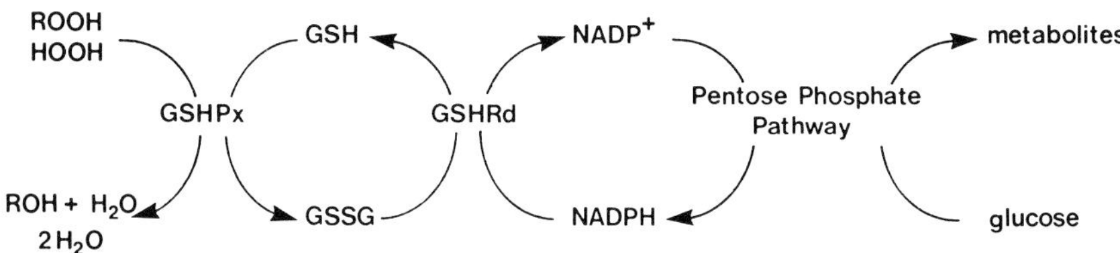

Fig. 7. Reduction of hydroperoxides by glutathione peroxidase. Glutathione peroxidase (GSHPx) catalyzes the reduction of both organic hydroperoxides (ROOH) and H_2O_2 using glutathione (GSH) as an electron donor. Glutathione is regenerated from its oxidized form (GSSG) through the action of the enzyme glutathione reductase (GSHRd). The latter enzyme uses NADPH as a reducing agent. NADPH is generated via glucose metabolism through the pentose phosphate pathway.

In addition to the selenium-dependent glutathione peroxidase, another enzyme, glutathione S transferase, is capable of acting as a peroxidase to catalyze the reduction of lipid hydroperoxides using glutathione as a reducing agent [20,21]. Glutathione S transferase does not reduce H_2O_2, as does glutathione peroxidase, but does catalyze the conjugation of glutathione to a wide variety of xenobiotics, an activity not displayed by glutathione peroxidase. The biologic importance of regulating tissue levels of lipid hydroperoxides is illustrated by the finding of Stone and Dratz [22] that tissue glutathione S transferase activities increase in response to a reduction in tissue glutathione peroxidase caused by selenium deficiency. In addition to the glutathione-utilizing peroxidases, mammalian tissues contain a variety of heme peroxidases that are capable of reducing H_2O_2 with a range of electron donors [23–30]. The existence of such a variety of peroxidase-metabolizing enzymes is strong evidence for the importance of regulating tissue hydroperoxide levels and thus preventing these hydroperoxides from decomposing nonenzymatically to generate free radicals. The heme peroxidases generally couple the reduction of H_2O_2 to the oxidation of a specific substrate whose oxidation product serves a useful biologic function. For example, thyroid peroxidase couples H_2O_2 reduction to the synthesis of thyroid hormone from tyrosine and iodide [23]. Thus the heme peroxidases are capable not only of preventing the potentially deleterious effects of H_2O_2 but of putting this compound to constructive uses.

Free Radical Scavengers

In addition to the antioxidant enzymes discussed above, tissues contain a variety of free radical scavengers capable of reducing free radical interme-

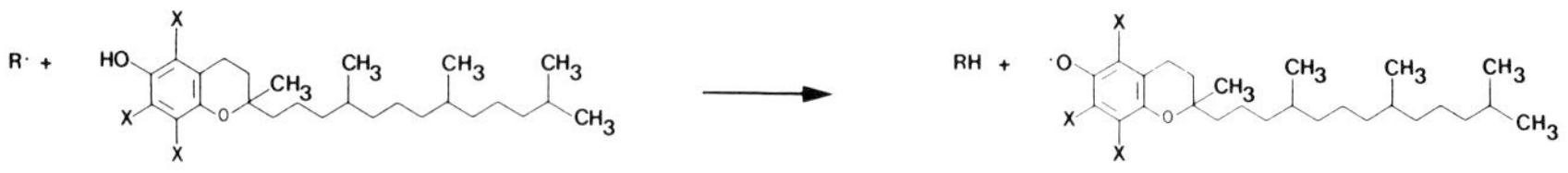

Fig. 8. Mechanism of free radical scavenging by vitamin E. The hydroxyl group of vitamin E can transfer a single electron to a lipid free radical (R•) to form the tocopheryl radical. The tocopheryl radical apparently does not propagate PUFA autoxidation reactions and eventually may dimerize or oxidize further. Various tocopherols that exist in biologic systems vary by whether the groups designated by Xs are methyls or hydrogens.

diates of autoxidation by what appear to be nonenzymatic mechanisms. By far the most thoroughly studied of these natural antioxidant compounds is vitamin E or tocopherol (Fig. 8). Despite the fact that the antioxidant activity of vitamin E has been recognized and studied for years [31], the precise mechanism of vitamin E action in vivo remains a matter of controversy. The most widely accepted theory is that an electron is transferred from the hydroxyl group of tocopherol to a free radical intermediate of autoxidation, thus terminating an autoxidation chain reaction (Fig. 8). Tocopherol, being a lipid, partitions into those parts of cells high in lipid content, such as plasma and organelle membranes, where it is ideally situated to impede autoxidation of phospholipid PUFAs. Apparently, the tocopherol radical, being less reactive than the free radical intermediates of lipid autoxidation, will not propagate autoxidation chain reactions. The ultimate fate of the tocopherol radical in vivo has not been well established, although several tocopherol derivatives, including tocopherol dimers [32] and oxidation products [33,34], have been isolated from animal tissues. Although tocopherol may be capable of terminating lipid autoxidation chain reactions, it is unlikely that it is effective in retarding the initiation of these reactions by the hydroxyl radical. The latter is so reactive that its likelihood of reacting with any molecule is dependent almost solely on the location and concentration of that molecule relative to the site of OH• generation.

POTENTIAL ROLE OF AUTOXIDATION IN ROP

A number of clinical trials have demonstrated that vitamin E treatment can be effective in impeding the development of ROP [1–3]. The only known biologic function of vitamin E is as an antioxidant [31]. Thus it is likely that the protective action of vitamin E in ROP is due to the antioxidant activity of this vitamin. Animal studies have clearly demonstrated the importance of vitamin E in protecting the retina, particularly the photoreceptor cells, from autoxidative damage [19,35–38]. The products and intermediates of lipid autoxidation are capable of diffusing from their site of generation in the photoreceptors and causing damage to nearby tissues in the eye [39]. In light of the fact that blood vitamin E levels, and therefore probably tissue vitamin E levels, are low in premature infants [1,2,39], it is possible that, in these infants, autoxidation of retinal components triggers the abnormal development of the retinal vasculature that characterizes ROP.

Kretzer and colleagues [40] have proposed that ROP is initiated by an increase in gap junction formation between spindle cells in the retina. Spindle cells are mesenchymal precursors of the inner retinal capillaries, and it is proposed that the increase in gap junction area between these cells resulting from premature birth halts their participation in the normal vasoformative process. Subsequent to this premature termination of retinal vascular development, an abnormal proliferation of retinal vessels, or neovascularization, takes place, probably in response to the release of angiogenic factors from cells of the abnormally avascular peripheral retina. Vitamin E supplementation of premature infants has been shown to suppress gap junction formation between spindle cells of the developing retina [39], suggesting that autoxidation is probably involved in triggering the proliferation of spindle cell gap junctions and thus the premature termination of retinal vascularization.

At present, we can do no more than speculate on the possible mechanism by which autoxidation in the retina triggers gap junction proliferation between spindle cells. As mentioned previously, many protective mechanisms against autoxidative damage are not fully developed in the premature infant [4–6]. Upon moving from the hypoxic environment of the womb to the normoxic or even hyperoxic atmosphere of the nursery, the infant's tissues are exposed to oxidative stresses they are not prepared to combat effectively. As a consequence, autoxidation products of retinal components are likely to be formed at a higher-than-normal rate. Certain of these autoxidation products, particularly malonaldehyde, are apparently capable of diffusing quite some distance from their sites of formation before reacting with retinal components [39]. Thus autoxidation in the retina, even if it does not take place to a significant extent within the spindle cells themselves, is capable of impinging on the latter if it occurs elsewhere in the retina. Apparently, cells have some mechanism of detecting the amount of autoxidative stress to which they are being subjected, since a number of adaptive responses to such stress have been demonstrated at the cellular and tissue levels [13,22,31,41]. It seems probable that gap junction formation between spindle cells, and the consequent termination of retinal vascularization, is such an adaptive response. Spindle cells, detecting a spurt of autoxidation product formation in the surrounding tissues consequent to premature birth, respond in a manner that would minimize autoxidation by reducing the access of oxygen to the retinal tissues. Since most oxygen consumed by tissues is delivered via the blood, reducing tissue vascularization is an effective means of reducing oxidative stress. Thus, in terms of protecting against autoxidation, termination of retinal vascularization is an adaptive response. It appears, however, that normal vascularization can only occur during a specific period of development. Later resumption of retinal vascularization in the premature infant, perhaps after alternative antioxidant mechanisms have developed, is typically abnormal.

SUMMARY

Oxygen can participate in a number of reactions that are potentially damaging to cells and tissues. Reactive forms of oxygen are generated during normal metabolic processes, and a variety of biologic mechanisms have evolved to protect organisms from damage by these compounds. Apparently these protective mechanisms are not fully developed in the fetus, which exists in a hypoxic environment in utero. Premature birth exposes the infant to a sudden increase in environmental oxygen content, for which it is not physiologically prepared. It is likely that this premature exposure to atmospheric oxygen triggers an elevation in the rate of autoxidative reactions in tissues and that the termination of normal retinal vascularization seen in ROP is the result of an attempt to minimize such reactions. This interpretation is supported by the finding that vitamin E, an antioxidant in vivo, reduces the severity of ROP when given at an early enough stage.

REFERENCES

1. Hittner HM, Godio LB, Rudolph AJ, Adams JM, Garcia-Prats JA, Friedman Z, Kautz JA, Monaco WA: Retrolental fibroplasia: Efficacy of vitamin E in a double-blind clinical study of preterm infants. N Engl J Med 305:1365–1371, 1981.
2. Finer NN, Schindler RF, Grant G, Hill GB, Peters K: Effect of intramuscular vitamin E on frequency and severity of retrolental fibroplasia: A controlled trial. Lancet 1:1087–1091, 1982.
3. Johnson L, Schaffer D. Boggs TR Jr: The premature infant, vitamin E deficiency and retrolental fibroplasia. Am J Clin Nutr 27:1158–1173, 1974.
4. Gallo-Torres HE: Transport and metabolism of vitamin E. In Machlin LJ (ed): "Vitamin E: A Comprehensive Treatise." New York: Marcel Dekker, 1980, pp 193–267.
5. Frank L, Groseclose EE: Preparation for birth into an O_2-rich environment: The antioxidant enzymes of the developing rabbit lung. Pediatr Res 18:240–244, 1984.
6. Wispe JR, Bell EF, Roberts RJ: Assessment of lipid peroxidation in newborn infants and rabbits by measurements of expired ethane and pentane: Influence of parenteral lipid infusion. Pediatr Res 19:374–379, 1985.
7. Chance B, Sies H, Boveris A: Hydroperoxide metabolism in mammalian organs. Physiol Rev 59:527–605, 1979.
8. Fridovich I: The biology of oxygen radicals. Science 201:875–880, 1978.
9. Cathcart R, Schwiers E, Saul RL, Ames BN: Thymine glycol and thymidine glycol in

human and rat urine: A possible assay for oxidative DNA damage. Proc Natl Acad Sci USA 81:5633–5637, 1984.

10. Hassan HM, Fridovich I: Enzymatic defenses against the toxicity of oxygen and streptonigrin in escherichia coli. J Bacteriol 129:1574–1583, 1977.

11. Fridovich I: Superoxide dismutases. Annu Rev Biochem 44:147–159, 1975.

12. DeRosa G, Keen CL, Leach RM, Hurley LS: Regulation of superoxide dismutase activity by dietary manganese. J Nutr 110:795–804, 1980.

13. Crapo JD, Tierney DR: Superoxide dismutase and pulmonary oxygen toxicity. Am J Physiol 226:1401–1407, 1974.

14. Percy ME: Catalase: An old enzyme with a new role? Can J Biochem Cell Biol 62:1006–1014, 1984.

15. Aebi H, Suter H: Acatalasemia. In Harris H, Hirschhorn K (eds): "Advances in Human Genetics." New York: Plenum Press, 1971, Vol 2, pp. 143–199.

16. Rotruck JT, Pope AL, Ganther HE, Swanson AB, Hafeman DG, Hoekstra WG: Selenium: Biochemical role as a component of glutathione peroxidase. Science 179:588–590, 1973.

17. Forstrom JW, Zakowski JJ, Tappel AL: Identification of the catalytic site of rat liver glutathione peroxidase as selenocysteine. Biochemistry 17:2639–2644, 1978.

18. Chow CK, Tappel AL: Response of glutathione peroxidase to dietary selenium in rats. J Nutr 104:444–451, 1974.

19. Katz ML, Parker KR, Handelman GJ, Bramel TL, Dratz EA: Effects of antioxidant nutrient deficiency on the retina and retinal pigment epithelium of albino rats: A light and electron microscopic study. Exp Eye Res 34:339–369, 1982.

20. Prohaska JR, Ganther HE: Glutathione peroxidase activity of glutathione-s-transferases purified from rat liver. Biochem Biophys Res Commun 76:437–445, 1976.

21. Prohaska JR: The glutathione peroxidase activity of glutathione-S-transferases. Biochim Biophys Acta 611:87–98, 1980.

22. Stone WL, Dratz EA: Selenium and non-selenium glutathione peroxidase activities in selected ocular and non-ocular rat tissues. Exp Eye Res 35:405–412, 1982.

23. Taurog A: The mechanism of action of the thioureylene antithyroid drugs. Endocrinology 98:1031–1046, 1976.

24. Kimura S, Jellinck PH: Studies on mammalian intestinal peroxidase. Biochem J 205:271–279, 1982.

25. Kanofsky JR: Singlet oxygen production by lactoperoxidase. J Biol Chem 258:5991–5993, 1983.

26. Olsen RL, Little C: Comparative studies on oestrogen-induced rat uterus peroxidase and rat eosinophil peroxidase. Biochem J 207:613–616, 1982.

27. Wever R, Kast WM, Kasinoedin JH, Boelens, R: The peroxidation of thiocyanate catalysed by myeloperoxidase and lactoperoxidase. Biochim Biophys Acta 709:212–219, 1982.

28. Patterson JR, Hood HT, Skellern GG: The role of porcine thyroid peroxidase and FAD-containing monooxygenase in the metabolism of 1-methyl-2-thioimidazole (methimazole). Biochem Biophys Res Commun 116:449–455, 1983.

29. Thomas EL, Jefferson, MM, Grisham MB: Myeloperoxidase-catalyzed incorporation of amines into proteins: Role of hypochlorous acid and dichloramines. Biochemistry 21:6299–6308, 1982.

30. Nauseef WM, Metcalf JA, Root RK: Role of myeloperoxidase in the respiratory burst of human neutrophils. Blood 61:483–492, 1983.

31. Katz ML, Robison WG: Nutritional influences on autoxidation, lipofuscin accumulation, and aging. In Johnson JE Jr, Walford R, Harman D, Miguel S (eds): "Free Radicals, Aging and Degenerative Diseases." New York: Alan R. Liss, Inc., 1986, pp. 221–259.

32. Csallany AS: A reappraisal of the structure of a dimeric metabolite of alpha-tocopherol. Int J Vit Nutr Res 41:376–384, 1971.

33. Csallany, AS, Draper, HH, Shah SN: Conversion of d-alpha-tocopherol-C^{14} to tocopheryl-p-quinone in vivo. Arch Biochem Biophys 98:142–145, 1962.

34. Mellors A, Barnes MM: The distribution and metabolism of alpha-tocopherol in the rat. Br J Nutr 20:69–77, 1966.

35. Katz ML, Stone WL, Dratz EA: Fluorescent pigment accumulation in retinal pigment epithelium of antioxidant-deficient rats. Invest Ophthalmol Vis Sci 17:1049–1058, 1978.

36. Katz ML, Robison WG, Dratz EA: Potential role of autoxidation in age changes of the retina and retinal pigment epitelium of the eye. In Armstrong D, Sohal RS, Cutler RG, Slater TS (eds): "Free Radicals in Molecular Biology, Aging, and Disease." New York: Raven Press, 1984, pp 163–180.

37. Robison WG, Kuwabara T, Bieri JG: Vitamin E deficiency and the retina: Photoreceptor and pigment epithelial changes. Invest Ophthalmol Vis Sci 18:683–690, 1979.

38. Robison WG, Kuwabara T, Bieri JG: Deficiencies of vitamins E and A in the rat. Retinal damage and lipofuscin accumulation. Invest Ophthalmol Vis Sci 19:1030–1037, 1980.

39. Zigler JS, Hess HH: Cataracts in the Royal College of Surgeons rat: Evidence for initiation by lipid peroxidation products. Exp Eye Res 41:67–76, 1985.

40. Kretzer FL, Mehta RS, Johnson AT, Hunter DG, Brown ES, Hittner HM: Vitamin E protects against retinopathy of prematurity through action on spindle cells. Nature 309:793–795, 1984.

41. Reddy CC, Thomas CE, Scholz RW, Massaro J: Effects of inadequate vitamin E and/or selenium nutrition on enzymes associated with xenobiotic metabolism. Biochem Biophys Res Commun 107:75–81, 1982.

Commentary and Questions: Session III

The classification of ROP is completed with the development of the classification of retinal detachment. Two stages (IV and V) are needed to classify end-stage disease completely: subtotal retinal detachment with or without macular involvement (stage IV) and total retinal detachment (stage V). The key question, however, is to what use this new classification will be put? Its obvious use (vide infra) will be in serving as the backbone of a study of the efficacy of newer methods of treatment of the late-stage ROP, a high-priority item on everybody's agenda for the disease.

Dr. Kalina began our journey back away from the microscopic details of ROP to address questions that, although they may seem mundane, are of extreme importance in today's environment in and outside the nursery. Which infants should be screened? When should they be screened? What criteria should we use to determine if rescreening is necessary? Dr. Kalina's paper goes a long way toward answering these difficult questions. The crux is that, the more incomplete the vascularization of the eye, the greater the need for observation of the fundus until the clinician is sure the process is achieving normalcy. How safely to examine? This is still another issue that needs our attention. Again Dr. Kalina provided common-sense guidelines for us to follow.

The next speaker, Dr. Kushner discussed the infant after discharge from the nursery to long-term follow-up for regressed ROP. If one can summarize his words, one would say that regression for us should be thought of as the end of the beginning rather than as the end of our concerns for the disease. For after the process of regression appears over, strabismus, amblyopia, and high refractive error occur even when one controls for brain damage and other neurologic processes in these infants. In those with milder forms of end-stage ROP, pseudodivergence of the eyes may occur because of heterotopia of the macula. Glaucoma, cataract, and rhegmatogenous retinal detachment (associated with a retinal tear or break) occur as well, as Dr. Kalina reminds us.

Questions regarding the incidence of rhegmatogenous retinal detachment surfaced again in the question and answer period. The consensus of the panel and other members of the audience with extensive experience in ROP is that retinal breaks are extremely rare in retinal detachments from acute prolifer-

Birth Defects: Original Article Series, Volume 24, Number 1, pages 249–251
© **1988 March of Dimes Birth Defects Foundation**

ative ROP. Such detachments are tractional, but there may also be an exudative component, and the relative contributions of traction and exudation may be difficult to separate. However, retinal breaks and subsequent retinal detachment are not at all uncommon in patients with regressed ROP, and they may occur during childhood or well into adult life. A further question was asked about what happens to intracranial pressure during ophthalmoscopic examination, reflecting concern for the safety of the infant in the nursery. Dr. Phelps was able to point out that, although elevation of intracranial pressure undoubtedly did occur, there is no reason to suspect any more than the rise expected from a host of procedures performed on the premature infant. A very pertinent question was asked by Dr. Sinclair regarding the reliability, reproducibility, and agreement among observers examining infants for ROP. Although the figures quoted by Dr. Schaffer in response seem to reflect a good agreement on this question, it is obviously an issue that needs constant update and must reflect the experience of the examiners performing the examination.

The next segment of this session was devoted to the oxygen hypothesis as seen from the perspective of the clinician as well as the basic researcher. Dr. Silverman began by questioning the sweeping nature of the hypothesis in its current form. As he pointed out, there are a number of glaring weaknesses in its current embodiment. For example, the linkage between oxygen and ROP has always been between duration rather than concentration. It is also important to recall in this regard that the risk of room air (21% O_2) is not zero. The real shape of the oxygen risk curve is unknown at this time.

Next came vitamin E as the only antioxidant "game in town." Dr. Phelps turned her considerable talents and experience as a clinician researcher into exploring the risk/benefit ratio of giving vitamin E to the forty-odd thousand premature infants in the doses recommended today for amelioration. (No one is claiming prevention of ROP with vitamin E.) This has consequences that are significantly different for infants born weighing above and below 1,000 grams. The key question is how many infants will get vitamin E, thereby needlessly exposing them to the risk of vitamin E therapy (which is not zero, in fact) vs the infants who will receive the vitamin E to their potential benefit against ROP assuming its efficacy in this regard. This is a vital question to ponder carefully before any large-scale therapy with the vitamin is recommended.

Dr. David Schaffer then reviewed the extensive experience of the University of Pennsylvania group with vitamin E for the prevention of ROP. He touched on the side effects of high doses of vitamin E (>3.5 μg/dl) in the premature infants and on a positive note he found a suggestion in reviewing the data on acute ROP that the infants receiving "early" vitamin E (first 24 hours of life) had a statistically significantly lower incidence of acute ROP than did infants receiving only placebo in this same group. This is the first time such an effect on the incidence of acute ROP has been shown, and if substantiated, is obviously important.

Dr. Martin Katz and coworkers then reviewed in detail the molecular mechanisms of autoxidative damage to cells, the protective mechanisms (primarily enzymatic) cells employ against autoxidative damage, and finally he related these two to ROP. The three oxygen miscreants are superoxide, hydrogen peroxide, and the hydroxyl ion, which can be generated when molecular oxygen is not fully reduced during oxidative metabolism. Enzymes that protect against cellular damage by these reactive oxygen species include superoxide dismutase and a variety of peroxidases and glutathione S transferases. Antioxidant protection is also provided by a variety of compounds, including vitamin E, that act without the apparent intervention of enzymes.

The question session produced a spirited discussion among clinicians about vitamin E. It turned on the apparent inconsistency between Dr. Schaffer's and Dr. Phelps's results regarding the efficacy of vitamin E therapy. In reply, Dr. Phelps cited the fact that the differences found by the Schaffer group in acute and end-stage ROP between treated and placebo groups were small and could fall well within the overlapping confidence intervals of the two data sets. Dr. Schaffer replied that he recognized that his data were only very preliminary and could serve only as underpinning for a testable hypothesis, not as providing a definitive answer to the question of vitamin E efficacy. Dr. Katz, replying to a question regarding vitamin E being a possible causal factor relating to necrotizing enterocolitis, called attention to the fact that vitamin E can impair protection against infection by inhibiting the bacteria-killing ability of inflammatory cells.

Probably the most imponderable question of the day was asked by Dr. Robert Machemer: If vitamin E was, in fact, acting as an antioxidant in preventing damage to endothelial cells, why don't we see more evidence of damage to neural elements, photoreceptors, ganglion cells, etc, than we do in these presumably vitamin E-deficient infants? Perhaps the answer is that there is such damage [1]; however, even that has been sharply questioned [2,3].

REFERENCES

1. Johnson BL, Ahdab-Barmada M: Hyperoxemic retinal neuronal necrosis in the premature neonate. Am J Ophthalmol 102:423–430, 1986.
2. Curtin VT, Bancalari E, Gass JDM et al: Hyperoxemic retinal necrosis in the premature neonate (correspondence). Am J Ophthalmol 103:343–344, 1987.
3. Brown HH, Glasgow BJ, Foos RY: Hyperoxemic retinal necrosis in the premature neonate (correspondence). Am J Ophthalmol 103:726–727, 1987.

VII. SURGICAL THERAPY OF RETINOPATHY OF PREMATURITY

Cryotherapy: Indications, Methods, and Current Status

Earl A. Palmer, MD

Department of Ophthalmology, Oregon Health Sciences University, Portland, Oregon 97201

DEVELOPMENT OF RETINOPATHY OF PREMATURITY (ROP)

It is a remarkable aspect of ROP that its appearance can be anticipated within a limited time window. Until we have more complete prospective natural history data, it may be useful to outline, in general terms, the time course of the clinical disease. The disorder runs its acute course very early in the life of affected premature infants.

ONSET OF ROP

It is rare to see severe retinopathy earlier than about age 6 weeks, although early evidence of ROP often can be seen by age 4 weeks. In 1979, I published data that led me to recommend age 7–9 weeks as the optimal time for a screening examination for ROP [1]. The rationale was that earlier examinations were unnecessary from the standpoint of ROP management, since damage to the macula was extremely unlikely before that, and I emphasized the fact that infants who end up blind from the disease may show little evidence of abnormality in the first month or so of life. The examinations on which the recommendation was based did not include scleral indentation, and it is safe to assume that some of the infants declared to be free of ROP actually had the disease in zone 3 (International Classification [2]) or far peripheral zone 2 (Fig. 1). It is virtually impossible to overlook zone 1 or posterior zone 2 ROP during a standard ophthalmologic examination with the binocular indirect ophthalmoscope.

At the Symposium on ROP sponsored by Ross Laboratories in December, 1981, after asserting my opinion that ROP rarely, if ever, develops after age 9 weeks [3], I asked the audience of professionals who had a special interest

Birth Defects: Original Article Series, Volume 24, Number 1, pages 255–263

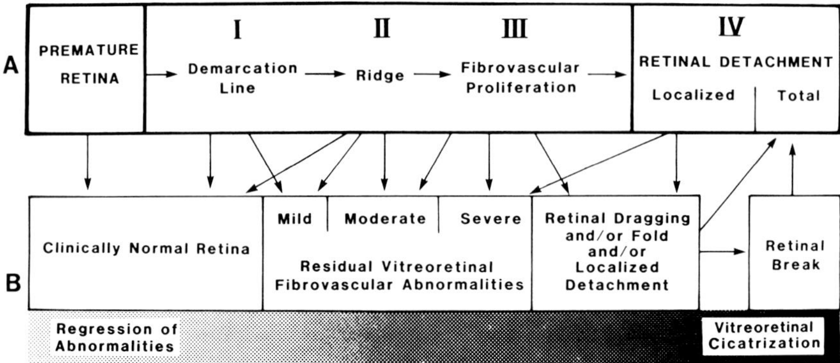

Fig. 1. Retinopathy of prematurity spectrum. A. Stages of disease. B. Possible outcomes.

in the disease if anyone had seen it develop later; no one raised a hand. I doubt if the disease ever makes its first appearance after age 3 months.

COURSE OF LESS SEVERE DISEASE

It is now commonly known that the great majority of patients with ROP do not develop retinal detachment. These less severely affected patients go into clinical regression at some stage short of stage 4. The final outcome for these patients appears to be clearly related to the degree of severity reached by the ROP at its maximum. Thus patients whose ROP never progresses beyond stage 1 seem never to develop macular damage, and consequently visual impairment, as a direct result of the ROP. Data are inconclusive as to vision outcome in relation to cases that never progress beyond stage 2 or 3.

APPEARANCE OF RETINAL DETACHMENT

Whenever ROP progresses acutely to stage 4, this ordinarily occurs during the third or fourth month of life [1], although it may occur somewhat later. Probability data on the timing of retinal detachment are not yet clearly defined.

RUSH DISEASE

This is an evocative term to describe zone 1 ROP that progresses rapidly to stage 4 without necessarily following a well-defined, stepwise progression through stages 1–3. It is described in a Japanese classification as type II (rapid-onset) ROP [4,5]. On the basis of clinical experience, it is clear that this is a relatively rare variant of ROP.

Tasman [6] recently reported two cases of zone 1 (''rush'') disease in whom the retina remained attached in one eye, yet the eye was apparently blind. This eye was the only one of the four among the two patients who had received cryotherapy. As the authors pointed out, it is possible that the infant was cortically blind or had suffered a retinal vascular occlusion. Still, this report raises the interesting and very important question of whether there is a form of ROP that damages the retina in a way that is independent of retinal detachment or severe retinal traction, conditions widely assumed to be prerequisites of blindness from acute ROP.

At the Oregon Health Sciences University Hospital, we recently observed the remarkable coincidence of two infants who simultaneously developed zone 1 ROP that went on to bilateral retinal detachment in both cases. As part of our local pilot study of cryotherapy, we had performed cryotherapy to the peripheral avascular retina of one eye in each case (unpublished observations). The failure of cryotherapy to prevent retinal detachment in these two eyes simply underscores the fact, already mentioned in published reports, that cryotherapy does not always prevent this adverse outcome. It is possible that future studies will indicate that interdictory surgical therapy is fruitless in cases of rush disease, or that techniques will be necessary that are different in some way from what has been attempted to date.

EARLY DEVELOPMENT OF INTERDICTORY THERAPY

In Japan, considerable experience has been accumulated with the surgical ablation of the avascular retina anterior to the ridge of ROP, and sometimes the ridge itself, by means of either a pulsed photocoagulation beam (directed in through the pupil) or cryotherapy (applied through the wall of the eye without surgically invading the integrity of the scleral coat of the eye) [4,5,7,8]. These two operations are relatively noninvasive, yet there are some potential complications that can damage vision or cause a medical setback for the infant. It is therefore important to evaluate carefully the effects of such interdictory therapy in relation to the risks of applying it. Such studies have not yet been completed, but I will later discuss a major clinical trial that began in the United States in 1986. Dr. Akio Majima has recently told me that there is already a clinical evaluation of therapy underway in Japan as well (personal communication).

The criteria for selecting patients for therapy in Japan are not always clearly stated in the reports; however, it appears that therapy is begun once the eye has reached stage III of the International Classification. Although photocoagulation for acute ROP is still popular in Japan, the Japanese have found that it cannot be done in all cases for technical reasons. Reasons militating against photocoagulation therapy in general include any physical factors making it difficult to aim and focus the light beam; for example, failure of the patient's pupil to dilate well from mydriatic eyedrops or haze within the refracting media of the eye. Furthermore, constant movements of the patient's eye would make photocoagulation impossible. Cryotherapy can be applied to a higher percentage of patients than can photocoagulation.

In addition to the question of risk vs benefit, uncertainty persists around the more fundamental question of whether cryotherapy works. The literature contains ample case reports and series to indicate that peripheral retinal ablation seems at least to shorten the time course of ROP [1–17]. The question of whether the eye is ultimately better off than an untreated eye is not as readily answered from a critical review of the literature. This issue has been reviewed elsewhere [18].

Existing studies can be summarized by stating that they are not rigorously designed clinical trials [19], complete with proper controls, unbiased assessment of outcome by independent evaluators, or even clearly stated outcome criteria. These issues are especially important in the case of ROP because of the very unpredictable course of the disorder and the fact that eyes can progress to advanced stage 3 and yet still undergo regression without serious damage to vision. When dealing with a disorder with a high rate of spontaneous regression, it is easy to credit that regression erroneously to a therapy. Since ROP frequently affects the two eyes differently, it is not sufficient to compare the two eyes unless large numbers of patients are studied. Finally, it deserves restating that it has not yet been adequately demonstrated that the earlier regression reported following cryotherapy indeed provides final benefit to the eye.

DEVELOPMENT OF THE CRYOTHERAPY TRIAL

To detect the maximum possible number of infants to randomize for cryotherapy in the Multicenter Trial of Cryotherapy for ROP (CRYO-ROP) [20,21], eligible infants will be examined at age 4–6 weeks, and then fortnightly, until each eye is beyond risk of progressing to the threshold for randomization or the threshold for randomization is reached. Provision has been made to analyze examination data for information about the natural course of ROP to permit optimal interpretation of the results of the cryotherapy trial.

At the time of initial contact with the parent or guardian of the premature infant, a brief informational leaflet about ROP is given, in which the result of the first examination is noted, and the plan for follow-up is stated. I have been using a hand-out like this for about 10 years. After refinement by members of the Executive Committee of CRYO-ROP, it was made a part of the study protocol. The version we are now using in Oregon is adapted from the study protocol model and is reproduced in Appendix I. It may be adapted for use by any who wish to do so in a nursery's screening program.

In the CRYO-ROP, scheduled to begin in January, 1986, allowance has been made for the asymmetric involvement of the two eyes that can occur. Asymmetric ROP would prevent using the fellow eye as a control. Thus, when only one eye reaches the stage of ROP that has been judged severe enough to warrant randomization for cryotherapy, then only that eye is studied, and the fellow eye is ineligible for the study. The randomized asymmetric eye is paired with another such eye in another patient. All the randomized eyes will therefore have a comparable level of severity of ROP. Half, randomly selected, will receive cryotherapy and half will serve as controls.

In the event that the fellow eye in such an asymmetric case progresses on to the level of ROP that would have qualified it for randomization, then that fellow eye is eligible for cryotherapy outside the study, if the parents so desire. In no case will cryotherapy be applied to both eyes, however, so that the risk of the investigational therapy will be thereby limited.

ENTRY CRITERIA FOR RANDOMIZATION FOR CRYOTHERAPY

It was the desire of the authors of the protocol for CRYO-ROP [22] that a threshold level of ROP be chosen that would represent a serious enough threat to vision to warrant the investigational therapy yet would not be so advanced that the chances of reversing the disease seemed remote. Statistical data on this issue were sparse, but, after considerable study and discussion, the following threshold level of ROP was chosen. The eligible eye must exhibit abnormal dilatation and tortuosity of the retinal blood vessels in the posterior pole of the eye and have stage 3 ROP occupying at least five contiguous clock-hour sectors or eight discontinuous sectors located in zone 1 or 2.

TECHNIQUE CHOSEN

It must be emphasized that none of the investigators in CRYO-ROP are advocating cryotherapy for ROP under any conditions outside a rigorously designed study involving risk-limiting randomization. The technique we have chosen to study is to ablate all the avascular retina peripheral to the ridge or demarcation line of ROP, without leaving any gaps between the ridge and the cryotherapy and without directly applying cryotherapy to the

TABLE I. CRYO-ROP Participating Centers

Alabama, Birmingham	Michigan, Detroit
California, Sacramento	Minnesota, Minneapolis
North Carolina, Durham	New York, Rochester
South Carolina, Charleston	Ohio, Cincinnati, Columbus
Florida, Miami	Oregon, Portland
Georgia, Atlanta*	Pennsylvania, Philadelphia; Pittsburgh
Illinois, Chicago	Tennessee, Nashville
Indiana, Indianapolis	Texas, Dallas, San Antonio
Kentucky, Louisville	Utah, Salt Lake City
Louisiana, New Orleans	District Of Columbia, Washington
Maryland, Baltimore	

*Withdrew before the study began.

ridge itself, while avoiding freezing the bays of the pars plana of the ciliary body anteriorly.

OUTCOME DETERMINATION

The primary aim of the investigational cryotherapy is to reduce the occurrence of damage to the macula of the eye through either retinal detachment or formation of a retinal traction fold that distorts the macula. In other words, for the purposes of CRYO-ROP, if the retina is detached only on the side of the optic disk opposite the macula, the eye is considered to have a favorable outcome so long as the macula itself is attached and smooth. In the world of stage 4 ROP patients, such an outcome is fortunate.

TIME LINE OF CRYO-ROP

In March, 1985, two sites were funded by the National Eye Institute: a Data Coordinating Center, located at the Center for Clinical Trials at the University of Texas Health Science Center in Houston, and a Study Headquarters, at the Oregon Health Sciences University in Portland. In September, 1985, 24 centers were awarded separate cooperative agreements by the National Eye Institute to serve as sites for this clinical trial. They are listed in Table I. In November, 1985, one or more Coordinators from each of the 24 Study Centers attended a training course at the Coordinating Center. In December, 1985, the principal investigator and a limited number of Coinvestigators from each of the 24 participating Study Centers attended a technical training course in Portland, Oregon. In January, 1986, infants born weighing 1,250 gm or less became eligible for entry into the multicenter study.

REFERENCES

1. Palmer EA: Optimal timing of examination for acute retrolental fibroplasia. Ophthalmology 88:662–668, 1981.
2. The Committee for the Classification of Retinopathy of Prematurity: An international classification of retinopathy of prematurity. Arch Ophthalmol 102:1130–1134, 1984.
3. Palmer EA: Natural history of retinopathy of prematurity. In "Retinopathy of Prematurity Conference Syllabus." Washington, DC, December 4–6, 1981, Vol 1, pp 441–448.
4. Majima A: Problems on retinopathy of prematurity. Statistical analysis of factors related to occurrence and progression of retinopathy, and fundus appearances and ocular functions in prematurely born subjects (authors translation). Acta Soc Ophthalmol Jpn 80:1372–1419, 1976.
5. Uemura Y: Current status of retrolental fibroplasia. Report of the Joint Committee for the Study of Retrolental Fibroplasia in Japan. Jpn J Ophthalmol 21:366–378, 1977.
6. Tasman W: Zone I retinopathy of prematurity. Arch Ophthalmol 103:1693–1694, 1985.
7. Nagata M, Kobayashi Y, Fukuda H et al: Photocoagulation for the treatment of the retinopathy of prematurity. Jpn J Clin Ophthalmol 22:419–427, 1968.
8. Yamashita Y: Studies on retinopathy of prematurity. III. Cryocauty for retinopathy of prematurity. Jpn J Clin Ophthalmol 26:385–393, 1972.
9. Payne JW, Patz A: Treatment of acute proliferative retrolental fibroplasia. Trans Am Acad Ophthalmol Otolaryngol 76:1234–1241, 1972.
10. Harris GS, McCormick AQ: The prophylactic treatment of retrolental fibroplasia. Mod Prob Ophthalmol 18:364–367, 1977.
11. Kingham JD: Acute retrolental fibroplasia. II. Treatment by cryosurgery. Arch Ophthalmol 96:2049–2053, 1978.
12. Hindle NW, Leyton J: Prevention of cicatricial retrolental fibroplasia by cryotherapy. Can J Ophthalmol 13:277–282, 1978.
13. Koerner FH: Retinopathy of prematurity: Natural course and management. Ophthalmology 2:325–329, 1978.
14. Mousel DK, Hoyt CS: Cryotherapy for retinopathy of prematurity. Ophthalmology 87:1121–1127, 1980.
15. Ben-Sira I, Nissenborn I, Grunwald E, Yassur Y: Treatment of acute retrolental fibroplasia by cryopexy. Br J Ophthalmol 64:758–762, 1980.
16. Stark DJ, Manning LM, Lenton L: The incidence and the results of active treatment of acute retrolental fibroplasia. Aust J Ophthalmol 10:135–140, 1982.
17. Keith CG: Visual outcome and effect of treatment in stage III developing retrolental fibroplasia. Br J Ophthalmol 66:446–449, 1982.
18. Palmer EA, Biglan AW, Hardy RJ: Retinal ablative therapy for active proliferative retinopathy of prematurity: History, current status and prospects. In Silverman WA, Flynn JT (eds): "Contemporary Issues in Fetal and Neonatal Medicine: Retinopathy of Prematurity," Boston: Blackwell Scientific Publications, 1985, Vol 2, pp 207–228.
19. Chalmers TC, Smith H Jr, Blackburn B, Silverman W, Schroeder B, Reitman D, Ambroz A: A method for assessing the quality of a randomized control trial. Controlled Clin Trials 2:31–49, 1981.
20. Palmer EA: The multicenter trial of cryotherapy for retinopathy of prematurity (Editorial). J Pediatr Ophthalmol Strabismus 23:56–57, 1986.
21. Palmer EA, Phelps DL: Multicenter trial of cryotherapy for retinopathy of prematurity. Pediatrics 77:428–429, 1986.
22. "Cryotherapy for Retinopathy of Prematurity Cooperative Group: Manual of Procedures." Portland: The Oregon Health Sciences University, 1985.

APPENDIX

TO: The Parents of Premature Infant ________________________

DATE: ________________

FROM: Infant Eye Specialist
             The Oregon Health Sciences University

ABOUT A PREMATURE BABY'S EYES

At the request of the pediatricians looking after your baby, an eye examination has been performed. Before explaining why this eye examination was necessary, the following brief description of the infant eye is needed.

The *retina* is the inner lining of the eyeball that receives light and turns it into visual messages that are sent to the brain. If one thinks of the eye as being like a camera, the retina functions as the film. Blood vessels that supply the retina are one of the last structures of the eye to mature, and have barely completed growing toward the front of the eye when a full term baby is born. This means that a premature infant's retina is still incompletely developed.

WHAT IS RETINOPATHY OF PREMATURITY?

For reasons not yet fully understood by medical science, the blood vessels in the immature part of the retina toward the front of the eye may develop abnormally in some very premature infants. This disorder is called Retinopathy of Prematurity (abbreviated ROP). It is more likely to develop in the smallest infants who have had the most complications during their Newborn Intensive Care Unit stay.

When ROP develops, one of three different things can happen:
1) In the large majority (80%) of babies who develop ROP, the abnormal blood vessels will heal themselves completely during the first year of life.
2) In some babies the abnormal blood vessels heal only partially.
   In these infants nearsightedness (myopia) develops and glasses may be required early in life. These children may be more prone to developing lazy eye (amblyopia) or a wandering eye (strabismus). Infants who develop any of these conditions need to have regular eye examinations

throughout childhood to assure the best possible vision. In some cases a scar may be left in the retina resulting in vision problems that are not entirely correctable with glasses or any other means; patients with these scars need life-long ophthalmic care. The scars of incompletely healed ROP are referred to as Retrolental Fibroplasia (RLF), and may be mild or severe, as described below.

3) In the most severe cases, the retinal blood vessels continue developing abnormally and form scar tissue which can pull the retina loose from its normal position in the back of the eye (retinal detachment). This severe problem results in serious loss of vision, and complete blindness can result. Fortunately, only a small percentage (less than 5%) of babies with ROP develop RLF.

If a baby's eyes appear to be developing the more severe forms of retinopathy or prematurity, important decisions have to be made about possible new surgical procedures to try to protect vision. This newborn center is conducting a study of ROP. If necessary we will be talking with you about whether you want to enroll your infant in this program.

WHAT ABOUT YOUR BABY'S EYES?

Your infant requires another examination because he/she

______   Has a normal examination but still could develop problems later, because the retinal vessels are still not fully developed.

______   Has early retinopathy of prematurity that will need further examinations to watch for serious developments.

Next eye examination recommended: ________________________________

Three copies: Parents
                Patient chart
                Research file

Surgical Approaches to Retinal Detachment in Retinopathy of Prematurity

William Tasman, MD

Wills Eye Hospital, Jefferson Medical School, Philadelphia, Pennsylvania 19118

Today, more and more premature babies who weigh less than 1,000 gm at birth are surviving. As a result, the incidence of active retinopathy of prematurity (ROP) is once again increasing, spurring renewed interest in the management of this potentially blinding disease [1].

Fortunately, in the majority of patients, ROP resolves without treatment. However, some progress to stage IV and stage V retinal detachment, a condition that may lead to blindness. It is important to realize that infants with stage III active ROP may have retinal detachment anterior to the ridge of mesenchymally derived tissue that separates vascularized from avascularized retina. This detachment of the nonvascularized retina disappears as retinal vessels grow into the avascular zone and is not an indication for surgical intervention. Detachment anteriorly is also not an indicator of stage IV disease, in my opinion.

SURGICAL ALTERNATIVES

To select properly those detachment patients for whom surgery is indicated, it is necessary to quantitate the degree of peripheral cicatrization and traction that is present. Eyes with progressive dragging of the retina do not necessarily fall into this category, since once dragging begins no form of therapy can reverse it (Fig. 1). On the other hand, some eyes develop progressive 360° cicatrization, which arises from the ridge, and the retina then begins to detach. Increasing traction leads to detachment posterior to the ridge (Fig. 2) and, as Machemer has pointed out, a trough anteriorly [2]. In addition, accompanying leakage of protein from the retinal vessels may lead to hazy media.

Both vitrectomy and scleral buckling have been used in the treatment of total retinal detachment in active ROP. Our preferred buckling technique includes dissecting a scleral bed temporally or nasally for 180° to a width of

Birth Defects: Original Article Series, Volume 24, Number 1, pages 265–274
© **1988 March of Dimes Birth Defects Foundation**

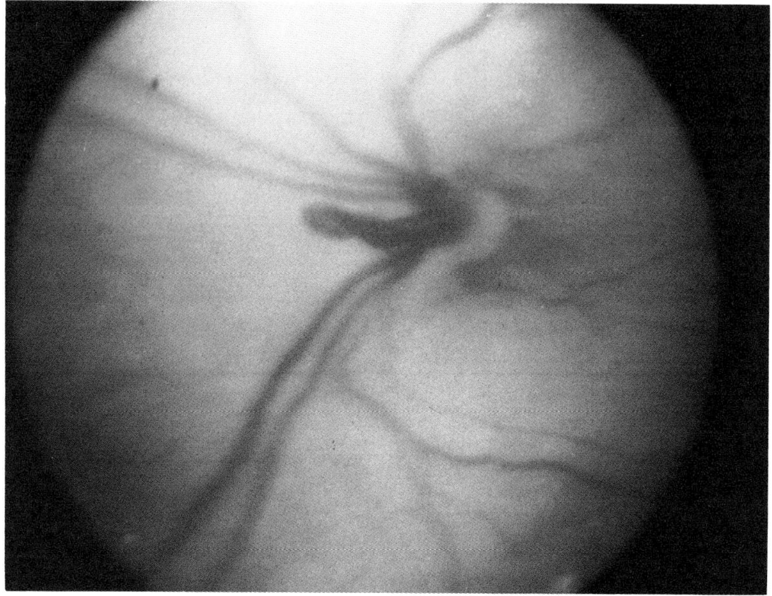

Fig. 1. Beginning temporal dragging of the retina in a premature with a persistent hyaloid vessel.

6 mm. A 4 mm silicone strip is placed beneath the scleral flaps, and a number 40 band is used as the encircling element (Fig. 3A–C). Cryotherapy is applied to any residual area of avascular retina. It is important to monitor these eyes carefully postoperatively to make sure that they maintain a satisfactory growth pattern, and removal of the encircling element 4–6 months after surgery is recommended.

Recently, Machemer [2] has advocated vitrectomy surgery in some cases of detachment with active ROP, but at present our experience with vitrectomy has been confined largely to the severe cicatricial stages after activity has subsided.

Most babies treated surgically for retinal detachment have a history of birthweight under 1,000 gm. Retinal detachment in these infants usually becomes apparent within 3–5 months of chronologic age. As experience in the natural history of this disorder has accumulated, and with the recognition that some detachments may resolve spontaneously (Fig. 4), only those eyes with a tractional component are treated surgically.

Over the last 5 years, progress has been made in surgery for stage V retinal detachment. These are usually eyes with white pupils that in the past have

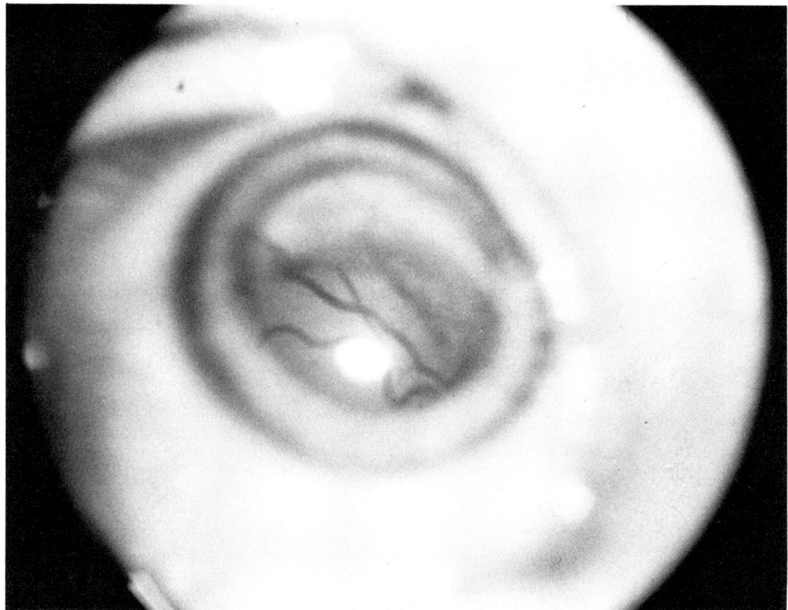

Fig. 2.   Traction retinal detachment.

been relegated to blindness (Fig. 5). Although surgery still yields less than a 50% reattachment rate and the visual results are poor, some eyes do obtain navigational vision postoperatively.

Two vitrectomy techniques have been advocated, closed- and open-sky. Charles [3] has advocated the former and has reported on over 400 cases treated by closed vitrectomy. Hirose and Schepens [4] have pioneered the open-sky approach in patients similar to those treated by Charles with closed vitrectomy. In this procedure, the cornea is first removed and stored during the operation in tissue culture fluid fortified with garamycin. After removal of the lens by intracapsular extraction with a cryoprobe, the membrane is dissected from the surface of the retina starting just posterior to the ciliary processes (Fig. 6). One is usually able to remove the membrane from the surface of the retina completely and in one piece (Fig. 7). Hyaluronic acid is injected to flatten the retina, and the corneal button is then sewn back into place. Hirose and Schephen's reattachment rate in well over 150 cases parallels that of Charles.

Unfortunately, as was mentioned above, even in those cases when the retina is successfully reattached, visual results can be disappointing. Of our 31 eyes treated by the open-sky technique, seven eyes (23%) were success-

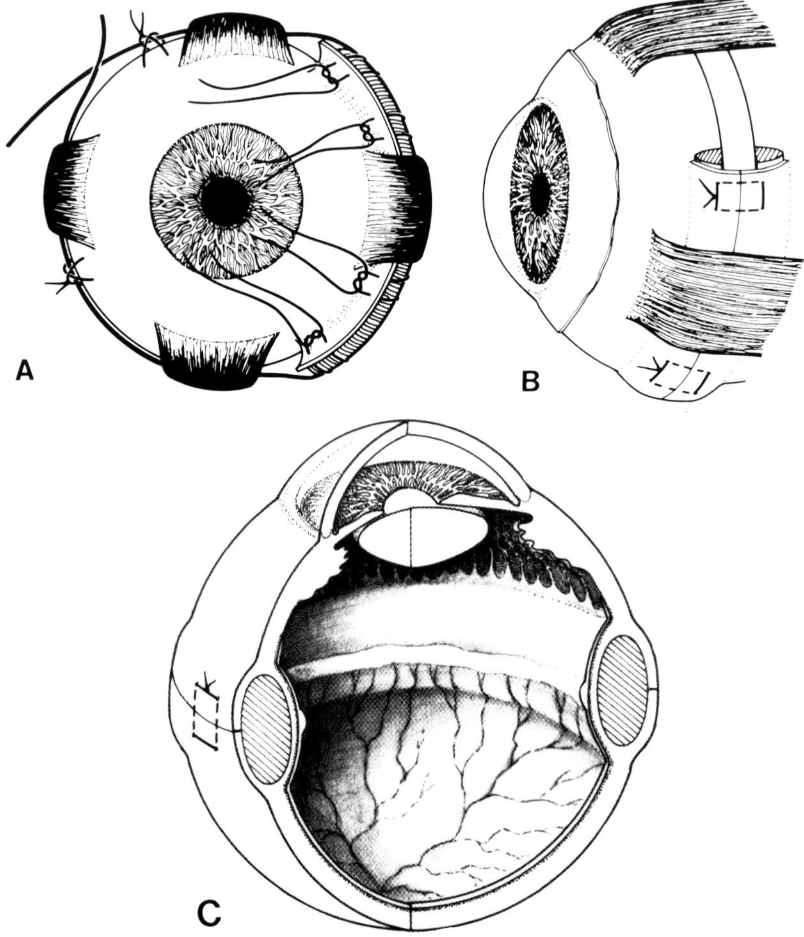

Fig. 3. A–C: Buried silicone strip in a 180° bed with encircling band.

fully reattached, but only two appear to have useful vision (Fig. 8). This may be due to the fact that some of the reattached retinas are avascular except in one quadrant. A period of months is necessary, however, before making a final determination about vision, since photoreceptor recovery may be extremely delayed.

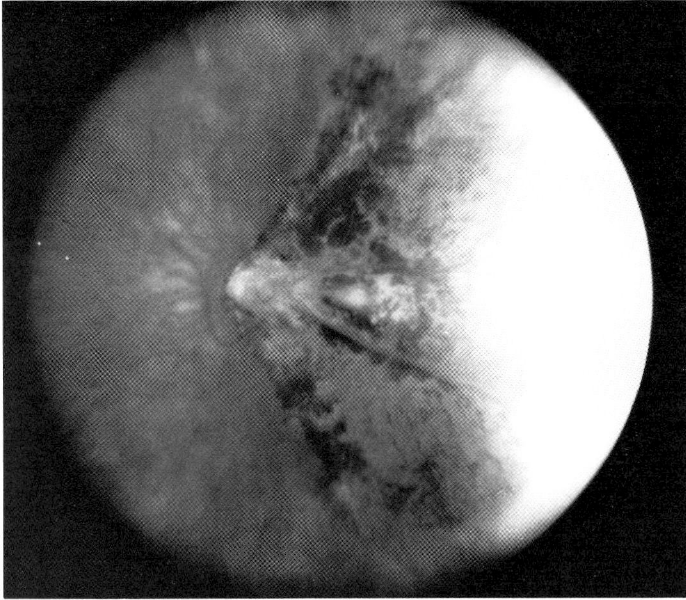

Fig. 4. Pigment in area of temporal dragging suggestive of spontaneously reattached retina.

LATE-ONSET RETINAL DETACHMENT

Retinal detachment may also occur in school-aged children and young adults who have had previous active ROP without blinding sequelae. Two types of detachments occur, tractional and rhegmatogenous. Tractional detachments may be localized or total and demonstrate telangiectatic vascular changes associated with subretinal exudation (Fig. 9). Whether localized or total, tractional retinal detachments may respond to scleral buckling coupled with cryotherapy to the abnormal telangiectasis.

Rhegmatogenous retinal detachments usually are seen with multiple rather than single retinal breaks. The most common age for onset of rhegmatogenous retinal detachment is 14 years, but we have seen them also in patients under 10 and over 20 years (Fig. 10).

The retinal breaks for the most part are round or oval in appearance and equatorial in location. They occur most commonly on the temporal side and may be associated with lattice-like degeneration, which is found twice as frequently in ROP patients (15%) compared to the 6–7% incidence in the

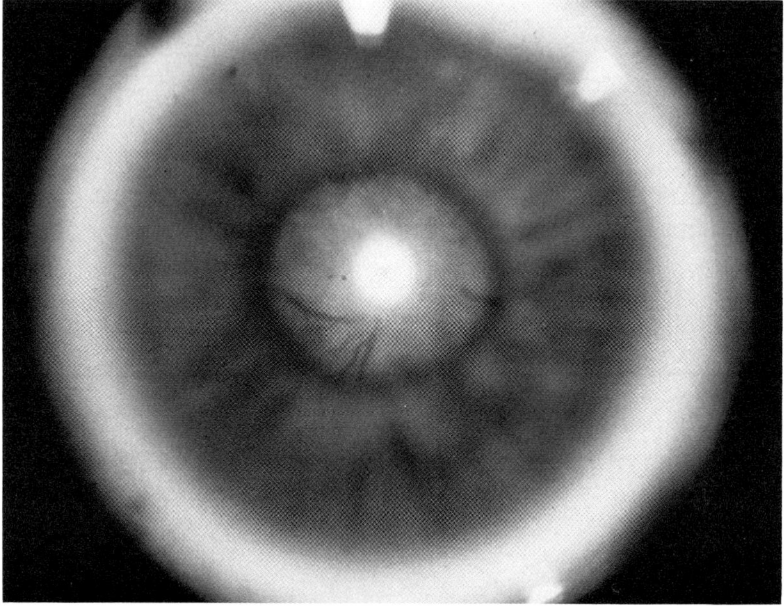

Fig. 5. Stage V retinal detachment. Retinal vessels can be seen beneath the retrolental membrane.

normal population (Fig. 11) [5]. These eyes respond well to conventional encircling scleral buckling procedures and closure of the retinal breaks. Fellow eyes with retinal breaks but no retinal detachment are usually treated prophylactically with cryotherapy, since posterior vitreous detachment is rare, and these eyes are at greater risk for detachment than eyes with asymptomatic retinal breaks but no vitreous traction.

SUMMARY

Outlined in this chapter are surgical approaches to retinal detachment in ROP. Technical details of the vitrectomy approach to stage V ROP are covered extensively in the chapters by Machemer and Charles. Late-onset retinal detachment is a rare complication. Two types of detachment, those associated with traction and those associated with retinal breaks or tears (rhegmatogenous), generally respond well to standard buckling procedures. The incidences of these complications provide reason for continued long-term follow-up of eyes with ROP.

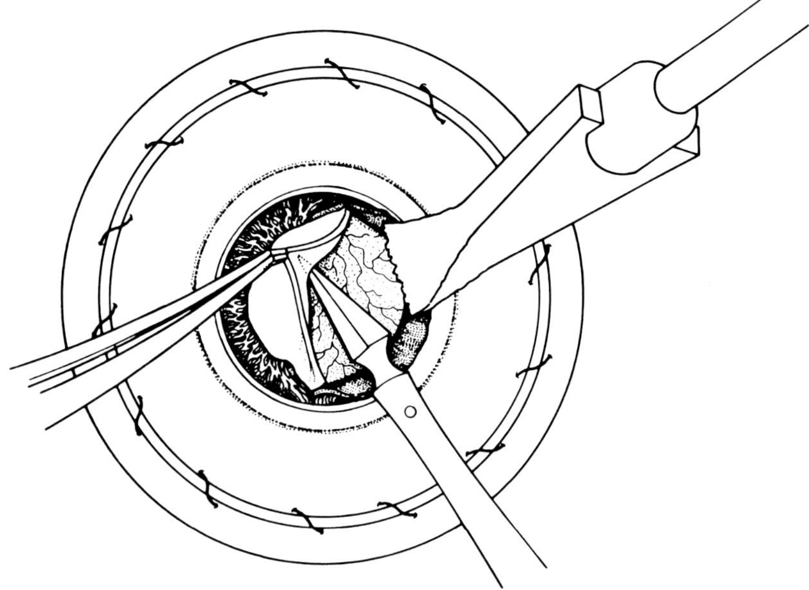

Fig. 6. Dissection of the retrolental membrane begins peripherally and continues toward the central funnel.

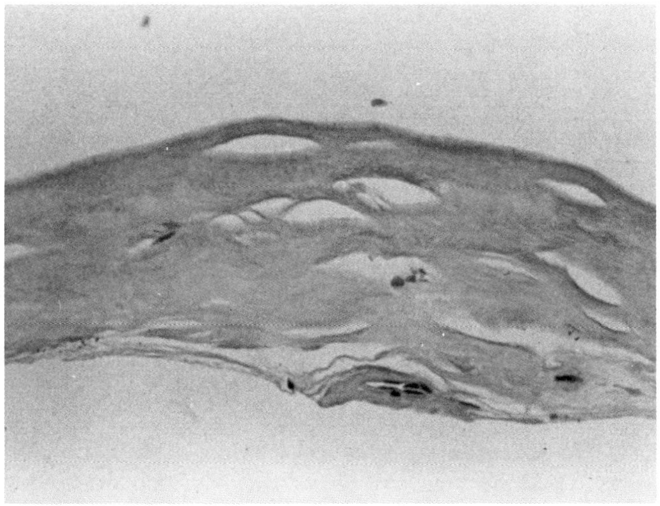

Fig. 7. Microscopic appearance of relatively avascular retrolental membrane.

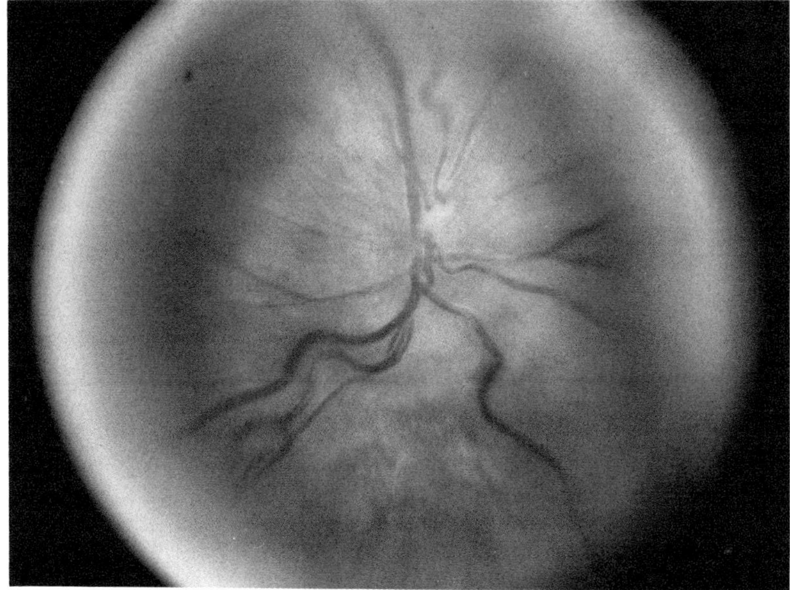

Fig. 8. Reattached retina after open-sky vitrectomy.

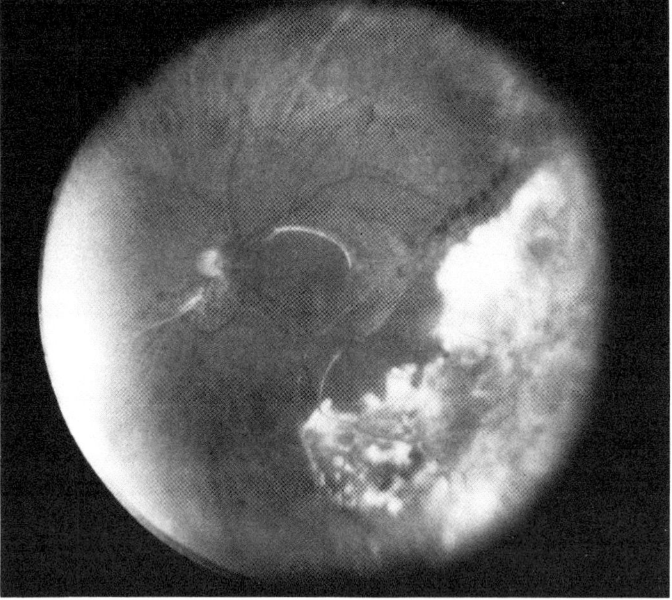

Fig. 9. Tractional retinal detachment in a 22-year-old girl with ROP.

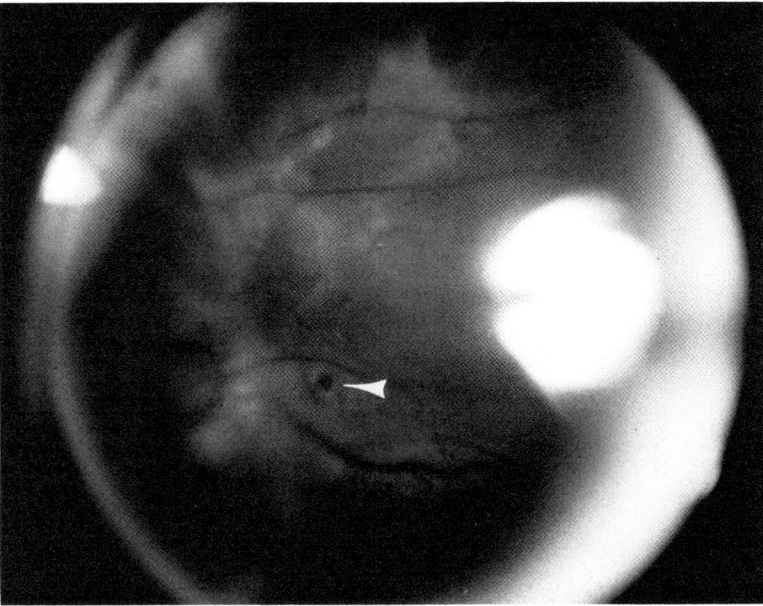

Fig. 10. Rhegmatogenous retinal detachment with temporal retinal hole (arrowhead) in a 2-year-old boy with ROP.

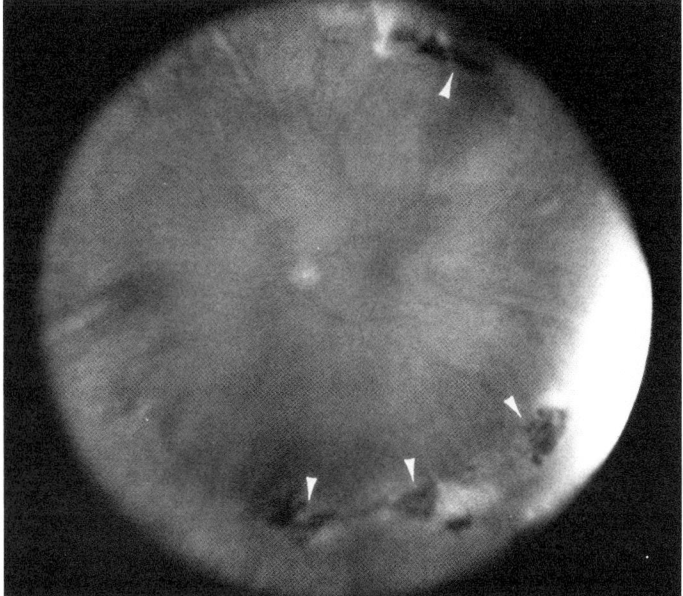

Fig. 11. Lattice-like degeneration (arrowheads) in the fundus periphery of a 16-year-old boy with minimal temporal dragging of the retina in the posterior pole.

REFERENCES

1. Patz A: Symposium on retrolental fibroplasia. Ophthalmology 86:1685–1689, 1979.
2. Machemer R: Description and pathogenesis of the late stages of retinopathy of prematurity: Description and therapy. Ophthalmology 92:1000–1004, 1985.
3. Charles ST: Vitrectomy for retrolental fibroplasia. Paper presented at the 1984 annual meeting of the American Academy of Ophthalmology, Atlanta.
4. Hirose T, Schepens CL: Open sky vitrectomy in retrolental fibroplasia. Paper presented at the 1984 annual meeting of the American Academy of Ophthalmology, Atlanta.
5. Tasman W: Late complications of retrolental fibroplasia. Ophthalmology 86:1724–1740, 1979.

Description and Pathogenesis of Late Stages of Retinopathy of Prematurity*

Robert Machemer, MD

Department of Ophthalmology, Duke University Medical Center, Durham, North Carolina 27710

The surgical treatment of severe retinopathy of prematurity (ROP) has afforded a unique opportunity to study the pathology of the late stages of this disease. The clinically visible changes of the early stages have been described in detail [1–3]. The late stages have been less fully described, however, because retrolental membrane formation has been a hindrance to observation.

Schaffer and coworkers [2], describing active ROP, classified as grade 4 those cases with partial retinal detachment posterior to the shunt and a 360° demarcation line, often with vitreous hemorrhages. They classified as grade 5 those cases with total retinal detachment or complete fibrovascular overgrowth into the vitreous and total destruction of the retina. Cicatricial ROP has been described by Tasman [3], who, although he described in detail findings in the early stages, gave very little description for grades 4 and 5 cicatricial ROP. His criteria for grade 4 are increased tortuosity of the retinal vessels in the posterior pole in infants and accumulation of subretinal exudation. He thought marked equatorial folds to be indicative of severe vitreous traction with lattice degeneration and breaks in the equatorial area. He classified as grade 5 those patients with organized retinal detachment.

It is apparent from these brief citations that very little has been described of the clinical picture or pathogenetic mechanisms of the late stages of ROP. Flynn [4] has described the various locations of the shunt areas; from his investigations, I conclude that the location of the proliferation is the key to understanding the various forms that late ROP may take.

*Originally reported in Ophthalmology 92:1000–1004, 1985; this chapter is an update.

Birth Defects: Original Article Series, Volume 24, Number 1, pages 275–280
© **1988 March of Dimes Birth Defects Foundation**

CONTRACTION OF SHUNT AREA WITH RETINAL STRETCHING

Neovascularization in ROP is preceded by proliferation of mesenchymal cells anterior to existing vessels and parallel to the ora serrata. This tissue provides the matrix for both new vessels and connective tissue. Just as with any other connective tissue, this new tissue contracts as it matures. The contraction produces traction on the retina around the lesion. Retinal tissue at the posterior edge of the proliferation is thus drawn toward the periphery. The effect will be more pronounced in the equatorial plane; the whole length of the shunt area is involved in the contraction. Thus retinal tissue that is the extension of the arc of the lesion will be pulled toward the shunt (Fig. 1A, B—See Color Section, pp. C4–5).

Avascular retina and vascular retina seem to respond differently to stretching. The vascular framework apparently offers resistance to stretch; avascular retina does not seem to be able to resist pull and begins to thin out. In that the vascular tree is not yet complete in these very young eyes, larger areas of the retina are avascular, and these areas and the areas between the major vessels (the raphe) are vulnerable to stretching. Vessels seem to serve as reinforcement for the retinal structure; they tolerate traction until they have been pulled straight, after which, with further pull, the retina becomes elevated and detaches.

Nonvascularized stretched retina does not detach. Normal suction forces of the choroid are apparently strong enough to keep the retina in adherence to the pigment epithelium despite the stretching forces.

Attraction of the retina to the pigment epithelium by the choroid is attributable to the osmotic pressure of the intravascular fluids of the choroid, which, being higher than those of fluids of the retina and vitreous, creates a net flow from the vitreous through the retina to the choroid. The blood flow in the choroid is very great in comparison with that of the retina, and there is, accordingly, a higher concentration of diluents in the choroidal vessels than in the retinal bloodstream, the net effect being that the retina is sucked toward the choroid.

A shunt area is usually located in the temporal periphery. As tissue in the shunt area shrinks, vessels are dragged toward the shunt area, increasing the gap between the superior and inferior vascular arcades nasally and leading ultimately to a temporal reorientation of all major retinal vessels. This contraction process may be so strong that finally all vessels pass in a straight line from the optic nerve head toward the temporal periphery. If contraction continues, the nonstretchable vascularized retina between the optic nerve head and the periphery becomes elevated, and folds develop between the disk and the temporal periphery. An additional factor for radial retinal folding in this area may be the overaccumulation of redundant retina (Fig. 2A,B—See Color Section, pp. C4–5).

The clinician may conclude that nasal retinal vessels have been dragged temporally when indeed nasal retina overlies the optic nerve head, causing a fold of retina completely covering it (Fig. 2B—See Color Section, pp. C4–5). Pigment epithelium under the avascular stretched and migrated retina is usually altered, as its mottled appearance indicates.

Tangential forces stretch and drag the retina toward the temporal periphery. Some transvitreal forces might also be operative, but this seems unlikely at this stage of the disease process. Although the mesenchymal ridge of tissue is elevated, it has not yet proliferated into the vitreous cavity, so direct pull on vitreous is probably very minor.

Stretching of retina and dragging of vessels toward the temporal periphery occur when a limited area of temporal retina is shortened through contraction of its proliferative tissue. The situation changes, however, when a proliferating shunt area involves the whole circumference. Since traction will be exerted relatively equally over all parts of the fundus, there may be some stretching and traction, but the vessels will remain close to their original locations in the posterior retina.

ELEVATION OF RETINA BY CONTRACTION OF PROLIFERATIVE TISSUE

A second factor contributing to the clinical picture of ROP is detachment of the proliferative tissue itself through its own contraction. As long as proliferative tissue involves only an area of a few clock hours, there will be no visible effect of contraction, but, as more of the circumference becomes involved (Fig. 3—See Color Section, pp. C4–5), the extensive contraction and shortening of the thick tissue produce peripheral detachment. When three or all four quadrants are involved, the shunt finally acts as a contracting ring, with resulting reduction of its radius. This contraction can be so considerable that a complete detachment of the retina anterior and posterior to the shunt area occurs (Fig. 4A,B—See Color Section, page C6). Often, the posterior retina exhibits a red reflex, appearing to be attached; nevertheless, there is a definite but shallow retinal detachment. As in any traction detachment, retina bulges outward, and a red reflex is retained. The heavy pigment mottling seen after reattachment in such cases testifies to the fact that the original retinal detachment was total (Fig. 5A,B—See Color Section, page C6).

INTRAVITREAL PROLIFERATION

A third and very important factor in the development of ROP is the proliferation from the shunt area into the vitreous. This proliferation is found only in the most severe types of ROP, usually with involvement of all four quadrants. The shunt is elevated and looks like a high ridge. The diffuse proliferation into the vitreous is apparent as collagen is deposited. The new tissue invades the anterior vitreous cavity to the limit of the anterior vitreous surface, which ultimately becomes white with collagen deposition. At vitreous surgery, the surgeon finds a gradual decrease of density of the tissue posteriorly, the more posterior vitreous being clear. The posterior vitreous is—as one would expect at this young age of the eye—mostly adherent to the retina, although small pockets of liquefied vitreous may be found. It is not known why proliferation is directed anteriorly, being densest just posterior to the lens and near the pars plana. Prominent remnants of the hyaloid artery system are often visible. They consist of fairly dense, whitish tissue containing vessels that originate at the optic nerve head. The tissue is usually dragged over to the temporal side in close proximity to the retina.

ANTEROPOSTERIOR LOCATION OF PROLIFERATIVE AREA

A fourth factor of importance in the clinical picture is the location of the shunt [4]. Depending primarily on the time at which oxygen exposure occurred, the more premature the baby, the more posterior is the development of the shunt. Thus a shunt may be found at any point from an area anterior to the equator to an area surrounding the posterior pole. Accordingly, the clinical picture differs.

If proliferations occur at or anterior to the equator, peripheral retina will detach and be contracted toward the axis of the eye (Figs. 3, 4A,B, 5A,B— See Color Section, pp. C4–6). In such cases, all the anterior retina is highly detached, but there is a high likelihood that the posterior retina, although stretched and shallowly detached, will be reasonably normal in terms of vessel distribution. Thus a red reflex is a good prognostic sign at surgery. Some neovascularization of the most peripheral retina is found.

If the initial proliferations occur posterior to the equator, a different picture develops (Figs. 6, 7A,B—See Color Section, page C7). The midperipheral retina is dragged centrally and anteriorly, exerting strong traction on the posterior retina. This portion of the retina is vascularized and cannot stretch; thus it detaches highly. A narrow funnel develops as the anterior progressively contracts. We may find a small area of red reflex, indicating a slight posterior bulge of streched retina. In this situation, the findings anterior to the ring of proliferation are notable. This retina, not yet vascularized, is therefore very stretchable. Two forces seem to have acted on it, one pulling it toward the axis of the eye (contraction of the proliferative ring) and the other one trying to keep the retina attached to the pigment epithelium ("suction pump" of the choroid). The peripheral retina is thus elongated in such a way that avascular peripheral retina may be found to be attached from the ora serrata to the equator. This retina then folds over anteriorly toward the contracting ring, producing a deep peripheral and often circumferential trough (Fig. 7A,B—See Color Section, page C7). New vessels can extend from the shunt into the trough and the peripheral retina.

In this situation, the surgeon must both remove a central plug of tissue and open the peripheral trough. These maneuvers will partially mobilize the retina and sometimes allow partial reattachment of the retina.

New vessels in young connective tissue are probably just as friable as new vessels in diabetic patients. When they are subjected to the traction forces of the surrounding connective tissue, they may rupture, with subsequent vitreous hemorrhages.

Intraocular proliferations affect the anterior segment only when they occur directly behind the lens. Contraction of peripheral intravitreal proliferations produces a forward movement of the lens (Figs. 4B, 7B). This makes the anterior chamber shallow and may even close off the chamber angle, causing glaucoma. The fact that anterior translocation of the lens occurs only in cases with retrolental proliferations and not with posterior proliferations supports the theory of mechanical origin of the glaucoma.

If the shunt is found very posteriorly along the superior and inferior vascular arcade, thus surrounding the posterior pole, a very peculiar picture develops (Fig. 8—See Color Section, pp. C8-9). The proliferative tissue remains essentially confined to the posterior part of the eye and does not gain access to the anterior vitreous cavity. Either of two pictures may develop.

In the first case, the posterior retina may remain attached between the disk and the temporal vascular arcades (Fig. 9A,B—See Color Section, pp. C8-9). A steep ridge of highly detached retina surrounds the posterior pole, giving it the appearance of a cup, whereas retina surrounding the cup is shallowly detached. On the nasal side, where vascularized retina is more peripheral, a high detachment will occur. Many new vessels proliferate into the vitreous from the height of the ridge in an anterior direction.

In the second situation (Fig. 10—See Color Section, pp. C8-9), the whole retina appears attached except for a whitish mound posteriorly. All the attached peripheral retina is avascular; the whitish mound is made up of connective tissue and collapsed retinal folds. This picture represents a late stage of the previously described situation. Connective tissue over the cup of detached retina has contracted, collapsing the walls of the cup. Surgical removal of the white scar tissue allows one to see, at the bottom of the cup, a small area of attached and vascularized retina. The optic nerve head is often not visible, because retina has been dragged over it, and it is covered by white scar tissue.

CONCLUSION

All retinal changes seen in ROP can be explained by proliferation and contraction of tissue originating in the shunt area. Stretching occurs in avascular areas and between vessels. Detachments occur when traction is exerted along the course of vessels and with concentric contraction of the proliferative shunt. Type and location of detachments vary with the amount and location of the contracting tissue. Detachments found in ROP are all initially traction detachments.

The late stages of ROP are apparently far less monotonous than the brief, previously published descriptions would suggest. These findings can be the basis for a more detailed classification of these stages. Understanding the underlying pathogenetic mechanisms will be a help to the vitreous surgeon attempting to remove scar tissue and eliminate traction.

Understanding the pathogenesis of the late stages of ROP helps in drawing some conclusions for the surgical therapy of this disease. It is my opinion that one should consider surgical intervention as soon as the retina shows a total detachment. This detachment may be shallow, but the advantages are that the retina is still unfolded and in the vicinity of the pigment epithelium and that removal of the proliferative tissue in the vitreous cavity can be performed more easily. There is probably a very narrow window of about 2 weeks, since the proliferative tissue tends to contract rapidly resulting in a narrow, funnel-shaped detachment. Once that stage is reached, surgery becomes difficult, with very little space in which to work. Dilated vessels bleed easily and are very difficult to diathermize without destroying retinal tissue. Once the retina is contracted, it is probably better to wait until active vascularization has subsided and the tissue is atrophic. Unfortunately, by this time, retina is severely damaged and little function can be regained in most cases.

REFERENCES

1. Flynn JT, Cassady J, Essner D et al: Fluorescein angiography in retrolental fibroplasia: Experience from 1969–1977. Ophthalmology 86:1700–1723, 1979.
2. Schaffer DB, Johnson L, Quinn GE, Boggs TR: A classification of retrolental fibroplasia to evaluate vitamin E therapy. Ophthalmology 86:1749–1760, 1979.
3. Tasman W: Late complications of retrolental fibroplasia. Ophthalmology 86:1724–1740, 1979.
4. Flynn JT: Notes on a model of acute proliferative retrolental fibroplasia as a guide to classification. Paper presented at the Workshop for the International Classification of Retrolental Fibroplasia, Calgary, September 9–11, 1982.

Surgical Pathoanatomy in Stage 5 Retinopathy of Prematurity

Eugene de Juan, Jr., MD, Robert Machemer, MD, John T. Flynn, MD, and W. Richard Green, MD

Department of Ophthalmology, Duke University Medical Center, Durham, North Carolina 27710 (E.d.J., R.M., W.R.G.); Bascom Palmer Eye Institute, University of Miami Medical School, Miami, Florida 33101 (J.T.F.)

It is estimated that over 500 infants per year will go totally blind from cicatricial retinopathy of prematurity (ROP) and retinal detachment [1]. Vitreous surgery may offer a hope for retinal reattachment and salvage of vision in this late stage [2,3]. The early stages of ROP have been described in some detail both clinically [4–6] and histopathologically [7–10]. Similarly, the late stages were described in early papers on the subject [11–14].

In contrast, relatively little has been written about the progression of stage 3 to stages 4 and 5 ROP [15]. The purpose of this chapter is twofold: first, to describe the histologic events leading from early extraretinal proliferation to retinal detachment; and, second, to describe specific aspects of stage 5 disease that are potentially important during vitreous surgery to remove proliferations and reattach the retina.

MATERIALS AND METHODS

Sixty-three enucleated and autopsy eyes with various stages of ROP were obtained from the eye pathology laboratories of Duke University, the Bascom Palmer Eye Institute, and the Wilmer Ophthalmological Institute. Since the eyes were obtained from multiple sources over a 30-year period, they were embedded in either paraplast, paraffin, or celloidin. All sections were stained with hematoxylin and eosin. A few additional sections were stained with periodic acid Shiff and Mallory trichrome. Clinical histories were obtained from the pathology records. Because the purpose of the study was to describe specific features in detail, no attempt was made to categorize the full spectrum of changes observed. Twenty-one of the eyes were obtained during the first 2 years of life. Thirteen of these 21 eyes were from the years

Birth Defects: Original Article Series, Volume 24, Number 1, pages 281–286
© **1988 March of Dimes Birth Defects Foundation**

1950–1959. The rest were from later periods. The 42 remaining eyes were enucleated after 2 years of age. These eyes were scanned for configuration of detachment and other findings but were not considered representative of earlier time periods.

RESULTS

Development of Retinal Detachment From Stage 3 Disease

Extraretinal proliferation (stage 3 disease) in the active phase often has a lush red border at the edge of vascularized retina (Fig. 1—See Color Section, pp. C10–11). Later, the proliferation extends toward the midvitreous cavity and often is directed slightly anteriorly and appears as a partially vascularized "veil." The veil in very early stages at its innermost tip is nearly invisible. In later stages, presumably as collagen formation increases, the proliferations become opaque and are more readily seen. Not only does the proliferation extend into the vitreous and toward the back of the lens, it can also course posteriorly along the retinal surface (Fig. 2—See Color Section, pp. C10–11). Posteriorly, the proliferations may or may not be directly connected with the retina by cellular proliferations. Histopathologic studies of these early proliferations reveal two things. 1) The angioblastic intravitreal proliferation is highly active, with many mitoses, immature cells, and primitive vessels. Along the posterior edge of this angioblastic proliferative mass are more developed vascular structures. These structures may or may not have a direct connection with the underlying retina. 2) The proliferations may course posteriorly along the surface of the retina, again with or without direct cellular intimate connection (Fig. 3—See Color Section, pp. C10–11).

In stage 3 disease, the proliferations tend to progress toward the lens (Figs. 3, 4—See Color Section, pp. C10–11). This is often interpreted clinically as a "vitreous veil." The veil is usually vascularized in active disease (Fig. 5—See Color Section, page C12). The proliferations extend directly into the vitreous, in contrast to diabetes mellitus, where they course along the posterior hyaloid surface.

As the intravitreal proliferation progresses, a contraction occurs, not only circumferentially but also in an anterior posterior direction. These cellular proliferations appear clinically as vitreous traction bands (Fig. 6—See Color Section, page C12). These bands often connect with each other, pulling these retinal folds to the equatorial lens region and to the pars plicata (Figs. 7, 8—See Color Section, pp. C12–13). Once the cells begin to mature in the vitreous cavity, their character changes from a very immature angioblastic appearance with a little surrounding cellular material to a more fibrous appearance typically described in retrolental fibroplasia. At this stage, vessels that were prominent arising from the ridge of active ROP into the vitreous cavity regress and leave a whitish glial scar behind the lens (Figs. 9, 10—See Color Section, page C13).

Surgical Pathoanatomy

Detachment of pars plana epithelium. In addition to having small eyes and soft sclera, the child with advanced stages of ROP presents special problems to the vitreoretinal surgeon. One of the most disturbing occurrences during the surgery for these infants is the appearance of xanthophillic (blood-stained) subretinal fluid early in the case. This often occurs from a source under the iris in the far periphery. Often, the exact location of the break cannot be determined. However, clues from histopathology indicate where the leakage may occur. As the peripheral traction detachment and intravitreal proliferative process continues, the peripheral retina is drawn in folds toward the lens and anterior vitreous structures (Fig. 11—See Color Section, pp. C14–15). This often continues until the pars plana epithelium separates as well.

The pars plana epithelium at this level is only one to two cell layers thick and communicates directly with the subretinal space. Since this tissue is so delicate, and is already under high tension, intraocular surgical manipulations often result in breaks communicating with the subretinal space. Additionally, since these are often at the posterior edge of the ciliary body, small, and covered by heavy fibrous tissue, they are difficult to locate. Understanding the peripheral anatomy is important for other reasons as well. We can see, even entering the eye through the pars plicata of the ciliary body, that one might easily inadvertently break through a pars plana detachment and thus begin the surgery with a peripheral retinal break that vastly worsens the surgical prognosis. It is for this reason that we recommend placing the instruments initially above the iris, including infusion cannulas, in an effort to prevent these tears. It should be noted that even an anterior chamber deepening procedure with movement of the lens iris diaphragm posteriorly can cause enough strain on the peripheral pars plana detachments that a tear and subretinal fluid can occur at the beginning of the operation. Once the eyes are entered anteriorly, the lens can be removed in a normal fashion. The lens is usually uninvolved in the proliferative process, and, although the proliferations do appear to course adjacent to the lens, they are rarely intimately connected to it.

Retinal and epiretinal vascular proliferation. A common question asked by people beginning to perform vitreous surgery for advanced retinal detachment associated with ROP is: How does one determine the difference between vascularized membrane and the retinal surface? With late proliferations, the membranes are whitish and often avascular so that they can be distinguished easily from the retina by color and texture. However, in earlier stages of development, this is a serious problem. The membranes are vascularized with branching vessels that resemble retinal vessels. The proliferations in ROP grow out from the retinal surface in broad, diffuse plaques (Fig. 12—See Color Section, pp. C14–15) and are intimately connected with the retinal surface with no anatomic planes between them, particularly among the areas of the most dense foci of the proliferative process. In certain areas, vessels appear to grow out of the substance of the retina and then diffusely along the plaques. These proliferations clearly lie within the substance of the retina and can be removed only at the risk of making at least partial-thickness retinal cuts (Fig. 13—See Color Section, pp. C14–15). Bleeding cannot be avoided in removing such proliferations. Additionally, the proliferations can grow posteriorly from the ridge along the retina. These proliferations are often avascular and can be removed by sharp cutting dissection, or some have used blunt dissection. It is our feeling that the posterior proliferations on the retinal surface occur, in part, from cells that originate from the retina more anteriorly.

Subretinal membranes and photoreceptor degeneration. The immature retina lacks full photoreceptor development. Therefore, it is somewhat difficult to evaluate the effect of detachment on outer retinal morphology. Additionally, we do not know the reversibility of these changes. However, subretinal membrane formation and outer retinal degeneration are common in stage 5 ROP. In the more severe cases of detachment, there is loss of recognizable outer retinal structures, with intraretinal gliosis and subretinal glial membrane formation (Fig. 14—See Color Section, pp. C16–17). These membranes are intimately connected with the retina, and anatomic planes cannot be distinguished histologically. In even more severe cases, subretinal blood is present (Fig. 15—See Color Section, pp. C16–17). In these cases, the retinal pigment epithelium proliferates where the retina inserts into the pars plana and posteriorly around the optic disk. In the most extreme cases, there is heavy pigmented proliferation along the entire subretinal surface, with no other recognizable retinal structures.

DISCUSSION

Despite recent advances in the surgical approach to stage 5 ROP, we are still a long way from having solved the surgical problems, much less the biological aspects, of the disease. Understanding the mechanism by which the retinal detachment occurs may lead to more effective treatment (Fig. 16A,B–Color Section, pp. C16–17). We believe the retinal detachment to be a cellularly mediated event beginning with immature angioblastic cells exiting the retina from the ridge of proliferative tissue. these cells migrate anteriorly to the back of the lens along fine collagenous strands in the vitreous. These cells also migrate posteriorly just above the retinal surface. As the angioblasts interact with the vitreous collagens, they produce new fibrous collagen and contract. The cells orient the randomly distributed collagenous strand in the vitreous along specific lines and then elongate and cause more traction along these same planes. This process is self-propagating, with more cells elongating along these traction bands and more traction then occurring, further feeding the proliferative stimulus. Once the traction becomes great enough, retinal detachment occurs.

As the proliferation becomes worse, more of the retina detaches, including the more anterior parts, particularly the pars plana epithelium. The pars plana epithelium is a delicate tissue, often one to two cell layers thick, that is very susceptible to intrasurgical trauma. Tears in the pars plana epithelium are often the reason why surgery for the severe cases of retinal elevation from ROP fail. Certain technical aspects of the surgery may minimize the risks to the pars plana epithelium, such as entering all instruments anterior to the iris into the anterior chamber. Additionally, lessening intraocular distortion of tissue will also minimize the risk of tearing the pars plana epithelium. Early surgery before detachment of the pars plana epithelium would decrease the chances of tearing it.

The proliferations that occur in ROP are different from the vascular proliferations that occur in other diseases, such as proliferative diabetic retinopathy and branch vein occlusion. In ROP, the proliferations course directly into the vitreous rather than along the hyaloid surface. It is not clear why this should occur; perhaps the immature primitive angioblasts have different extracellular matrix restrictions than more mature cells.

The proliferations in ROP occur over broad areas of the retina and often form intimate connections with it at multiple locations. Histologically, there often is no clear plane between the proliferations and the retina. Peeling or cutting attempts to remove the epiretinal proliferations are often accompanied by bleeding and partial-thickness retinal wounds. Both increase the chance of reproliferation postoperatively.

Finally, although photoreceptor degeneration and subretinal membrane formation are quite common in the later phases of the stage 5 disease, they are relatively uncommon in the earlier, less severe phases. This might indicate a more favorable prognosis if the retina could be attached before these severe changes occur in the outer retina. However, since the retina is immature, it may be able to reverse the severe changes seen histologically once it has reattached. It is hoped that an understanding of the peripheral anatomy as well as the epiretinal proliferations will result in a better understanding of the surgical aspects of the disease and its development.

REFERENCES

1. Phelps D: Retinopathy of prematurity: An estimate of vision loss in the United States—1979. Pediatrics 67:924–926, 1981.
2. Trese MT: Surgical results of Stage V retrolental fibroplasia and timing of surgical repair. Ophthalmology 91:461–466, 1984.
3. Machemer R: Closed vitrectomy for severe retrolental fibroplasia in the infant. Ophthalmology 90:436–441, 1983.

4. Flynn JT, O'Grady GE, Herrera J et al: Retrolental fibroplasia. I. Clinical observations. Arch Ophthalmol 95:217–223, 1977.

5. Tasman W: The natural history of active retinopathy of prematurity. Ophthalmology 91:1499–1503, 1984.

6. Flynn JT: Acute proliferative retrolental fibroplasia: Multivariate risk analysis. Trans Am Ophthalmol Soc 81:549–591, 1983.

7. Kushner BJ, Essner D, Cohen IJ, Flynn JT: Retrolental fibroplasia. II. Pathologic correlation. Arch. Ophthalmol 95:29–38, 1977.

8. Foos RY: Acute retrolental fibroplasia. Albrecht von Graefes Arch Ophthalmol 195:87–100, 1975.

9. Kalina RE, Forrest GL: Proliferative retrolental fibroplasia in infant retinal vessels. Am J Ophthalmol 76:811–815, 1973.

10. Kretzer FL, Hittner HM, Johnson AT et al: Vitamin E and retrolental fibroplasia. Ultrastructural support of clinical efficacy. Ann NY Acad Sci 393:145–166, 1982.

11. Friedenwald JS, Owens WC, Owens EU: Retrolental fibroplasia in premature infants: III. The pathology of the disease. Trans Am Ophthalmol Soc 49:207–234, 1951.

12. Reese AB, Payne F: Persistence and hyperplasia of the primary vitreous. Am J Ophthalmol 29:1–24. 1946.

13. Reese AB, Blodi FC: Retrolental fibroplasia. Am J Ophthalmol 34:1–24, 1951.

14. Foos RY: Chronic retinopathy of prematurity. Ophthalmology 92:563–574, 1985.

15. Machemer R: Description and pathogenesis of late stages of retinopathy of prematurity. Ophthalmology 92:1000–1004, 1985.

Vitreoretinal Surgery for Retinopathy of Prematurity

Steve Charles, MD

Vitreoretinal Research Foundation, Memphis, Tennessee 38119

The purpose of this chapter is to outline the state of the art in the surgical management of ROP stage V and to highlight its many problems. An outline form has been chosen to emphasize areas requiring further research.

Successful trans ciliary body surgical management of stage V cases began with the author's work in early 1977, reported subsequently at the Retina Society Meeting (34 cases). Lightfoot and Irvine [1] reported success in four cases with open funnels using a trans limbal approach. Hirose and coworkers [2] have continued to develop an open-sky approach, which has the problems of bleeding, longer operating times, and the anterior segment complications of corneal transplantation.

PRESURGICAL EVALUATION
Office Examination

Lid retractors and speculums should never be used; they traumatize the lids and have the risk of inducing ptosis as well as emotional trauma. Similarly, restraints should never be used. The frequent apnea spells in these children mitigate against the use of any sedation in the office environment. The children should be comfortable in the parent's lap and examined without touching the lids if they spontaneously open their eyes. It is never necessary to restrain the lower body or place them with their head on the mother's knee, which is an uncomfortable position for most children. Gentle thumb pad pressure from the physician and an additional person are used to open the lids if this does not occur spontaneously. By holding the $+20$ diopter indirect ophthalmoscopy lens still, the eye can be seen as the patient moves the head back and forth.

Examination Under Anesthesia

Many physicians around the country perform examination under anesthesia just to acquire information. Because of anesthesia risk, this should be

Birth Defects: Original Article Series, Volume 24, Number 1, pages 287–293

done only if surgery is anticipated at the same time. In this way, undergoing two anesthesias, one for examination and a subsequent one for surgery, is avoided. The electroretinogram (ERG) is nonrecordable in all cases, even in successfully operated cases, making it of no value. In spite of this, many physicians put patients to sleep without any anticipation of surgery just to perform ERG and ultrasound. The visual evoked potential (VEP) is of no more value than objective determination of light perception in these infants. Because of its cost and complexity, it is certainly unnecessary as well. Contact B-scan ultrasound is of great value if the cornea is opaque, or in the rare instance of an opaque retrolental membrane. In most cases, the apparent retrolental mass is in fact a closed funnel retinal detachment, and indirect ophthalmoscopy is all that is required. Retinal drawings and photographs prolong anesthesia, increase risks, and do not benefit the patient, only data accumulation for the doctor. A useful plan is to anesthetize the patient with a mask, verify the need for surgery, choose the eye with the better prognosis, intubate, and proceed with definitive vitreoretinal surgery.

SURGICAL CRITERIA
Timing

Early cases (3–6 months) have bleeding, fibrin leakage, more reproliferation, and greater anesthesia risks. In contrast, if successfully repaired, the eyes should have better vision because of duration of detachment and an easier anatomic dissection in contrast to later cases (6–18 months). It is the hope that the use of thrombin [3] to prevent bleeding will permit successful surgery in some earlier cases without bleeding. It is thought, however, that the activity of the proliferative disease process in these early cases will cause a higher reproliferation rate if early surgery is performed.

Funnel Geometry

Funnels that are narrow both anteriorly and posteriorly carry a worse prognosis than those that are wide in both regions. Because many narrow-narrow cases are successfully repaired, it appears to be indicated to continue surgery on these babies.

Anesthesia Risks

Because successful cases have resulted from surgery performed as late as 18 months of age, it is better to wait if cardiopulmonary status is unstable. Many of these babies will improve with time, making surgery possible with reduced anesthesia risk.

Bilaterality

Successfully operated unilateral cases uniformly have profound amblyopia. Surgery then should be limited to those unilateral cases with excellent medical and neurologic status in the context of prevention of phthisis and retention of low-grade ambulatory vision and a "reserve" eye.

Angle Closure Glaucoma

Lensectomy and chamber deepening within a few days' onset of flat chamber with glaucoma and early corneal edema can result in a clear cornea, permitting later vitrectomy.

Corneal Opacity

Corneal decompensation occurs rapidly in areas of corneal-iris contact secondary to pupillary block. After a period of approximately 1 month, penetrating keratoplasty with open delamination techniques replaces chamber deepening and subsequent vitrectomy.

SURGICAL MANAGEMENT
Comparison of Alternative Methods

Some surgical techniques create problems significant enough to merit mentioning in this report. Larger instruments with a three-port cannula system result in bleeding from low intraocular pressure and high risk of dialysis when the cannula is introduced and are inflexible in that many instruments will pass through the cannula system. The bimanual approach with scissors in one hand and forceps in the other is unnecessary and requires either a three-port system or a Healon-filled eye. Hyaluronic acid promotes reproliferation, obscures the view of bleeding if present, is costly, and is impossible to remove completely at the end of the surgery.

All surgeons remove the lens, remove most or all of the epiretinal membrane, and relieve anterior loop traction [4]. Scleral buckling has many complications and few if any advantages, and its use is on the decline.

Current Method

A bent 20-gauge blunt cannula is used for infusion through an incision made approximately 0.5 mm posterior to the limbus. This is through the iris root or anterior ciliary body and frequently necessitates a sector iridectomy with the vitrectomy instrument. Infusion cannulas sewn to the sclera strike the lid margin and rotate into the subretinal space. The use of an all-20-gauge system permits changing the infusion cannula from the usual nasal entry to a temporal entry to permit the introduction of the scissors nasally for a better dissection angle.

Endoillumination and a fundus contact lens are not required because of the extreme anterior location of this pathology, seen well with coaxial illumination. Sphincterectomy is frequently necessary to permit visualization of the dissection of the anterior loop traction. Lensectomy with a 20-gauge aspirating ultrasonic fragmenter saves considerable anesthesia time, in contrast to the use of a vitrectomy probe. It is essential to remove all lens capsule utilizing scleral depression to reduce the incidence of postoperative inflammation.

The retrolental membrane (RLM) is minimally vascular and appears to be a single layer, although composed of the anterior and posterior hyaloid faces, with further cellular contraction and proliferation. The posterior hyaloid face is adherent to the retina over an extensive but quite variable area in stage V cases. Although others use the term "membrane peeling or stripping," this type of dissection is never possible. Scissors segmentation that retains some epicenters of epiretinal (retrolental) membrane (developed by the author in 1975) has been largely supplanted by scissors delamination.

Initial entry into the retrolental membrane is usually made centrally, with extreme care to avoid displacement of this rigid structure and subsequent dialysis. Radial cuts are made to produce a stellate incision extending to the anterior loop region. Circumferential cuts in the anterior loop traction usually extend 360° but occasionally spare the nasal area if the gap is very narrow. Delamination of the triangular pieces produced by these radial and circumferential cuts can be accomplished with the modified 45° or 90° Sutherland 20-gauge manual scissors. Delamination is continued until all epiretinal membrane is removed from the retinal surface, extending down into the posterior apical portion of the funnel. The delaminated epiretinal (retrolental) membrane is then removed from the eye with the vitrectomy probe.

Bleeding is controlled with thrombin infusion [3]. A transient elevation of intraocular pressure can control bleeding, but care must be taken not to infarct the retina. Minimal diathermy is utilized to reduce the retinal necrosis/breaks and tissue destruction leading to reproliferation.

Extreme care must be taken to avoid retinal breaks; they markedly worsen the prognosis. Retinal breaks are extremely difficult to approximate to the retinal pigment epithelium because of residual retinal stiffness. Cyanoacrylate retinal patching with a power glue injector shows the most promise in the management of these posterior breaks. Scleral buckling is seldom possible with these breaks. Air is used for surface tension management, for retinal breaks, or if subretinal fluid is observed in the vitreous cavity. The continuous-infusion air pump is utilized for air infusion through the cannula, so fluid is removed with an extrusion needle and delta (linear) suction.

Subretinal fluid is drained in all cases with retinal breaks and high detachments using the 25-gauge needle trans scleral drainage method [5]. Drainage is terminated when fluid initially stops flowing, and increased transretinal pressure gradients are never used to avoid relief tears in the thin posterior retina.

Encircling bands are not used; they intrude into the sclera; require traction on the muscles, which induces bradycardia; and increase the risk of iris-retinal adherence. Antibiotics and steroids are injected subconjunctivally at the conclusion of all surgical procedures.

PROBLEMS

Reproliferation

There is a 30–40% incidence of reproliferation in these patients. It seems to be proportional to the amount of dissection required and the bleeding that occurs in the postoperative period. Iris-retinal adherence is a particularly common form of reproliferation and seems to occur because of surgical trauma to the iris and peripheral retina in the presence of residual lens material. Air or gas frequently create iris-retinal adherence, and hyaluronic acid increases the chance of reproliferation.

At this time, minimization of surgical trauma, avoiding diathermy and retinopexy, and the use of thrombin and normotensive wound closure to prevent bleeding are the only measures to reduce reproliferation. Subconjunctival intraocular 5-fluorouracil has not been effective in the author's hands. It is hoped that polypeptides that block the receptors by which glial cells attach to collagen, fibrin, and elastin (Glaser et al, this volume) will become useful to halt reproliferation. It is apparent that the migration/contraction phase is more important than a true proliferative mitotic phase. Tightening and bundling of preexisting collagen such as the retinal surface by cellular elements is the essential mechanism to block. Although colchicine pharmacologically is appropriate for this use, it may have serious systemic risks in these infants.

Iron Toxicity

Iron toxicity from subretinal blood, photoreceptor loss from long-term detachment, and vasoocclusive disease all seem to play a role in the poor acuity that is the rule rather than the exception. Disorderly migration of retinal spindle cells theoretically can lead to permanent visual loss.

Management of Aphakia

Spectacle correction is required because of the difficulty of fitting contact lenses in these highly hyperopic ($+22.00$ to $+30.00$ D) eyes. Epikeratophakia [6] shows promise in the management of these patients but has the added problems of anesthesia risks.

Poor Acuity

The vast majority of successful cases have only ambulatory vision. Only two of the author's ICROP stage V cases have 20/200 vision, and none are better than that. There is evidence that failure to have a normal visual stimulus during the period of development of the visual pathways in the central nervous system results in permanently decreased vision. This can be thought of as bilateral amblyopia and is similar to the slow development these children may manifest in other neurologic areas. It is essential that full aphakic correction, even without demonstrated vision, should be kept in place for a period of at least 2 years to allow visual stimulation to play a role in visual system development. In many instances, doctors try on the glasses, quickly check the patient's vision in the office, many times after indirect ophthalmoscopy has been used, and conclude that they have no vision and so do not prescribe glasses.

FUTURE DIRECTIONS

It is hoped that a new physical means of dissection, not using peeling or scissors, will reduce retinal break formation and surgery time. It is hoped that cyanoacrylate will get approved by the FDA and that a power glue injector developed by the author can be utilized to treat retinal breaks and improve the prognosis in these desperate cases. The author believes that randomized trials to assess the role of surgical timing have no merit because of bleeding, anesthesia risks, and confusion as to what constitutes an early case.

Research findings should emphasize prevention of prematurity or prevention of retinopathy, by as yet unknown medical means. In these cases, coming to stage V, emphasis should be placed on funding programs for research in pharmacologic means to block the migration/contraction process that results in redetachment.

REFERENCES

1. Lightfoot D, Irvine AR: Vitrectomy in infants and children with retinal detachments caused by cicatricial retrolental fibroplasia. Am J Ophthalmol 94:305–312, 1982.
2. Hirose T, Schepens CL, Lopansri C: Subtotal open-sky vitrectomy for severe retinal detachment occurring as a late complication of ocular trauma. Ophthalmology 88:1–9, 1981.
3. Blacharski PA, Charles S: Thrombin infusion to control bleeding during vitrectomy for stage V retinopathy of prematurity. Arch Ophthalmol 105:203–205, 1987.

4. Charles S: ''Vitreous Microsurgery, 2nd Ed.'' Baltimore: Williams and Wilkins, 1987, pp 137–138.
5. Charles S: Controlled drainage of subretinal and choroidal fluid. Retina 5:233–234, 1985.
6. Morgan KS, Stephanson GS, McDonald MB, Kaufman HE: Epikeratophakia in children. Ophthalmology 91:780–784, 1984.

VIII. CONTINUING ISSUES THROUGH LIFE FOR THE RETINOPATHY OF PREMATURITY PATIENT

Retinopathy of Prematurity Over the Patient's Lifetime: A Clinician's Perspective

William A. Silverman, MD

Columbia University College of Physicians and Surgeons, New York, New York 10032

A few years ago, an articulate medical researcher wrote a disturbing article in the *New England Journal of Medicine* describing his personal experience of becoming blind and the shortcomings of his doctors in providing needed advice and support during the ordeal [1]. He summarized his impression of ophthalmologists' attitudes toward patients whose eye conditions have progressed beyond specific medical help: "We are interested in vision, but we have little interest in blindness." In one of many letters to the editor written in reply to the angry article, a reader commented on the unhappy situation by recalling Shakespeare's horrifying scene in which King Lear's monstrous daughter, Regan, incites Cornwall into tearing old Gloucester's eyes from their sockets [2]. Regan then commands her servants,

> *Go thrust him out the gates,*
> *and let him smell his way to Dover.*

The damning poetry reminded me of the experience with pediatricians described by some parents of children who became blind in the 1942–1954 retinopathy of prematurity (ROP) epidemic. In interviews, parents told me that doctors (they were not yet called "neonatologists") were very attentive and supportive during the stormy early neonatal period after premature birth but that, when the diagnosis of blindness was established, a chill developed in the relationship. "Just when we needed him most," parents reported, "our doctor began to behave very formally, he avoided us, and we felt abandoned." Much of the anger of parents of retrolental fibroplasia (RLF)-blinded children can be traced to the feeling that their doctors were saying, in effect, "Sniff your way to Dover."

The embittered parents faced a succession of frustrating misunderstandings and difficulties in the 1950s. Few if any of the families knew what to expect in rearing a blind infant, and professionals provided little guidance.

Birth Defects: Original Article Series, Volume 24, Number 1, pages 297–300
© **1988 March of Dimes Birth Defects Foundation**

Many of the children developed stereotyped hand motions, rocking, swaying, mutism, or echolalic speech. The children sat for hours sucking on objects, rocking, detached, and unresponsive to the mother or to anyone else. A label of "autism" was frequently applied, and the abnormalities of behavior and development were blamed on parents for not providing adequate sensory and emotional stimulation in early infancy. However, later studies comparing RLF-blinded with children blind from other causes revealed behaviors (which came to be called "blindisms") and delayed development of RLF-blinded preschool children that were not strikingly different from those observed in others with early loss of vision (ie, before mobility, acquisition of language, and feeding and toilet habits were established) [3–9].

When the blind children were old enough to go to school, families frequently encountered hostile attitudes from the past: "parents are the worst enemies of their blind child." [10]. In the 1950s, most blind children (88%) in the United States were enrolled in residential schools away (often in a different part of the state) from their families [11]. The parents of thousands of RLF-blinded children could see no valid reason why separation from the family during the school years was necessary. The families (now battle-hardened, articulate, of largely middle-class status) pressed school boards to provide day classes for blind children within the community school facilities. It is generally acknowledged that it was, in large measure, the influence of the RLF-blind "wave" that forced a change in school arrangements: By the 1970s, two-thirds of all blind children attended day school classes and less than one-third were in residential schools, and it was this "mainstreaming" movement that led the way for acceptance of other handicapped children in public school classes.

Thousands of medical malpractice suits (the exact number has never been determined) preoccupied the time and attention of many families with RLF-blinded children over the past 30 years (as near as I have been able to find out, the first suit was filed in November, 1954). I strongly suspect that many of these actions were triggered by the anger of parents as described above. Many of them have told me that they were able to understand the limitation of medical knowledge at the time their children were born, but they could not forgive doctors for failing to help with advice when parents needed it so desperately. However, tort lawyers have played a major role in fueling the parents' anger. In one particularly cruel instance, the parents were advised by lawyers to delay a program of home counseling for fear that improvement in the infant's development and responsiveness would ruin chances of a large cash award from a sympathetic jury!

I have interviewed many RLF-blinded young adults and have been surprised to find that they seem to know very little about the eye disorder. In September, 1977, a young RLF-blinded law student sat through days of testimony in her own malpractice suit against the treating pediatrician (the action was initiated by the parents in their daughter's name). For the first time in her life, the young woman heard the details of her birth and of the care given in the premature nursery. At the end of the trial, the student wrote this letter to her lawyer and sent a copy to the presiding judge:

> . . . I have decided that I do not wish to pursue my cause of action against ______.
>
> Having consulted with several distinguished attorneys and with my own ophthalmologist, I have reached the conclusion that my case is without merit and its continuation would perpetrate a fraud on the judiciary and the public.
>
> I thus revoke your authority to represent me in this matter.

Her parents were enraged by this move and the attorney filed suit against his (now former) client. The complaint was thrown out of court.

The reluctance of parents and of doctors to discuss, with the child or, later, the young adult, the details of birth and the subsequent development of blindness has led many of the affected to conclude that there was something very shameful about their affliction. One young man told me that he usually lied about it, telling questioners that he was blinded in the war or as the result of some "honorable" accident.

At the request of a number of RLF-blinded adults who wished to learn about premature infant care, I have taken small groups on field trips to a modern neonatal intensive care unit. Nursing staffs have been very cooperative in allowing these now adult ex-premature infants to "see" the incubators and other hardware used in the care of small neonates, and "to see" the newborn patients themselves. The experiences have led to some instructive dialogues between nurses and now vocal former patients. Some of the exchanges have been quite startling: When asked by a nurse whether (given the ever-present risk of blindness) the heroic efforts to keep very small infants alive were justified, one blind man said "No."

The most disturbing finding in my crude efforts to understand the long-term social costs of the 1942–1954 ROP epidemic is the note of discouragement expressed by many of the parents (now in their 60s and early 70s). After fighting for decades against entrenched attitudes [12], they seem exhausted and bitter. Many see, at this late stage in the unrelenting battle, that most of the children have not yet achieved independence. Less than one-third of the working age, severely visually impaired population in the United States is found in the labor force [13].

REFERENCES

1. Stetten D Jr: Coping with blindness. N Engl J Med 305:458–460, 1981.
2. Gilchrist JH: Coping with blindness (letter). N Engl J Med 305:1475–1476, 1981.
3. Parmelee AH Jr: The developmental evaluation of the blind premature infant. Am J Dis Child 90:135–140, 1955.
4. Norris M et al: "Blindness in Children." Chicago: University of Chicago Press, 1957.
5. Keeler WR: Autistic patterns and defective communication in blind children with retrolental fibroplasia. In Hoch PH, Zubin J (eds): "Psychopathology of Communication." New York: Grune & Stratton, 1958, pp. 140–144.
6. Parmelee AH Jr et al: Mental development of children with blindness due to retrolental fibroplasia. Am J Dis Child 96:641–654, 1958.
7. Parmelee AH Jr et al: The development of ten children with blindness as a result of retrolental fibroplasia. A four-year longitudinal study. Am J Dis Child 98:198–220, 1959.
8. Chase JB: "Retrolental Fibroplasia and Autistic Symptomatology." New York: American Foundation for the Blind, 1972.
9. Fraiberg S: "Insights from the Blind: Comparative Studies of Blind and Sighted Infants." New York: Basic Books, 1977.
10. Lowenfeld B: "Our Blind Children: Growing and Learning With Them." Springfield, IL: Chas. C Thomas, 1971.
11. Lowenfeld B: "The Changing Status of the Blind: From Separation to Integration." Springfield, IL: Chas. C.Thomas, 1975.
12. Goffman E: "Stigma, Notes on the Management of Spoiled Identity." Englewood Cliffs, NJ: Prentice-Hall, 1963.
13. Kirchner C et al: "Data on Blindness and Visual Impairment in the U.S.: A Resource Manual on Characteristics, Education, Employment, and Service Delivery." New York: American Foundation for the Blind, 1985.

Development of the Blind Infant and Child With Retinopathy of Prematurity: The Physician's Role in Intervention

Stuart W. Teplin, MD

Clinical Center for the Study of Development and Learning, Child Development Institute, University of North Carolina at Chapel Hill, Chapel Hill, North Carolina 27514

Research regarding retinopathy of prematurity (ROP) continues to proliferate, yielding new information about pathophysiology, prevention, and treatment modalities. Unfortunately, however, this progress has little to offer for the young child whose severe ROP is irreversible, resulting in blindness or severe visual impairment. When confronted with such an infant, what can and should the pediatrician and ophthalmologist do to help him or her reach an optimal developmental potential despite the loss of vision, and to help the family cope and provide the opportunities such development requires?

Despite the usually prompt diagnosis of severe visual problems in infancy, educational and supportive interventions are often absent or delayed until the child is of school age. Parents often voice their frustration regarding their perception of their physician's attitude: ''I'm sorry. Your child is blind. There's nothing more that can be done at this time.'' Even when this message is presented in a sympathetic manner, the parent is needlessly left with many unanswered questions and fears.

Although no studies have documented this ''hands-off'' style as a prevalent approach by physicians, such parental perceptions, particularly among families of ROP babies, have been previousiy cited [1–3], suggesting

This work was supported in part by the USPHS MCH Project grant 916, by the U.N.C. Biological Sciences Research Center, by the Clinical Center for the Study of Development and Learning, and by the North Carolina Council on Developmental Disabilities and the funds it receives through Public Law 98–527, the Developmental Disabilities Act of 1984.

This chapter is an updated adaptation of a previously published article [27] and chapter [38]. Portions of this chapter have been reproduced with permission of *Pediatrics* and Blackwell Scientific Publications, Inc., respectively.

Birth Defects: Original Article Series, Volume 24, Number 1, pages 301–323
© **1988 March of Dimes Birth Defects Foundation**

a relative lack of medical interest in or awareness of the developmental, emotional, and social implications of congenital blindness. Apart from the strictly medical aspects of an infant's eye condition, a physician's management approach toward an infant blinded by ROP (or by any other cause of early blindness) is molded primarily by two factors: general style in communicating with parents and knowledge about the effects of blindness on children's development and intervention approaches. The remainder of this review will focus primarily on the latter, ie, what is known about the development of blind and severely visually impaired young children, particularly those with prematurity and cicatricial ROP, and how such knowledge can be used by physicians. The topic of physician communication with parents is no less important and will be addressed again in the final section. A quotation at this point, however, will serve to illustrate this issue.

Silverman [1], in his interviews of parents of children blinded by ROP many years after the neonatal events, described the intensity with which they expressed anger and bitterness toward physicians:

> . . . most were convinced that physicians had rendered excellent care and had used supplemental oxygen liberally in well-meant efforts to improve the chances of the small babies for intact survival. But, almost without exception, parents recalled (with rancor) that once the diagnosis of RLF was made, a chill in relationships developed. At the very time when they needed support and advice, their physicians became distant and defensive, the parents recalled. Most blamed their doctors for failing to maintain interest and concern, not for failure of clairvoyance! (p 111.)

Although professionals other than the neonatologist, ophthalmologist, and pediatrician may have greater expertise in working with the blind infant and his or her family toward a goal of optimal functioning, the fact is that many families first turn to their physicians for direction and support.

To provide this help, it is not necessary for the physician to become an expert in the development and education of blind children. What is important are three actions:

1. A willingness to supportively discuss the parents' questions and concerns.

2. A recognition that early intervention and parent education are important for later normal development.

3. A recognition that, unless the physician takes the initiative in referring to the appropriate agency or resource service, the family may flounder needlessly, while the infant misses valuable opportunities for cognitive, motor, and emotional development.

The rationale for these actions lies with an understanding of a few principles about the development of blind infants, which is the main focus of this review. What follows is a brief overview of the impact of blindness on an otherwise normal infant's development. Then more specific aspects of the unique developmental patterns of premature infants blinded by ROP will be reviewed. Finally, specific intervention issues and the role of physicians in their implementation will be discussed. Although this chapter focuses specifically on children with ROP, the principles of intervention also apply for other causes of severe visual impairment and blindness in young children.

DEVELOPMENTAL PATHWAYS OF BLIND VERSUS SIGHTED YOUNG CHILDREN

The developmental progress of a normal, sighted infant is intimately tied to the superior perceptual organization conferred by the sense of vision [4,5]. For example, by 6 months of age, repeated visual experiments of tracking the movements of valued people and objects allow the sighted infant to learn about such important concepts as object permanence and cause/effect relationships. Similarly, visually mediated imitation becomes a significant tool for learning, facilitating advances in mobility, language, and social skills.

Such are the future parental expectations for any newborn baby. Suddenly, when the parents are confronted with the fact that their 3-month-old baby is permanently blind, expectations evaporate. In addition to overwhelming grief, the parents are left with tremendous uncertainty about their child's (and their own) entire future. For example, they may be wondering: Will his vision get better? How will he know who I am? How will he learn? What will I tell the baby's grandparents, the neighbors, my friends? Will he ever be able to live independently, get married, have a job? How can I help him? Why did this happen to me?

Generalizations about the developmental routes of congenitally blind young children tend to obscure the extreme variability of styles and timing in adapting to the absence of vision. Other factors that confound research attempts to learn and chart the "typical" developmental pathways of blind infants and children include the variable presence of chronic illness (eg, respiratory illness and cardiac disease) and associated handicaps, including mental retardation, cerebral palsy, hearing impairment, and epilepsy. These additional impairments occur in approximately 35–70% of severely visually inpaired children [6,7]. Furthermore, many visually impaired infants require repeated hospitalizations, including some for surgical procedures, which can have at least temporary adverse effects on children's development.

Fraiberg [4] attempted to avoid these covariables in intensive studies of the impact of congenital blindness in otherwise healthy and normally developing infants. Her study sample was very small (N = 10), highly selected, and therefore not necessarily representative of most blind children. Nevertheless, the following generalizations, adapted from Fraiberg's work [4], are useful guidelines by which to view the young blind child's development. They can provide information on which to base parent counseling, with appropriate modifications for any individual child's unique strengths and problems.

Blind infants without other handicaps, and with the benefit of actively involved parents as initial mediators of the environment, are capable of developing through the same stages and along remarkably similar timetables as sighted infants. However, some important differences in timing and sequence are observed.

Attachment and Social Development

Perhaps most crucial for parents in the early months are signs that their baby recognizes them and enjoys their nurturing. Parents need to be reassured that the important milestones of attachment and bonding do occur, and at approximately the same time as for sighted babies. For example, by 6 months of age, a blind baby, just like one who is sighted, can recognize his parents and cries or tenses when picked up by a stranger. Parents may also be worried about their baby's frequent vacant or "dull" facial expression and paucity of smiling. They can be reassured that this is likely to be a function of the child's not being able to see, and therefore not imitating, other facial expressions and is not necessarily an indication of sadness or mental deficiency. Parents need to learn to watch for cues of attention and emotion in addition to the infant's facial expression, eg, subtle hand and body movements [4,8]. They can also facilitate their infant's abilities to recognize them by encouraging him or her to feel their faces with his hands.

Connections Between Motor and Cognitive Development

Motor and cognitive development are closely linked. Reaching out for a sound cue follows the blind infant's preliminary awareness of object permanence (ie, that objects can exist independently of one's immediate perception of them), occurring at the age of about 9 months [4]. This developmental sequence, as described by Fraiberg [4], differs from that occurring in sighted infants, in which visually mediated, almost automatic, reaching out and grasping of objects at 4 months of age promotes an eventual understanding of object permanence. For the blind infant, sound becomes a motivator for reaching and then for mobility toward objects out of reach. Thus mobility is often "delayed." Unassisted walking, for example, often does not emerge until 18–24 months of age. On the other hand, motor

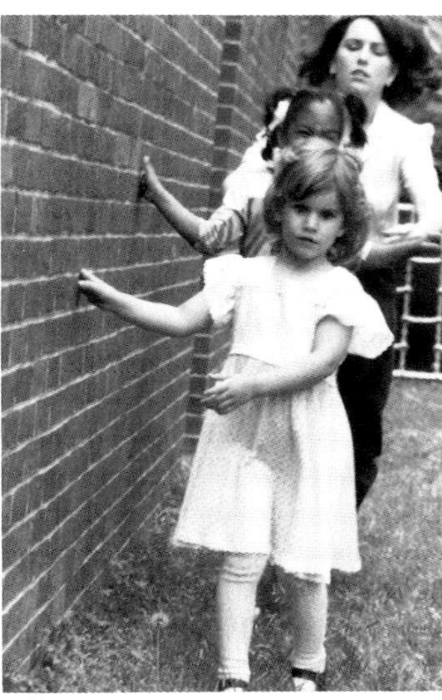

Fig. 1.   Early acquisition of mobility and orientation skills enhances independent exploration of the environment.

milestones that do not require active movement through space (eg, independent sitting balance) occur at roughly the same age as for sighted infants. Once mobile, the child can explore his environment and independently expand his awareness of the world around him (Figs. 1 and 2).

Inasmuch as hands, ears, and proprioceptive sense must become imperfect substitutes for eyes, it is crucial that parents and other early caretakers take the time to expose these infants actively to a variety of meaningful tactile, auditory, and kinesthetic experiences, eg, games emphasizing discrimination of shape, orientation in space, and auditory attention (Figs. 2–5).

Language Development

Fraiberg [4] noted that language skills matched those of sighted infants, except during the second and third years, when there was often confusion regarding personal pronouns ("I" vs "you"). Many young blind children become skillful at imitating sounds and words, sometimes to the point of becoming echolalic. Well meaning but poorly informed parents may have the child listening for hours to radio or television as a form of "stimulation." This also happens inadvertently in many hospital rooms, where the television remains on most of the day whether or not it is appropriate for the pediatric patient. Such input for the blind young child, lacking in the crucial aspect of contingent responsiveness, can be detrimental, teaching the infant and young

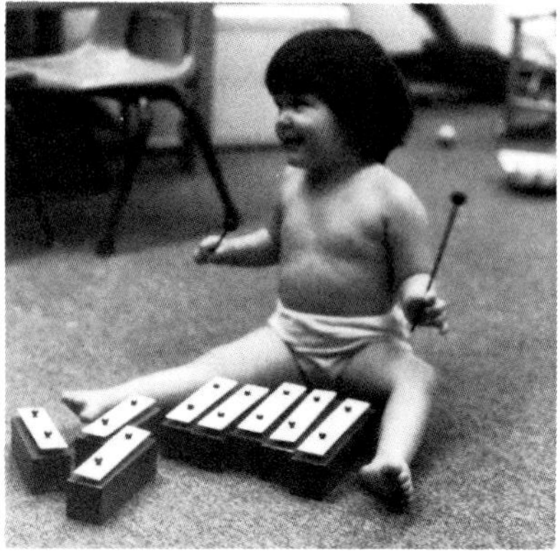

Fig. 2.   Music facilitates auditory discrimination and listening skills.

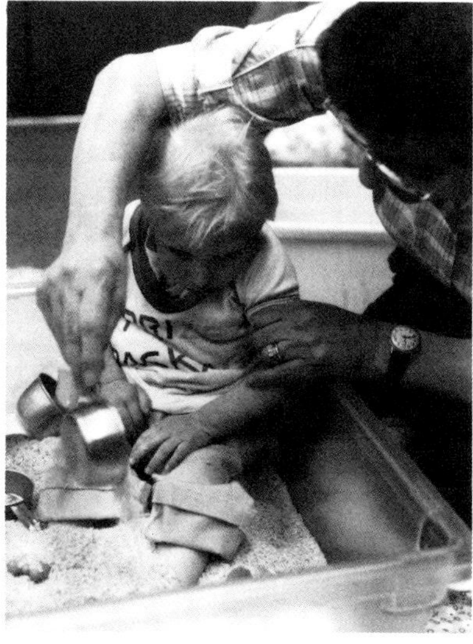

Fig. 3.   The tactile sensation of uncooked rice (or sand, water, etc) promotes body awareness and tactile discrimination skills.

child that sounds are meaningless and are unrelated to his own efforts to communicate.

Parents, sibs, and others can promote the meaningful use of language by frequently talking to and verbally responding to the baby's vocalizations. They can also help by providing consistent verbal labels to body parts, everyday objects, feelings, and activities. When new words are introduced to

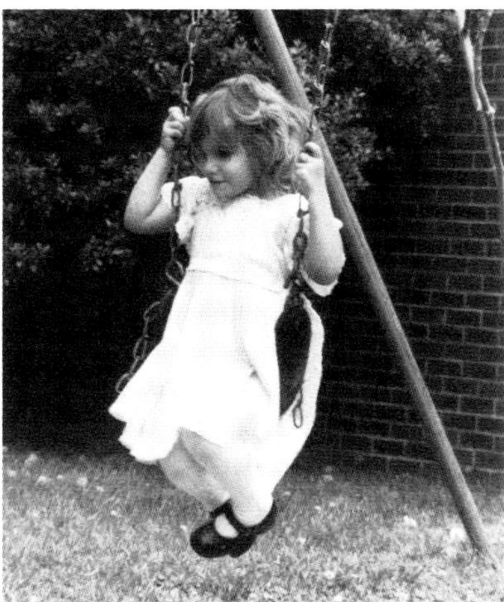

Fig. 4. The joy of swinging can also promote language and orientation concepts (eg, up/down, fast/slow).

the young child, efforts should be made to pair them with the appropriate experiential referents [9] (Fig. 5). To minimize echolalia and facilitate the young blind child's attempts to understand the "whys" and "hows" of his or her environment, parents should not only label objects but describe their functions and properties as well [10].

Mannerisms

Young blind children frequently engage in a variety of stereotypic mannerisms, sometimes referred to as "blindisms." These include eye-rubbing or poking, head-swaying, body-rocking, and hand-flapping. All involve repetitiveness and are often associated with periods of decreased attention to environmental stimuli. Most authorities hypothesize that these disturbing behaviors represent a form of self-stimulation and may arise out of a need for increased sensory or social stimulation [11]. Parents can be encouraged to try behavioral modification approaches, such as diverting the child's attention from himself or herself to objects or people in the environment.

Overprotectiveness

The potentially devastating effects of parental overprotection cannot be overemphasized. Even when parents are appropriately counseled about the inevitable need for their child to experience "bumps and bruises" as he learns about getting around, they must often contend with well meaning

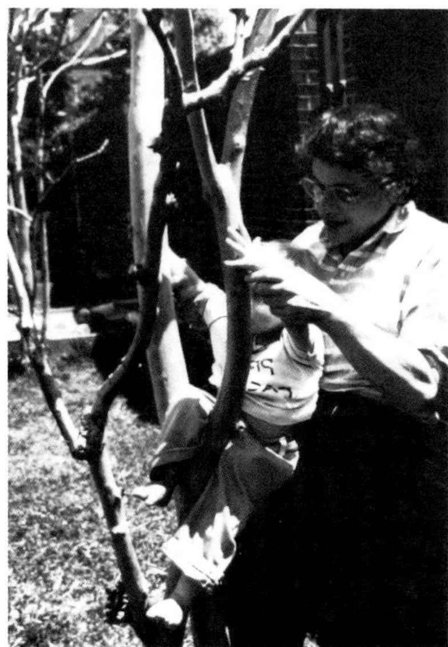

Fig. 5. Experiencing the texture, shape, size, and position of a tree fosters meaningful understanding of the word "tree."

grandparents, neighbors, etc, who chastise the parents for "mistreating" the "poor child." Such attitudes are difficult to overcome and therefore deserve specific and repeated discussions by physicians and other parent counselors, preferably to the extended, as well as to the immediate, family. The effects of understimulation, often aroused by guilt and fear and disguised as "protecting" the infant and young child from harm, are potentially even more pronounced among ROP-blinded children, as will be discussed in the next section.

DEVELOPMENT OF INFANTS WITH BLINDNESS FROM CICATRICIAL ROP
Studies on Children Born in the 1940s and 1950s

Considerable interest has been aroused regarding the possibility of unique developmental profiles of infants and children who are blind from the scarring stages of ROP. Much of this literature, with reference to the older term retrolental fibroplasia (RLF), has been succinctly summarized by Warren [9].

Methodologic Considerations

These studies were sometimes flawed by methodologic weaknesses, eg, comparing blind children who have different associated handicaps, comparing blind children with partially sighted children, and comparing children with early vs later onset of blindness. The cognitive tests used sometimes lacked the rigorous standardization of comparable tests for sighted children. Also, most of these studies occurred in the 1950s and 1960s, on children born during the initial RLF "epidemic" (1942–1954), when neonatal intensive care standards differed significantly from those of today. The following is a very brief review of results from these early investigations.

IQ and Cognitive Development

The conclusions regarding intellectual outcome of blind RLF children varied among studies. Many ex-premature infants with RLF attained normal or superior IQs [9,12–20]. Some authors noted no significant differences between mean IQ or percentage of retarded children among RLF and non-RLF blind, school-age children [12–15]. However, others noted a skewing toward lower IQs for RLF groups, although control groups varied [16–19]. Lower IQ scores among RLF children tended to be associated with lower birthweights [18–20]. Although developmental testing proved useful to parents and professionals during the child's infancy [19], long-term predictions of IQ or eventual neurologic impairments from such testing in the second year were often unreliable [20,21].

Emotional Factors and Autism

Ex-premature infants with RLF tended to be at higher risk for emotional and behavioral problems, including autistic-like features, than children with non-RLF causes of blindness [2,3,9,15,22]. These problems were sometimes associated with the appearance of mental retardation; such "pseudoretardation" seemed to be linked to parental underexpectations and emotional withdrawal [2,3,9,15,22] as well as preconceived negative attitudes about blindness by professionals [23].

Parental Factors

The parents of babies with RLF had usually already contended with daily "life and death" crises as their babies battled through the multiple complications of prematurity. Frequently, physicians had already braced parents for the possibilities of death or survival with eventual severe mental and/or neurologic impairments. Although such discussions are often appropriate, the child who survives may become even more "special" and consequently

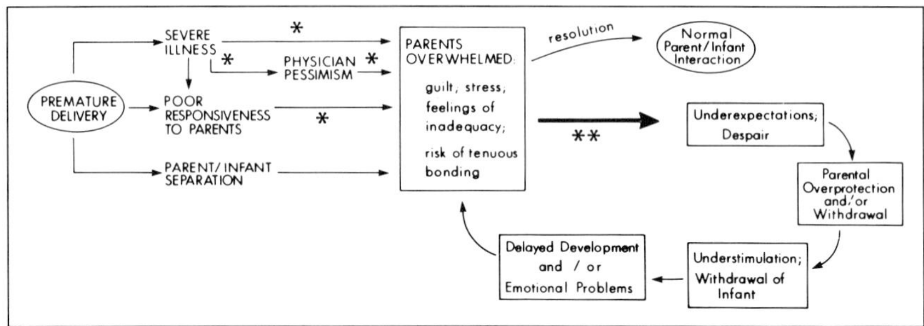

Fig. 6. Suggested causes and outcomes of altered parental attachment to premature infants with blindness from RLF. *Factors affecting attachment of all premature babies that are exacerbated by discovery of blindness. **Onset of "vicious cycle" leading to emotional/developmental problems (pseudoretardation). This cycle may be prevented by providing parents with information about developmental expectations, infant intervention programs, and parent support services. (Reproduced from Teplin SW: Development of blind infants and children with retrolental fibroplasia: Implications for physicians. Pediatrics 71:6–12, 1983, with permission of the publisher.)

"vulnerable" to negative alterations in parent-child interactions (Fig. 6) [24].

Parental fostering of continued dependency is thus a double hazard for the blind infant who has survived a crisis-ridden neonatal period. The adverse effects of early parent-infant separation and parental despair, overprotection, and withdrawal from the blind infant can be potentially more handicapping in the long run than the blindness itself (Fig. 6) [2,22,23,25,26].

Recent Studies of Blind ROP Infants

Despite the increased incidence of ROP and its reemergence as a focus of medical attention in recent years, there continues to be a dearth of information regarding developmental follow-up of those visually impaired ROP children who were in neonatal intensive care units during the 1970s and 1980s [27,28]. Several recent reviews have summarized the above-mentioned literature from earlier years and provided recommendations for developmental interventions for blind and partially sighted young children with ROP [27–30]. Nelson [30] also stressed the importance of appropriate psychologic testing, the availability of both mainstreamed and residential educational programs, and the increasing role of technologic advances in helping visually handicapped young children.

Recent Evidence of Increased Risk for Multiple Handicaps

Only one study has specifically examined neurodevelopmental sequelae and psychosocial variables in ROP infants from a "modern" intensive care setting [31]. During the years 1975–1981, of 645 surviving neonates with birthweights less than 1,500 gm, 14 (2.2%) had stage III–IV "RLF" in one or both eyes. These 14 infants and 14 matched controls were followed for 2–7 years. A significantly greater number of the RLF babies had required at least 2 weeks of oxygen therapy compared to controls, and the RLF infants required more days on assisted ventilation. Sequential developmental assessments revealed that ". . . the RLF survivors had a significantly higher incidence of neurologic abnormality, lower developmental quotients, increased requirements for special education, increased number of hospitalizations for illness, and more maternal stress . . ." (p 287) [31]. The authors did not comment on the validity of comparing scores from the IQ tests used for the visually impaired subjects (tactile and/or verbal portions of the Psychological Stimulus Response test and of the Wechsler Preschool and Primary Scales of Intelligence) to the Stanford-Binet scores obtained for the sighted controls. Nevertheless, their findings were striking. For ages 3, 4, and 5 years, the mean IQs of the RLF group were 53, 66, and 70, respectively, compared to IQs of 92, 98 and 105, respectively, for the control group. Seven RLF vs two control children had definite cerebral palsy or seizure disorders. The prevalence of intraventricular hemorrhage in the two groups could not be adequately assessed, but it was speculated that this complication might be more common in the RLF group.

The emotional/behavioral characteristics of these infants were not reported. However, the authors did observe higher stress levels in the families of the RLF group, with four of the 14 families showing major disintegration. Although the degree of family social support was similar for the RLF and control groups, the stresses in the former group imposed a need for additional sources of support. Corroborating recommendations from previous reports [27,29,30], these authors stressed the importance of physicians taking an active role in making early referrals of such infants for comprehensive intervention and family support services.

Additional controlled studies of the developmental follow-up of blind ROP infants born in the 1970s and 1980s have not yet been published. This author has been following 12 blind children with ROP at North Carolina Memorial Hospital in Chapel Hill. As of 1985, they range in age from 1 to 7 years. Among these children, preliminary findings indicate that four have cerebral palsy, seven appear to be mentally retarded on tests designed to look at cognitive development in blind children, and three are autistic, ie, showing distorted, echolalic language; perseverative, stereotypic play; and limited social relatedness to people. Only four of the 12 children have no apparent handicaps in addition to blindness. These early findings are consistent with those of Vohr and Coll [31]. It is difficult to know, however, the extent to which these results are affected by an ascertainment bias in this small sample.

This author has also informally polled a number of teachers of visually impaired preschool children from a variety of centers in the United States. When they were asked whether, in their experience, those children with ROP have distinctive developmental characteristics, there was no uniform answer. There appears to be considerable variability in opinion on whether current blind preschool ROP children have a higher or lower incidence of multihandicaps than their RLF counterparts from 20–30 years ago.

Several teachers have independently noted that blind children with ROP tend to have more difficulty with understanding the positions of their own bodies in space than children who are blind from other conditions. However, no formal research has focused on this issue, leaving this an undocumented speculation.

Summary of Developmental Studies on ROP Children

Conclusions from earlier studies were somewhat inconsistent but tended to suggest that blind infants with cicatricial ROP born in the 1940s and 1950s were at increased risk for cognitive and emotional problems. However, several studies documented a number of such children whose IQ was normal to superior. A recent study [31] of a "modern" cohort of ROP infants implies that associated neurodevelopmental handicaps are definitely more prevalent among the ROP infants than in matched, control infants.

Speculation as to reasons for the increased risk of cognitive and emotional problems among ROP-blinded children focuses on environmental factors (isolation, understimulation, parental emotional withdrawal, overprotectiveness, lack of sufficient social support) as well as biologic variables in the perinatal period. The latter remain poorly understood. As with most other questions about developmental outcome, it seems reasonable to assume that complex interactions between biology and environment are at work. Further research in these areas should help to clarify the nature of these interactions.

IMPLICATIONS FOR PHYSICIANS

According to a nationwide survey in 1965, cicatricial ROP accounted for 9% of all blindness in preschool children [32]. Currently, ROP is reported to occur in 1.8–4% of all premature infants weighing less than 1.5 kg at birth [32]. It was estimated that in the United States in 1979, 546 infants were blind due to cicatricial ROP [33].

Although the physician's traditional role has been to provide medical or surgical preventive measures and treatments for RLF, these have only limited value to those infants and children whose vision is already irreversibly lost. As was noted above, the physician also needs at least some information about relevant developmental issues and services and must work toward effective communication of this information with the families of affected infants.

OBSTACLES TO EFFECTIVE PHYSICIAN–PARENT COMMUNICATION
Parental Needs and Physician Attitudes/Unawareness of Services

In the poignant account of his own deteriorating vision, Dr. DeWitt Stetten, Jr, [34] recalled multiple examinations by several eminent ophthalmologists. He lamented the fact that they attended much more to the pathologic condition of his eyes than to him as an individual in need of help:

> . . . No ophthalmologist has at any time suggested any devices that might be of assistance to me. No ophthalmologist has mentioned any of the many ways in which I could stem the deterioration in the quality of my life . . . . If after all [of the diagnostic and therapeutic manipulations of the patient's eyes] the patient still has a serious visual impairment, the ophthalmologist is missing an extraordinary opportunity if he or she fails to direct the patient's attention to . . . the aids and agencies designed to improve the quality of life of the visually handicapped person (p 458) [34].

Dr. Stetten's feelings are similar to those expressed by parents of ROP-blinded children in the Silverman quotation [1] in this chapter's introduction. They are directed not only to ophthalmologists but to all physicians who have withdrawn from truly helpful involvement with the blind child and his family. The reasons for this, aside from uncertainty about how to help, may stem in part from the very human trait of discomfort in confronting one's "failures" and the pessimism many feel regarding a blind young child's potential capabilities [3] (Fig. 6). Neonatologists may find it difficult to deal with the parents of a baby who was blinded iatrogenically, even though it may have been the unavoidable "cost" of saving the baby's life [1]. As noted, ophthalmologists may feel they have no more to offer once their treatments have "failed" to restore vision. These feelings, coupled with the stereotyped underexpectations for blind individuals, often prevent the communication and counseling with parents necessary for early and continuing intervention with their visually impaired children, yet most parents turn to the "experts," their doctors, including ophthalmologists, neonatologists, pediatricians, and family physicians. Frequently, the pediatrician or family physician assumes that, since the ophthalmologist is the "eye specialist," he or she will know how to answer the mother's questions about how optimally to raise her blind child and where intervention services are located. However, most ophthalmologists, rigorously trained as surgical subspecialists, have little or no training in counseling parents on these developmental issues. Furthermore, they may hesitate to bring up potentially upsetting intervention needs to a family when uncertainty still exists as to the child's ultimate visual function. Although it may be true that, with time or after surgery, a child's vision may improve, it is usually appropriate to make early referrals for developmental services, with the understanding that they can always be discontinued or revised at a later time.

Communication Styles and Timing

Frequently when such discussions regarding blindness and its developmental implications do take place, inadequate time is scheduled for the physician to really encourage the parents to express their questions and fears. This may be particularly true when the physician has limited information to provide or is uncomfortable admitting "I don't know" to some of the parents' questions (many of which have no other realistic answer). However, simply knowing that the chiid's doctors allowed these questions to be aired is of great relief to most parents and provides a basis on which the parents and doctor can be partners in seeking answers and services.

The early emotional shock, denial, or anger associated with learning about their child's blindness may render some parents temporarily unable to discuss developmental interventions or the child's future needs. On the other hand, some parents deal with these feelings best by aggressively pursuing information and services. Physician awareness of these needs can help determine more optimal pacing for physician–parent discussions.

Without appropriate counseling and referrals by physicians, parents are left to fend for themselves. Often, they are remarkably resourceful and successful in raising their blind children, but the support of professionals would clearly enhance the process. The ongoing relationship that a pediatrician or family physician develops with these children and their families can often provide an optimal framework for the needed communication [26].

PRACTICAL ASPECTS OF DEVELOPMENTAL INTERVENTION

Once this communication exists, what information needs to be conveyed? As noted earlier, some developmental issues may be more relevant to ROP than to other causes of severe visual impairment. In general, however, the information and guidance needed by the family are universally appropriate, regardless of etiology. Table I and Figures 7–9 provide an overview of some major developmental tasks for blind infants and children and examples of the types of practical activities that the parent can carry out at home to help in achieving these goals. This listing is not complete, but indicates how knowledge of the development of these children can be translated into

TABLE I. Developmental Goals and Sample Activities for Blind Infants and Children (Partial listing)

Goal	Sample activities to help in reaching goal
Infants (0–2 years)	
Parent–infant emotional attachment	Early positive parent-infant contact during newborn-infant hospitalization [36]
	Promotion of maximal holding, carrying, and talking to infant
	Social/emotional support of parents by family, professionals, parent groups
Active exploration of environment; improving tactile/auditory discrimination	Strengthening neck and trunk by encouraging prone position; discouraging prolonged supine lying
	Repetitive games to encourage reaching for sound cues
	Liberal exposure to new textures, sounds, smells, and sights (to encourage residual vision; Figs. 2,3,9)
	Encouraging hands together in midline
Increasing independence and mobility	Encouraging self-feeding (despite mess; Fig. 7)
	Encouraging tactile search for dropped toys
	Expecting/tolerating minor bumps, bruises
Language development	Parent's contingent "talking" to infant vocalizations
	Consistent and repetitive use of labels for objects, activities, body parts (Fig. 5)
	Prevention of prolonged exposure to noncontingent sound (eg TV, radio)
Preschool (2–5 years)	
Social interaction	Encouraging interaction with peers, including nonhandicapped (eg, nursery school)
	Setting behavioral limits
Self-help skills	Teaching specific techniques for toileting, dressing, bathing, etc (Figs. 7,8)
Mobility and orientation	Games that teach directional concepts (eg, up, down, under; Fig. 4)
	Concrete techniques for safely walking (Fig. 1)
Concepts/"real-world" experiences	Frequent exposures to sounds/textures of everyday environments (eg, yard, grocery store, gas station; Fig. 5)
Early school age (6–10 years)	
Reading	Determination of optimal mode(s), ie, Braille, large-print, use of optical aids, recorded books
Improved orientation and mobility	Individualized orientation and mobility training

From Teplin SW: Development of blind infants and children with retrolental fibroplasia: Implications for physicians. Pediatrics, 71:6–12, 1983, reproduced with permission of the publisher.

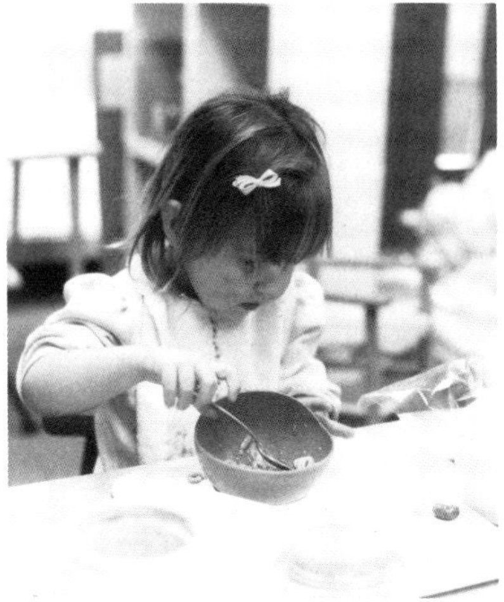

Fig. 7.   Self-feeding encourages confidence, independence, and improved fine-motor skills. Parental perseverance and tolerance of messiness are necessary.

appropriate interventions. Such "treatments" have been documented as beneficial [4,9]. Physicians both comfortable and uncomfortable in discussing these concepts with parents can more completely meet the child's needs by making an appropriate referral to the person, center, or agency in his or her region who is most knowledgeable in this area. Such referrals are listed in Table II along with other suggested roles for physician advocacy for the blind child's optimal development.

Each state, or region within a state, varies with regard to the organization of these educational and supportive services. Sometimes, unfortunately, the fact that an agency providing services for blind individuals exists does not necessarily imply that the services are specifically adapted or appropriate for young children. The physician-as-advocate needs to find out from the parents and the agency whether this is the case. If so, he or she can help to "lobby" for the needed services. Since congenital blindness is a relatively low-incidence handicap, and fiscal belt-tightening currently threatens all human service programs, services for blind children may be unavailable or insufficiently staffed. However, with the assistance of professionals and the teaming together of concerned and persistent parents, program improvements can be created.

Innovative professionals have devised individualized ways to improve services to blind children. For example, at the University of North Carolina, one pediatric ophthalmologist has a teacher for visually impaired children periodically see each child and family in his clinic to provide guidance

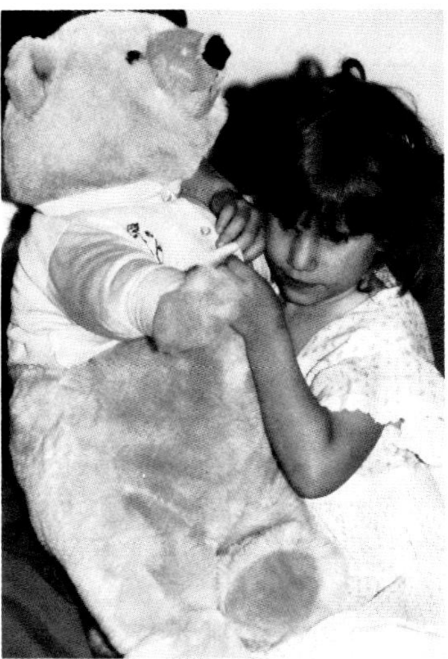

Fig. 8.   Buttoning a shirt and other self-help skills involve fine-motor dexterity and promote independence.

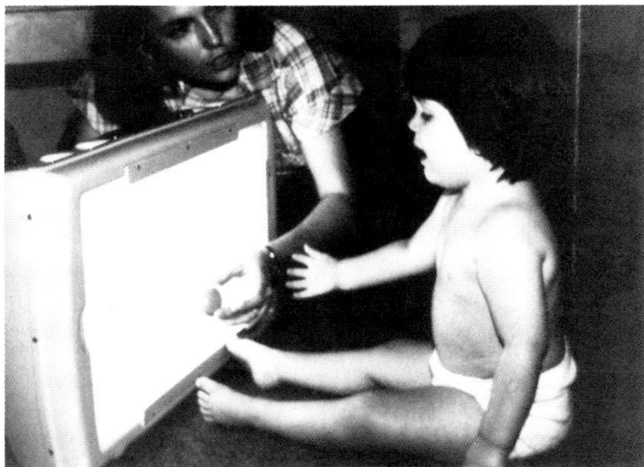

Fig. 9.   A light box in a dim room is one of many low-vision aids. It provides enough contrast to promote a young child's use of any residual vision.

regarding materials, state services, and counseling on questions about everyday activities. At a major teaching hospital in Massachusetts, one nurse in the neonatal intensive care unit was particularly interested in visually

TABLE II. Roles of Physicians in Promoting Optimal Development of Blind Infants and Children

1. Consider as *child* who is blind, not *blind* child
2. Encourage questions and comments from parents about their child's developmental progress
3. Know about and refer to community resources, eg, developmental preschools, interdisciplinary evaluation centers, state agency for blind, home early intervention programs for infants; maintain communication with programs in which one's visually handicapped patients participate and be available to clarify to teachers and parents the practical, functional implications of the child's impairments [35]
4. Provide or refer for genetic counseling when indicated or requested (not applicable for ROP).
5. Provide emotional support for child and family; refer to parent groups; explore impact on siblings
6. Help family integrate information from multiple "experts" who evaluate the child; attempt to "demystify" medical jargon for parents
7. Consider use of low-vision aids and games to encourage child's use of any residual vision (Fig. 9) [30]
8. Arrange for in-service training for hospital-based personnel (eg, nurses, aids, etc) regarding optimal ways of interacting with blind young children who are hospitalized [36,37]
9. Help family prepare for child's enrollment in school; encourage their early exploration of availability of special classrooms, teachers, materials; Advocacy when needed [35]
10. Refer parents to written books, pamphlets, and materials that will provide further information and ideas for home activities and adapted toys (see Appendix)

From Teplin SW: Developmental issues in blind infants and children with retinopathy of prematurity. In Silverman WA, Flynn JT (eds): "Retinopathy of Prematurity." Boston: Blackwell Scientific Publications, Inc, 1985, reproduced with permission of the publisher.

impaired babies and infants and became a consultant to the ward teams regarding appropriate counseling and initiation of intervention services.

Many parents are eager to read about blind children's development and ways they can work with their own child. In the past 5 years, there has been an "explosion" of excellent written materials specifically aimed at guiding parents in raising their visually handicapped children. The Appendix contains a listing of suggested books and agencies that physicians can recommend to parents. The physician, too, can learn from these publications.

Blindness is a tragic handicap. However, physicians can greatly enhance the quality of the lives of their visually impaired young patients and their families. An appreciation of the impact of blindness on normal development, a knowledge of community and national services available, and a willingness to confront and overcome physician attitudinal barriers are the ingredients necessary for effectively helping parents in encouraging optimal development of their visually impaired children, including those with ROP.

ACKNOWLEDGMENTS

The author thanks Janice Jarrell for secretarial assistance, and the staff, students, and families participating in the C.D.L. Project for Visually Impaired Preschoolers.

REFERENCES

1. Silverman WA: "Retrolental Fibroplasia—A Modern Parable." New York: Grune and Stratton, 1980, p 111.
2. Hallenbeck J: Pseudo-retardation in retrolental fibroplasia. New Outlook for the Blind 48:301–307, 1954.
3. Blank HR: Psychiatric problems associated with congenital blindness due to retrolental fibroplasia. New Outlook for the Blind 53:237–244, 1959.
4. Fraiberg S: "Insights From the Blind: Comparative Studies of Blind and Sighted Infants." New York: Basic Books, Inc, 1977.
5. Gesell A, Ilg FL, Bullis GE: "Vision—Its Development in Infant and Child." New York: Hafner Press, 1949.
6. Robinson GC: Causes, ocular disorders, associated handicaps and incidence and prevalence of blindness in childhood. In Jan JE, Freeman RD, Scott EP (eds): "Visual Impairment in Children and Adolescents." New York: Grune and Stratton, 1977.
7. Fine SR: Incidence of visual handicap in childhood. In Smith V, Keen J (eds): "Visual Handicap in Children." London: Spastics International Medical Publications, 1979.
8. Als H, Tronick E, Brazelton TB: Affective reciprocity and the development of autonomy: The study of a blind infant. J Am Acad Child Psychiatr 19:22–40, 1980.
9. Warren DH: "Blindness and Early Childhood Development, 2nd Ed." New York: American Foundation for the Blind, 1984, pp 184–188, 209, 261–262, 266–269.
10. Kekelis LS, Andersen ES: Family communication styles and language development. J Vis Impair Blind 78:54–65, 1984.
11. Eichel VJ: Mannerisms of the blind: A review of the literature. J Vis Impair Blind 72:125–130, 1978.
12. Hayes SP: "First Regional Conference on Mental Measurements of the Blind." Watertown, MA: Perkins Publications, 1952, No. 15.
13. Gore GV: Retrolental fibroplasia and IQ. New Outlook for the Blind 60:305–306, 1966.
14. Norris M, Spaulding PJ, Brodie FH: "Blindness in Children." Chicago: University of Chicago Press, 1957.
15. Parmelee AH, Cutsforth MG, Jackson CL: Mental development of children with blindness due to retrolental fibroplasia. Am J Dis Child 96:641–654, 1958.
16. Cohen J, Boshes LD, Snider RS: Electroencephalographic changes following retrolental fibroplasia. Electroencephalogr Clin Neurophysiol 13:914–922, 1961.
17. Cohen J, Alfano JE, Boshes LD, Palmgren C: Clinical evaluation of school-age children with retrolental fibroplasia. Am J Ophthalmol 57:41–57, 1964.
18. Cohen J: The effects of blindness on children's development. New Outlook for the Blind 60:150–154, 1966.
19. Parmelee AH, Fiske CE, Wright RH: The development of ten children with blindness as a result of retrolental fibroplasia. Am J Dis Child 98:198–220, 1959.
20. Genn MM, Silverman WA: The mental development of ex-premature children with retrolental fibroplasia. J Nerv Ment Dis 138:79–86, 1964.

21. Gillman AE, Goddard DR: The 20 year outcome of blind children 2 years old and younger: A preliminary survey. New Outlook for the Blind 68:1–7, 1974.

22. Keeler WR: Autistic patterns and defective communication in blind children with retrolental fibroplasia. In Hoch PH, Zubin J (eds): "Psychopathology of Communication." New York: Grune and Stratton, 1958.

23. Elonen AS, Zwarensteyn SB: Appraisal of developmental lag in certain blind children. J Pediatr 65:599–610, 1964.

24. Green M, Solnit A: Reactions to the threatened loss of a child: A vulnerable child syndrome. Pediatrics 34:58–66, 1964.

25. Omwake EB, Solnit AJ: It isn't fair: The treatment of a blind child. Psychoanal Study Child 16:352–404, 1961.

26. Parmelee AH, Liverman L: Blindness in infants and children. In Green M, Haggerty RJ (eds): "Ambulatory Pediatrics." Philadelphia: WB Saunders, 1968.

27. Teplin SW: Development of blind infants and children with retrolental fibroplasia: Implications for physicians. Pediatrics 71:6–12, 1983.

28. Scharf LS, Adams KM: Long-term neuropsychological impact of retrolental fibroplasia: Review and implications. J Pediatr Psychol 9:303–316, 1984.

29. Porat R: Care of the infant with retinopathy of prematurity. Clin Perinatol 11:123–151, 1984.

30. Nelson LB: The visually handicapped child. Pediatr Rev 6:173–182, 1984.

31. Vohr BR, Coll CT: Increased morbidity in low-birth-weight survivors with severe retrolental fibroplasia. J Pediatr 106:287–291, 1985.

32. Hatfield EM: Blindness in infants and young children. Sight Sav Rev 42:69–89, 1972.

33. Phelps DL: Retinopathy of prematurity: An estimate of vision loss in the United States—1979. Pediatrics 67:924–926, 1981.

34. Stetten D Jr: Coping with blindness. N Engl J Med 305:458–460, 1981.

35. O'Brien R: Education of the child with impaired vision. Pediatr Ann 9:434–440, 1980.

36. Lovelace BM: The blind child in the hospital. AORN/J 31:256–270, 1980.

37. Harrell L: "Touch the Baby: Blind and Visually Impaired Children as Patients—Helping Them To Respond To Care." New York: American Foundation for the Blind, 1984.

38. Teplin SW: Developmental issues in blind infants and children with retinopathy of prematurity. In Silverman WA, Flynn JT (eds): "Contemporary Issues in Fetal and Neonatal Medicine: Retinopathy of Prematurity." Boston. Blackwell Scientific Publications, 1985, Vol 2, pp 267–288.

APPENDIX: RESOURCES FOR PARENTS OF VISUALLY IMPAIRED YOUNG CHILDREN

Books/Pamphlets

Brennan M: Show me how: A manual for parents of preschool visually impaired and blind children. 1982, American Foundation for the Blind, 15 W. 16th St., New York, NY 10011.

*Chernus-Mansfield N, Hayashi D, Horn M, Kekelis L: Heart to heart—Parents of blind and partially sighted children talk about their feelings, 1986, Blind Children's Center, 4120 Marathon St., P.O. Box 29159, Los Angeles, CA 90029-0159 [a frank and

---

*Best general references.

empathetic description of common feelings aroused in families when confronting their young child's blindness, with many quotations from parents].

Corn AL, Martinez I: When you have a visually handicapped child in your classroom: Suggestions for teachers. 1977, American Foundation for the Blind, 15 W. 16th St., New York, NY 10011 [Practical ideas regarding visually handicapped children in classroom settings; written for teachers but helpful for parents as well; single copy, free].

*Ferrell KA: Parenting preschoolers: Suggestions for raising young blind and visually impaired children. 1984, American Foundation for the Blind, 15 W. 16th St., New York, NY 10011 [Excellent and practical answers to most common questions asked by parents, including references and agency lists; single copy, free].

*Ferrell KA: Reach out and teach: Materials for parents of visually handicapped and multihandicapped young children. 1985, American Foundation for the Blind, 15 W. 16th St., New York, NY 10011 [An excellent, field-tested handbook for familiarizing parents with the development of blind young children, along with a workbook for parents to monitor their child's progress (Combination $25.00). Also available are eight illustrative slide/tape presentations ($150)].

*Fraiberg S: Insights from the blind. 1977, Basic Books, Inc. New York, NY 10022 [Written more for child development professionals, this is a somewhat technical but fascinating research study of early development of blind children].

Harrell L: Touch the baby: Blind and visually impaired children as patients—Helping them to respond to care. 1984, American Foundation for the Blind, 15 W. 16th St., New York, NY 10011 [Practical guidelines for helping blind and visually impaired newborns and preschoolers in medical settings; single copy, free].

*Heiner D: Learning to look. A handbook for parents of low vision infants and young children. 1986, International Institute for Visually Impaired, 0–7, Inc. (Blind Children's Fund), 1975 Rutgers Circle, East Lansing, MI 48823 [practical suggestions regarding toys, lighting, contrast, colors, and seeking help with assessing visual function].

Instructional Materials Center, Illinois Supt. of Public Instruction: Preschool learning activities for the visually impaired child. ERIC Documents, P.O. Box 190, Arlington, VA 22210. [Good book giving very specific toys, games and activities a parent or teacher can use].

*Kastein S, Spaulding I, Scharf B: Raising the young blind child. 1980, Human Sciences Press, 72 Fifth Ave., New York, NY 10011 [Excellent and practical guide for parents and teachers on providing a stimulating environment for the visually impaired infant and preschooler].

*Kekelis L, Chernus-Mansfield N: Talk to me. 1984, Blind Children's Center, 4120 Marathon St., P.O. Box 29159, Los Angeles, CA 90029-0159 [Language guide for parents of blind children; single copy, free for parents].

Kronheim JK: Learning pillows. P.O. Box 631 New Town Br., Boston, MA 02258 [pillows which depict stories in tactile and colorful materials to promote exploration; accompanied by audiotaped stories. Prices range from $8 to $20].

*Lowenfeld B: Our blind children: Growing and learning with them. 1971, Charles C Thomas, 301-327 E. Lawrence Ave., Springfield, IL 62717 [A renowned expert in the area of education for preschool blind provides developmental guidelines for parents].

Moore, PM: Toilet habits: suggestions for training a child who is blind. 15 W. 16th St., New York, NY 10011 [Advice and encouragement for parents on toilet training a blind child].

Muste J, Fellows RR: Moving and doing: How to help visually impaired children know their world. 1982, Comprehensive Eye Center, Children's Hospital, 700 Children's Drive, Columbus, OH 43205 [Guidelines for parents to promote gross and fine motor skills, body awareness, balance; includes songs and rhyming games].

*Nousanen D, Robinson L: Take charge! A guide to resources for parents of the visually impaired. 1980, National Association for Parents of the Visually Impaired, Inc., 2011 Hardy Circle, Austin, TX 78657.

*Raynor S, Drouillard R: Get a wiggle on. AAHPER Publication Sales, 1201 16th St., NW, Washington, DC 20236 [Easy-to-read booklet with practical suggestions for parents of visually impaired infants up to the walking stage].

*Raynor S, Drouillard R: Move it. AAHPER (same address as above) [Sequel to Get a wiggle on, with suggestions for preschool visually impaired child from stages of walking to kindergarten].

*Recchia S: Welcome to the world—Toys and activities for the visually impaired infant. 1986, Blind Children's Center, 4120 Marathon St., P.O. Box 29159, Los Angeles, CA 90029-0159 [tips on encouraging learning through play for blind and visually impaired infants; single copy free for parents; available in English and Spanish].

*Recchia S: Learning to play—Common concerns for the visually impaired preschool child. 1987, Blind Children's Center, 4120 Marathon St., P.O. Box 29159, Los Angeles, CA 90029–0159 [explores toys/materials, making transitions between activities, and peer play; free for parents and professionals].

*Scott EP, Jan JE, Freeman RD: Can't your child see? 1979, University Park Press, Chamber of Commerce Building, Baltimore, MD 21202 [Excellent book for both parents and professionals on all aspects of raising a blind or visually impaired young child; includes chapter on multihandicapped blind child].

*Ulrich, SE: 1972, University of Michigan Press, 615 E. University, Ann Arbor, MI 48106 [A mother's account of the first 5 years of raising her blind daughter, who had retinopathy of prematurity; describes how she learned to cope with her daughter's blindess and guide her into becoming a happy, independent child; highly recommended by many parents of blind children].

Webster R: The road to freedom: A parent's guide to prepare the blind child to travel independently. 1977, Katan Publications, 2012 Cedar St., Jacksonville, IL 62650 [Practical suggestions to promote mobility and orientation for the young child].

Willoughby DM: A resource guide for parents and educators of blind children. 1979, National Federation for the Blind, Baltimore, MD 21230.

Yates V: Tune In! 1980, Delta Gamma Foundation for Visually Handicapped Children of St. Louis, 9313 Manchester Rd., Suite 101, St. Louis, MO 63119 [Parent guide for facilitating listening skills in young visually impaired children].

Newsletters for and by Parents of Visually Impaired Preschool Children

Awareness: School-age and preschool. National Association for Parents of the Visually Impaired, P.O. Box 180806, Austin, TX 78718 ($5).

Future Reflections: School-age and preschool. National Federation of the Blind, Box 1947, Boise, ID 83701 ($3).

National Newspatch: Preschool only. Oregon State School for the Blind, 700 Church St, SE, Salem, OR 97310 ($4).

VIP Newsletter: Preschool only. IIVI, 0–7, Inc., 1975 Rutgers, East Lansing, MI 48823 ($5).

Agencies

American Foundation for the Blind, 15 W. 16th St., New York, NY 10011 (212-520-2000). Provides a variety of services, products, and publications. Catalogs available. Publishes *Journal of Visual Impairment and Blindness.*

American Printing House for the Blind, Inc., 1839 Frankfort Ave., Louisville, KY 40206

(502-895-2405). Provides a variety of products, including specially adapted toys and materials for infants and preschool-age visually impaired children. Catalogs available.

The Blind Children's Center, 4120 Marathon St., Los Angeles, CA 90029 (213-664-2153). In addition to providing a variety of programs for blind children in the Los Angeles area, the Center also offers an Educational Correspondence Course for any parent of a visually impaired child. Individualized home-program ideas are suggested, based on parents' descriptions of their child's developmental status. Developmental checklists available.

Division for the Blind and Physically Handicapped. Library of Congress, Washington, DC 20542 (202-287-5100). A national resource for recorded books, records, cassette books, and other materials; many states also have similar libraries with free service and postage.

International Institute for Visually Impaired, 0–7, Inc. 1975 Rutgers Circle, East Lansing, MI 48823 (517-332-2666). Provides resource references and consultation with regard to education for blind and visually impaired infants and preschoolers and support for their families. Publishes the *VIP Newsletter* for parents.

M.C. Migel Memorial Library and Resource Center, American Foundation for the Blind, 15 W. 16th St., New York, NY 10011 (212-620-2160). Reference and circulating inkprint materials relating to nonmedical aspects of blindness; consultative services; references can be borrowed through the mail at no charge.

National Association for Parents of Visually Impaired, Inc., 2011 Hardy Circle, Austin, TX 78657 (512-459-6651). A national parent organization. Publishes the parent newsletter, Awareness.

This is an updated revision of the Appendix in Teplin SW: Development of children with retrolental fibroplasia. Pediatrics 71:6–12, 1983, reproduced with permission of the publisher.

Continuing Issues Through Life for the Retinopathy of Prematurity Patient: Medical Expert Testimony in a Court of Law

David Rutstein, MD,[†] and Marshall Simonds, PC

David Rutstein, M.D.

I am here today because I am worried about what goes on in our courts of law; I am only going to worry about the doctor's side, because Mr. Simonds can worry about the lawyer's side, and he can defend himself. In any event, I would like to read one paragraph of a paper I drafted some time ago to give you a focus on where I feel we are.

This is the background on the legal aspects of what you now call "ROP." We are concerned with this, but we are also concerned with a whole host of other problems—suits against corporations or other defendants on questions relating to things like toxins, environmental hazards, drugs, or carcinogens. With that as a background let me read this paragraph to you:

> There is growing confusion regarding the value of medical expert testimony in a court of law. What I mean by that is very simple. I see some of my distinguished confreres making statements in courts of law, under oath, which obviously are not true, or which, obviously, are not documented. They provide information that is not completely documented. It is very disturbing to see what really goes on. Disagreements, interpretations and conclusions by expert witnesses, concerning subjects as disparate as insanity and the toxicity or carcinogenicity of an environmental exposure to a particular substance are cases in point. Indeed, concern has been expressed that the opinions of the expert witness may, at times, depend more on the needs of the party calling the expert rather than on the existing medical knowledge relevant to the question at hand.

[†]Deceased.

This summary was prepared by the editors from tapes of the presentations of Dr. Rutstein and Mr. Simonds.

Birth Defects: Original Article Series, Volume 24, Number 1, pages 325–333
© **1988 March of Dimes Birth Defects Foundation**

The situation is exacerbated by the general lack of appreciation on the part of the public, within the legal profession, and perhaps within the medical profession that there are gradations of reliability and validity of medical testimony depending on whether a particular conclusion is based on a scientific fact, a clinical impression, or a guess. These are three very different standards we have to think about.

Further, the confusion is difficult to correct because there is no procedure or rule during a trial in a court of law to guide the fact finder in an understanding of these three gradations of medical expert testimony. When I ask you to look at a trial, I am focusing on two groups of participants. I am talking about the so-called experts testifying and the lawyers examining and cross-examining those experts. They think quite differently from each other. They have different backgrounds. As you well know, the courts are a lot older than scientific medicine. They take you back to the English common law, and who knows how far back that goes? Scientific medicine isn't more than about a century old. It is all relatively new, and much has occurred during my lifetime. Some of these radical changes we now call medical science are really very young. What I am trying to do is, within the walls of this established legal structure, to see whether anything can be done without disturbing the structure, or disturbing it as little as possible, to develop some formal procedures to deal with these three grades of medical testimony.

What is a scientific fact? That is the first of these three types of medical testimony. When I was a freshman at Harvard, a man by the name of Lawrence J. Henderson told us very simply what a scientific fact was. He called it a reproducible observation. I've never seen a better definition of it. You do an experiment; I do an experiment; we do the same experiments; we have the same protocol; we work in two different cities; and, if we follow the rules, we are going to get answers that are exactly the same within certain limits of experimental error. That's what a *scientific fact* is. Now, if the fact is documented, and by documented I mean put in the form of a paper and judged by peers, and if after that it is published and it stands up repeatedly to testing, that is what we mean by a scientific fact. Unfortunately, a very small percentage of what we do as physicians is based on scientific facts.

Next, we go to our clinical impressions, and, of course, there are all kinds of gradations of reliability here. There is the information a colleague told me yesterday about findings or symptoms in his patient that turn out to be similar to findings or symptoms in one of my patients; or information that may be set forth in a paper that I saw, which wasn't really very well written but, nevertheless, seemed to point in a certain direction. Or, on ward rounds, I may see a group of patients that exhibit a particular set of symptoms, but it is really not scientifically documented. These are the kinds of things we call clinical impressions.

Finally, we have guesses. A practicing physician, when he does his job, has to take care of the patient. He cannot say to a sick person, ''I don't have a fact, and, therefore, I can't take care of you.'' He gets what facts he can, and he uses the facts in the best way possible. He adds to those facts whatever clinical impressions he has, and finally he's forced in many cases to make guesses. That is what you have to do if you are a clinician. And that is what you are faced with when you think about what is being said in a court of law as well, because it is the same kind of thing. And you have problems with the guesses.

When I have defined a scientific fact for you, is it different from a legal fact? Yes, it's entirely different from a legal fact, because most legal facts are historical and by definition nonreproducible. This is what we are all trapped with. It is a dilemma with which I am very sympathetic, but I have no solution to this problem. In the end, what we finally have is an individual ''expert,'' called an expert witness, on the witness stand and under examination by two lawyers who are opposed to each other with the judge sitting as a referee. Whatever conclusions a jury may reach from his testimony are the facts—legal facts, not scientific facts. This is what really happens in a court of law; the procedure is to attack the witness from both sides and out will come the truth. The lawyers do this because they work in an adversarial system.

The question is, can anything be done to improve this process? First of all, we do have a procedure in medicine by which an evaluation is made of the validity of asserted facts, establishing whether the matter asserted can be accepted as a fact and whether such fact is worth reproducing and reporting. This is what happens in the offices of a good medical journal. The medical editor and his referees, in effect, make a judgment concerning the reliability of the facts in any article submitted for publication to the journal. If the job is done right, then what is published in the journal represents facts. We all know that this is not always the case, particularly when we get our papers turned down! But I wonder if it wouldn't be possible to follow the same kind of procedure in a court of law. For example, from a manuscript, the editor is able to evaluate the quality of the design and the conduct of the experiment. The reliability of the data collected and how the data are analyzed in relation to relevant existing knowledge in the medical literature are evaluated next. The reproducibility of the scientific fact makes it possible for the editor to compare the new evidence in the manuscript with scientific facts reported in the references appended to the manuscript and in the medical literature in general. How could we apply this to the legal process? My suggestion (and my colleague, Mr. Simonds, doesn't like it at all) is that if an expert witness states that he has some facts about which he is going to testify and knows what they are, he should be required prior to the trial to provide a brief listing of medical references and the literature he is going to use for documentation of his testimony and have that distributed to the other side, and have the other person's expert testimony distributed to his side, so that they can both get these things straightened out before testifying. The lawyers will tell you that one of the big problems with all this is that somebody (the jury) has finally got to decide whether the experts are telling the truth. Lawyers present evidence but don't decide the truth of that evidence; judges enforce procedural rules but do not find facts; and the jury, who decide who is telling the truth, obviously aren't trained for the job.

All I propose is that we try a different approach on an experimental basis and see how it works. To this end, I've recommended two things. First, that we have simulated trials of cases before large groups of physicians, lawyers, judges, and potential jurors and try this kind of an experiment. The American Academy of Arts and Sciences and the American Bar Association seem interested in this, but the difficulty, as always, is getting the money to carry out the experiment. The second thing I would like to do is establish a study group of medical and legal scholars to explore questions such as procedures for recognition and identification of a scientific fact in the course of a trial, procedures for grading and evaluating the validity of clinical impressions, and, finally, some rules by which the courts can deal with and control expert testimony that falls into the category of pure guesses.

Marshall Simonds, Esq.

It is with appreciation but some trepidation that I stand here as the only representative of my profession in a hall full of doctors. Communications between our professions are not always warm and friendly. For the most part, I work on your side and some of the most impressive people I have ever met have been in your profession, but I also have to tell you that, in the course of my work, some of the biggest fools I have ever met have come from your profession. Where I hope I can be of help today is in talking about the law in terms that will help you to listen and in trying to persuade you that there are at least some of us in the legal profession who would like to listen to you too. We do not think that the present antagonism between our professions is in the least desirable.

Let me start by telling a joke, if you will permit it. Obviously, I have to tell a joke about lawyers. You have probably all heard endless jokes about us, none of them flattering; I think I've heard even more. I have picked out one of the most flattering to tell you. If you've heard it, indulge me nonetheless. Three professionals, a biologist, a physicist, and a lawyer, were discussing which profession was the oldest. The biologist pointed out that when the primeval ooze began to ooze, life and biology began. The physicist pointed out that prior to living matter there was the problem of creating order out of chaos in the universe and that order was the business of the physicist. The lawyer merely smiled and asked of the physicist and the biologist, "Who do you think was responsible for the chaos?"

If we can take that story as a point of departure for my comments about what happens in a court of law when a doctor is a defendant, let me see if I can both demystify the process and make some suggestions about why it goes wrong when it goes wrong. ROP is an example, and a useful example, of a subject on which I understand there is scientific and medical uncertainty. You do not yet know the truth about the causal mechanism. There is no agreement within your profession about the single best course of treatment to prevent ROP. The disagreement about causative factors presumably reflects a lack of knowledge, because you have not yet had the opportunity to make the needed studies, or perhaps because those studies simply cannot be performed. The disagreements about the best treatment modality typically arise in such circumstances and can be seen in a number of areas. For example, we do not know much about the toxicity of the 60,000 or 80,000 chemical substances that have been identified to date. Health effects from exposure to those chemicals are increasingly a major issue in the courtroom. The scientific community simply does not yet know the correct answers to many of these questions. Indeed, in many instances, you may not have even identified the right questions to ask.

The problem is that the courts are in the dispute-resolution business. Even though science does not know the answer, a court is confronted with the claims of an injured party and seeks to decide now whether there should be remediation for those claims. The pressure on the court may derive in part from the ambitious lawyer who sues you and earns your intense dislike, but those pressures derive from a number of other circumstances as well, and you must recognize that. They derive from a growing expectation that perhaps everyone should be entitled to a risk-free life. They derive from the notion that there should be accountability every time there is an adverse circumstance. Whether you are a doctor, a manufacturer, a lawyer, an engineer, or an architect, that notion of accountability is a phenomenon that did not originate with the plaintiff's lawyer in a medical malpractice case; it is a phenomenon of our society. And perhaps it is useful to observe some of the changes that have occurred in the court system in response to that. Traditionally, and this is still true for doctors in malpractice cases but not for drug manufacturers, for example, a plaintiff has to do the following things under our *fault* system: The plaintiff has to show: first, I have been injured; second, my injury was caused by conduct of Dr. Smith; and third, his medical treatment of me was negligent or careless and not in accordance with the contemporary standards of physicians in this community. And the plaintiff has to prove each of these elements to a reasonable degree, not beyond a reasonable doubt, but by what lawyers call a preponderance of the evidence. That means that if the scale on which the evidence is weighed tilts ever so slightly toward the plaintiff, you lose; but until that happens, you win.

The plaintiff has to prove certain elements such as causation and standard of care by producing expert testimony. Who is expert on the issue of medical malpractice in a particular area? If it's ophthalmology, it's ophthalmologists. If it's pediatrics, it's pediatricians. Ophthalmologists have to take the stand and testify against the defendant doctor, and other ophthalmologists have to come and give their expert opinions on behalf of that doctor. From the lawyer's viewpoint in malpractice cases, and the record will bear me out, however you think your malpractice premiums are moving, there has been a relatively low percentage of wins for plaintiffs. I understand that the record in ROP cases is more favorable to the plaintiffs. I suppose that may be explained by the scientific uncertainties that have split your ranks coupled with the dramatic courtroom impact of a blind baby.

Have the rules in our court system changed in ways that impact on the future of ROP? Let me use as an example the problems confronting a defendant drug manufacturer. And let me use the specific drug I have been defending for the past 10 years, diethylstilbesterol. The plaintiff must prove today that she was exposed in utero to this drug and that there is a causal relationship between the drug and her claimed injury. She must prove that her injury was caused by her exposure to that drug and not by something else. In many jurisdictions plaintiff must also show that the drug company, some 30 years earlier, should have known or foreseen that the drug would or might cause such an injury. Over the course of the 10 years I mentioned, however, foreseeability has dropped out as an issue in a number of jurisdictions. In those jurisdictions, it no longer matters whether the drug company could have foreseen the risk. That's irrelevant. All that is necessary is proof that the company made the product and that there is a causal relationship to the claimed harm. This formulation of accountability is called strict liability. Under this legal theory, the focus is not on fault but on compensation. Now that is not the rule in malpractice cases, but I think it is useful to recognize that the malpractice claim today arises in a court in which the emphasis and, indeed, the expectations are increasingly focused on compensation, not fault.

This pressure on the courts reflects, in part, a failure of the legislative and executive branches to respond to the pleas for compensation. Since the court is increasingly seen as the best recourse for the injured party and fault is seen as increasingly irrelevant, the judges are under compulsion to say, "Shouldn't the parents of that blind baby, shouldn't that blind baby, be entitled to some compensation for that lifelong injury?" And there is a natural human instinct to answer "Yes."

Let us turn to how the court deals with the expert testimony that is offered to show that Dr. Smith did wrong when he provided oxygen at what may have been an absolutely prudent level to a premature baby. The court deals with it in the same way it deals with expert testimony in any case. It expects the adversary process to test the validity of that testimony. It expects me as defense counsel to cross-examine the plaintiff's expert and to demonstrate, if I can, that what the expert says is not credible and should not be relied on by the jury.

I think that many of you believe that, if you face a blind baby claim, you are a loser; that the system simply doesn't work. I have a contrary belief from my own experience in defending catastrophic injury claims, including blindness. That is, if the evidence is made available and is effectively used, jurors will more often than not reach a right, scientifically sound decision. Let me go back to a point David Rutstein made. I think that there is another difference between a scientific fact, which I am going to call a scientific truth, and a legal fact, which I am going to call a legal truth. A scientific truth may be a reproducible observation or it may be a conclusion based on an accumulation of research that seems to be overwhelmingly credited by scientists in the field, so much so that it has become generally accepted. But a legal truth in this context is what a jury finds in a particular case, based on the evidence of that case and nothing else. A doctor is or is not negligent in his treatment of ROP based on the evidence presented in his trial, and that evidence is presented through human beings who are cross-examined— expert witnesses who present their opinions with reference to the medical literature they rely on and who are cross-examined on that medical literature. These expert witnesses are seen as good witnesses, as credible witnesses, or as shifty and unreliable witnesses. They are presented and cross-examined by lawyers of varying skills. The jury takes a snapshot; they elect a ''queen for a day,'' and it is either the defendant or the plaintiff, but it has nothing to do with the truth in the next case, that involves a new jury and is a new ballgame. You have to understand that difference if you want to be prepared for the realities of the courtroom.

Cross-examination is an enormously important tool in the trial court. Let me give you an illustration, current and truthful. Two people were in a taxicab leaving from Washington National Airport to come to this NIH auditorium this morning. I was one of them, David Rutstein was the other one. I am not going to ask these questions to David but I represent to you that this is a truthful exposition of what the testimony would be, were he under cross-examination. The hypothetical case is one in which Dr. Rutstein has been called as an expert and has given an opinion that the particular taxicab in which he rode had broken springs in the backseat and was unfit for passenger use. Indeed, since he is an aggressive plaintiff's expert, he has gone farther; he has persuaded his plaintiff's lawyer to bring a class action suit against all Washington taxicabs and has extrapolated from this single event that all cabs operating out of the National Airport have broken springs in the backseat and are unfit for human use. And he seeks class action damages. No more exaggerated than what might be said of some of the suits that are launched against the medical profession.

Cross-examination: "Doctor, what is the basis for your assertion that the cab you were in had broken springs?"

Dr. Rutstein: "I felt them; they were sticking in; I commented on them to the driver. He did not deny it. I have had 76 years of experience sitting in taxicabs and I know a broken spring when I sit on one."

Next question: "Dr. Rutstein, what investigation did you undertake beyond feeling something with your bottom before you reached this conclusion?"

Dr. Rutstein: "None was necessary; it was so clear."

Conclusion to cross-examination: "Well doctor, isn't it a fact that when you got out of the cab I removed from the seat directly under where you were sitting your umbrella, and isn't it a fact that you had been sitting on this umbrella all the way from the airport to the NIH?"

Credibility of the witness is destroyed. The jury will no longer believe him about anything to do with Washington taxicabs. Effective cross-examination based on superb preparation by defense counsel: Namely, observing the umbrella. This is what happens. It happens in a way only a little different in the courtroom when you examine the expert who is overreaching and asserting a conclusion that cannot be justified by the medical literature.

Now, what puzzles me is why in areas like ROP the medical community that is concerned with ROP has not engaged in what I would call minimal self-help. The medical profession has engaged in a number of self-help efforts: activities at the legislative level, public education about the depressing effect of malpractice risks on the willingness of a clinician to exercise innovative judgment when, without that willingness, the patient suffers. However, strident attacks on the plaintiffs' bar are not the most effective use of your voices, your prestige, or your money. They will only draw equally strident attacks by plaintiffs' lawyers against the medical profession, and, since most legislators are lawyers, not doctors, you are probably fighting in a forum where you will lose.

Let me suggest some things that you might consider. There is a phrase in the accounting profession called "GAAP." It is short for "generally accepted accounting principles." For your benefit alone, with great imagination, I created another acronym, "GAPS," for "generally accepted practice standards." When I read the literature, or when, to be candid with you, I read Dr. Flynn's chapter summarizing the status of learning about

ROP, which I did only last night, I discovered that there is a great paucity of data; that we are talking about a disease, or condition, that was described as an epidemic between 1940 and 1950; that, thereafter, the incidence of blindness in premature babies declined sharply, apparently because of reduced use of oxygen; but that the incidence of brain damage or death of the premature babies increased; and now, with use of oxygen back in vogue, you are keeping the prematures alive, but ROP has come back and again approaches epidemic levels. You still need to collect data; you need to do multicenter studies. I am all in favor of that. When the data are sufficient to solve the uncertainty, you will not have problems in the court. You will not have witnesses who come in with wild-eyed theories, or it will be easy to shoot them down. You haven't reached that resolution yet. You are still dealing with uncertainty. Each of you deals with uncertainty every day when you treat these patients. Why don't you develop in your literature practice standards that recognize the realities that you are dealing with? Why don't you enunciate and publish those standards? This would make it possible for good defense counsel to conduct effective cross-examination and much more difficult for the fringe elements of my profession and yours to put forth unworthy cases. That step is within your power. That would be in addition to the kind of steps David Rutstein is talking about in terms of improving the requirements that an expert really be an expert with effective credentials and with reasonable reliance on the literature before he is credited by the courts.

Commentary and Questions: Session IV

The first of the two modules constitutes a remarkable advance in our notions about ROP. A decade ago, no one would have considered a serious discussion of various forms of surgical therapy as part of a symposium on the disease, yet the subject today is a natural part of our conception of what we should be thinking about and perhaps doing in relation to ROP.

The technical details of the surgical procedures are not of interest to us here. The authors of the individual chapters covered those topics well. It is important to point out that the therapies themselves are for entirely different phases of the disease and as such have almost no overlap. Cryotherapy as described by Dr. Palmer is applicable only in the early stages of the disease, when the retina is in contact with the pigment epithelium (ie, no retinal detachment has yet occurred). Once a detachment has occurred, surgical maneuvers designed to treat it, described by Dr. Tasman, become the approach of choice. It needs emphasis, however, that these detachments, for the most part, are late in occurring and are associated with a retinal break or tear. They then represent an entity completely different from the end-stage catastrophic funnel-type traction detachments, a description of the surgical anatomy of which is the subject of Dr. de Juan's paper. The technical details of its treatment are the contents of Drs. Machemer's and Charles's chapters. This type of surgery is probably at the very limits of the technical capabilities of the retina-vitreous surgeons. It poses questions for us that go beyond its technical success/failure rate. Do these infants see better as a result of these operations or not? Resolving this question is one of the knottiest of problems on our agenda today, touching as it does visual development early in life and accurate quantitative measurements at very low levels of visual function. These are challenges sufficient to keep the very best young minds in both specialties occupied for the next decade.

The questions put to the panelists revolved around two issues primarily, the mechanics of the application of cryotherapy during the course of ROP and when we should start to look at these babies? Is age 28 days too late in some cases? To this Dr. Palmer replied that, when all the factors were considered, including haze of the intraocular media, fragility of the infant's condition, and the time required to develop the disease, the 28-day window seemed appropriate. The rationale of the application of cryotherapy to 360° of the

Birth Defects: Original Article Series, Volume 24, Number 1, pages 335–337
© **1988 March of Dimes Birth Defects Foundation**

avascular retina was essentially a decision arrived at by consensus. It was made primarily on the basis of what was safest for both the eye and the infant as a whole. Since cryotherapy carries many unknowns, it was thought that this form of ablative therapy would most likely accomplish the goal in the fewest possible treatment sessions. The cryotherapy trial progress has many provisions built into it for safety, including stopping the trial early should the therapy prove beneficial or harmful beyond reasonable statistical boundaries.

The questions directed at the retina/vitreous surgeons, Drs. Tasman, Machemer, and Charles, revolved around two issues: Questions of operative technique, which are of interest only to those doing the surgery, and questions of visual outcome, which are of interest to all. Although all three have many cases of documented retinal reattachment, the visual acuity results are far more nebulous and less certain. This reflects the state of our art more than the perspicacity of the involved surgeons.

The final session was appropriately opened by Dr. Bill Silverman who, reflecting on some 40 years of experience following a now fully grown adult group of patients with more severe forms of the disease, finds that our society has made little progress in helping these individuals cope with their ROP. Fully two-thirds of them have failed to find gainful employment. This represents, at best, an enormous waste of human potential and, at worst, rebuke to our society's care and compassion. Dr. Teplin next covered the stresses a family encounters in coping with a blind or visually handicapped child. Needless to say, this is a problem for which most physicians need constant education because of the crucial role we play in the whole support system.

Dr. Rutstein and Mr. Simonds then discussed at length the differences between medical and legal truth, how the boundaries of medical truth had become, increasingly blurred over the years, and they proffered some suggestions as to how these boundaries might be restored and with them the confidence of the people. In the question and answer session, Mr. Simonds, in replying to how informed consent might be obtained to treat ROP, stated that, although there may be some liability involved here, "common sense" factors were also involved. The issue for the law regarding informed consent is, in essence, did you represent the information concerning the procedure correctly? Did you make the person fully aware of the risks and benefits of the proposed treatment? Did you conform in your informed consent to all state regulations, to hospital rules, and to what is known about the disease and its course and complications? He emphasized the fact that lawyers do not testify in court, doctors and experts do. Juries do not decide on the basis of the lawyer's testimony but rather on the basis of the doctor's testimony.

At this point, Dr. Steve Charles commented on the legal and social issue involved here, saying that the commonly adopted attitude today is "don't mess around with politics because they are dirty and this inevitably leads, to dirty politics when people feel this way.'' He believes that the same may hold true for legal testimony. It is essential that doctors do testify as experts. Mr. Simonds commented that, instead of scorning the tort system, doctors should understand it and work with it. It is really the best system we have, and any other system of experts sitting in judgment is bound to become biased or politicized.

Mr. Simonds was then asked if anybody looked at how frequently judgments in trials were right. He responded again that, although the trial system is not perfect, there is no better way to resolve charges of negligent conduct than to let lawyers skilled in the adversary system use the methods they know to get at that truth.

Dr. Anderson from Fort Worth, Texas, spoke for the practitioners not involved in the ongoing CRYO-ROP study and asked what liability they might have for withholding or giving this experimental treatment in the light of the fact they were not involved in the CRYO-ROP study. Mr. Simond's response was that, when treatment is clearly experimental, a private practitioner would be well advised to be very careful about giving it. Dr. Rutstein pointed out that any clinical trial, if conducted properly, is looking not only for whether the treatment is beneficial but for harmful side effects.

Finally, Dr. Teplin was asked two questions, one in reference to whether, in fact, there were IQ or psychologic tests that were specifically prepared for and truly tested blind children. Dr. Teplin responded that there were several tests and checklists that have been devised or adapted for blind children. However, these tests, particularly those for preschool blind children, are not adequately standardized or validated; thus they cannot be considered equivalent to the IQ tests used for sighted children. In response to another question, he asserted that all blind children are probably not covered by the Social Security System.* On that note, this session, and the meeting as a whole adjourned.

*However, children with handicaps, including those with blindness, whose families have an income level below specified thresholds are eligible for Supplemental Security Income (S.S.I.). S.S.I. has been part of the Social Security Program since 1974.

Index